Health promotion research

Towards a new
social epidemiology

WHO Library Cataloguing in Publication Data

Health promotion research : towards a new social
    epidemiology / edited by Bernhard Badura and Ilona
    Kickbusch

    (WHO regional publications. European series ; No. 37)

    1.Health promotion 2.Research 3.Socioeconomic factors
    4.Life style 5.Community health services 5.Europe
    I.Badura, Bernhard II.Kickbusch, Ilona III.Series

    ISBN 92 890 1128 9   (NLM Classification: WA 20.5)
    ISSN 0378–2255

World Health Organization
Regional Office for Europe
Copenhagen

WHO Regional Publications, European Series, No. 37

Health promotion research
Towards a new
social epidemiology

Edited by

Bernhard Badura

and

Ilona Kickbusch

ISBN 92 890 1128 9
ISSN 0378-2255

PRINTED IN ENGLAND

CONTENTS

Part III. Families, workplaces and hospitals as settings for health promotion

Part IV. Population-oriented health promotion

Part V. Community intervention in health promotion

Contributors

Bernhard Badura
Technische Universität Berlin, Germany

Sven Bjørk
Psychiatry Department A, Ullevaal University Hospital,
Oslo, Norway

Neil Bracht
School of Public Health, University of Minnesota,
Minneapolis, MN, USA

Ralph Catalano
Program in Social Ecology and Public Policy Research
Organization, University of California, Irvine, CA, USA

Geneviève Cresson
Sociologist, Centre régional d'analyse des mouvements sociaux
et des modes de vie, Université de Lille I, France

Odd Steffen Dalgard
Psychiatry Department A, Ullevaal University Hospital,
Oslo, Norway

Kathryn Dean
Institute for Social Medicine, University of Copenhagen,
Denmark

Christiane Deneke
Research Staff, Projekt Gesundheitsselbsthilfegruppe,
Medizinische Soziologie, Universitäts-Krankenhaus Eppendorf,
Hamburg, Germany,

David Dooley
Program in Social Ecology and Public Policy Research
Organization, University of California, Irvine, CA, USA

Lesley Doyal
Department of Nursing Health and Applied Social Studies,
Bristol Polytechnic, Redland Hill, Bristol, United Kingdom

Mary Ann Elston
Department of Community Medicine, University College
London, United Kingdom

Michael Faltis
Research Staff, Projekt Gesundheitsselbsthilfegruppe,
Medizinische Soziologie, Universitäts-Krankenhaus Eppendorf,
Hamburg, Germany

Helmut Hildebrandt
Research Staff, Projekt Gesundheitsselbsthilfegruppe,
Medizinische Soziologie, Universitäts-Krankenhaus Eppendorf,
Hamburg, Germany

Bjørn E. Holstein
Institute for Social Medicine, University of Copenhagen,
Denmark

James S. House
Survey Research Center, and Departments of Sociology and
Epidemiology, University of Michigan, Ann Arbor, MI, USA

Ilona Kickbusch
Regional Officer for Health Promotion, WHO Regional Office
for Europe, Copenhagen, Denmark

Manolis Kogevinas
Department of Community Medicine, University College,
London, United Kingdom

Michael G. Marmot
Department of Community Medicine, University College,
London, United Kingdom

Alan Maynard
Director, Centre for Health Economics,[a] University of York,
United Kingdom, *and* Co-director, Addiction Research Centre,
Universities of York and Hull, United Kingdom

Nancy Milio
Professor, Health Policy and Administration, University of
North Carolina, Chapel Hill, NC, USA

---

[a] The Centre for Health Economics is a WHO collaborating centre (in conjunction with the Institute for Health Studies, University of Hull and the Department of Health Education, Leeds Polytechnic) in psychosocial and economic aspects of health.

Aulikki Nissinen
Medical Officer, Cardiovascular Diseases, World Health
Organization, Geneva, Switzerland

Horst Noack
Department of Social and Preventive Medicine,
University of Berne, Switzerland

Roisin Pill
Department of General Practice, Welsh National School of
Medicine, University of Wales Health Centre, Cardiff,
United Kingdom

Agnès Pitrou
Director, Sociological Research — CRNS, Laboratoire
d'économie et de sociologie de travail, Aix-en-Provence,
France

Lois Pratt
Professor of Sociology, Jersey City State College, NJ, USA

Pekka Puska
Director, Department of Epidemiology, National Public Health
Institute, Helsinki, Finland

Ann Richardson
39, Glenmore Rd, London NW3 4DA, United Kingdom

Neil Sol
Director, Department of Health Promotion, Methodist Health
System, Memphis, TN, USA

Carolyn I. Speros
Director, Department of Patient and Community Education,
Methodist Hospitals, Memphis, TN, USA

Tom Sørensen
Psychiatry Department A, Ullevaal University Hospital,
Oslo, Norway

Töres Theorell
National Institute for Psychosocial Factors and Health,
Stockholm, Sweden

Alf Trojan
Research Director, Projekt Gesundheitsselbsthilfegruppe,
Medizinische Soziologie, Universitäts-Krankenhaus Eppendorf,
Hamburg, Germany

Holger Ursin
   University of Bergen, Norway

David R. Williams
   Department of Sociology, Yale University, Newhaven, CT,
   USA

Erio Ziglio
   Research Fellow, Research Unit in Health and Behavioural
   Change, *and* Lecturer in Social Policy, Department of Social
   Policy, University of Edinburgh, United Kingdom

Introduction

Bernhard Badura & Ilona Kickbusch

The influence of social factors on health has been recognized for centuries. Everyone is probably familiar with Robert Virchow's oft-quoted statement that "medicine is a social science, and politics is nothing else than medicine on a large scale". The psychosomatic hypothesis of Sigmund Freud that personality factors and emotions can affect physical illness is now established common sense.

Substantial contributions, however, on how health and illness may be related to psychological and social processes are of a more recent origin. Even though research dealing with the relevance to health of social support, psychosocial stress and lifestyle may be traced back to the nineteenth century, findings that are conceptually convincing as well as empirically valid and reliable are not much older than perhaps 30 or 40 years. Today, sociologists, psychologists, economists and policy analysts contribute both to the understanding of health and illness and to the solution of health problems. The time has come for a fruitful and close collaboration between the natural and social sciences, particularly as regards the social origin and distribution of health and illness, the readjustment of existing health services to the health needs of the population, and the development of healthy public policies and health promotion programmes.

During the period of industrialization, both social policy and traditional public health were remarkably effective in modifying the physical and social environment in a beneficial way. A modern public

1

health policy ought to be capable of similar achievements in regard to the social and environmental risks in industrialized societies. René Dubos was among the first who made this claim. In his *Mirage of health* published in 1959 he considers how in the nineteenth century the concern with social reform rapidly evolved into public health practices with "spectacular" improvements in the sanitary and nutritional condition of the western world *(1)*. Social reformers began to improve the health of populations by "cleaning up the mess" caused by industrialization "long before the modern era in medicine". The great microbiological epidemics were brought under control, Dubos states, "not by treatment with drugs" but "largely by sanitation" and by "the raising of living standards". He recommends the same public health strategy to fight the great epidemics of today: the vascular diseases, the cancers, the mental disorders. In his belief, people are wrongly advised today that "the royal avenue" to the control of today's epidemics is through "scientific knowledge" and "medical technology". What they need instead is "to discover and to reform" those aspects of the physical and social environment that have brought about the present pattern of disease.

Some 20 years later, Thomas McKeown picked up these issues again in his now famous work *The role of medicine (2)*. He summarizes his results on the history of medicine and on its present situation as follows:

> Medical science and services are misdirected, and society's investment in health is not well used, because they rest on an erroneous assumption about the basis of human health. It is assumed that the body can be regarded as a machine whose protection from disease and its effects depends primarily on internal intervention. The approach has led to indifference to the external influences and personal behaviour which are the predominant determinants of health. It has also resulted in the relative neglect of the majority of sick people who provide no scope for the internal measures which are at the centre of medical interest.

General statements such as that quoted above raise two fundamental questions as to how to improve our understanding of the social determinants of health and disease and how to transform existing knowledge into action.

Within the last 30 years, social scientists have contributed to stress research, analysing the effect on health of personal crises, chronic strain and stressful transitions, as well as coping styles such as the well known type-A behaviour pattern. More recently, they have done research on the different effects of social support on health and illness. The evidence is now overwhelming that social factors influence the body system independently from and/or in addition to well known risk factors and risk behaviours such as cigarette smoking, excessive alcohol consumption, use of illicit drugs, certain dietary habits, insufficient exercise, reckless driving and inappropriate response to social pressure. It is accepted now, for example, that acute stress may lead to an increase in catecholamines and a marked rise in blood pressure. It is likewise accepted that social factors affect the immune system. Social epidemiology and psychophysiology therefore need each other, since the interpretation of statistical relationships between social factors and medical end-points has to be built onto the knowledge of sociopsychosomatic mechanisms. There are two basic paths leading from social factors to health, one involving positive or negative emotions and the central nervous system, the other involving behaviour that is either beneficial or detrimental to health.

Perhaps the most subtle and most comprehensive picture of the present state of stress research has been presented by Richard Lazarus and his collaborators at the University of California, Berkeley. According to his view, understanding the stress process depends as much on a rigorous understanding of social and psychological processes as it does on a sound knowledge of physiology. Lazarus agrees with Dubos that stress is an "inevitable aspect of the human condition". It is the "cognitive appraisal" of potential stressors and individual "ways of coping" that "make the big difference" in adaptational outcomes (3). There is thus no objective way of predicting psychological stress without reference to the properties of the person concerned. Cognitive appraisal determines emotions and consequently physiological reactions and behaviour that are dangerous or beneficial to health.

Do people today experience more stress than people in pre-industrial society? Lazarus admits that social change may lead to a loss of the "anchors" on which people have long depended, such as religion and ascribed social relations that are stable and available throughout the life cycle, thereby creating "a sense of foundering in a world that no longer seems predictable or even familiar" (3). But he does not believe that the degree of stress is greater today. Whether this is true or not is certainly difficult to assess. We do know, however, that in all industrialized societies health and illness are still

3

distributed unequally among different social strata in spite of well developed welfare institutions. Even in societies with free access to highly sophisticated medical services, social factors such as status, income and education are among the best predictors of premature death. One explanation of these findings might be that the degree of stress is distributed unequally. Another might be that social support is distributed unequally, thus increasing the vulnerability of people with lower incomes to psychological and physical damage.

As early as 1897, the famous French sociologist Emile Durkheim published *Suicide*, in which he presented data suggesting that people who lack social bonds are more vulnerable to self-destructive behaviour than people who are socially well integrated *(4)*. Among sociologists, positive social bonds within the family and community and at the workplace have long been considered fundamental to high self-esteem and psychological wellbeing. In recent epidemiological literature, the concept of social support has begun to appear as a major contributor to positive health and as a major intervening variable between potential stressors and disease outcomes *(5,6)*. To learn more about the causes underlying epidemiological findings that suggest that social support promotes health, a better understanding is needed of social relations and communication processes.

Research on stress and on social support constantly remind us that today's health problems are rooted in an environment shaped by people. Prospects for the health of societies are therefore determined by social, political and economic forces that shape this environment.

Social trends such as technological change, migration, unemployment and changes in values, norms and social relations constantly influence living conditions, which are themselves either positively or negatively related to the health of societies, regions or communities. To create a healthy society people should understand these trends and their implications for health and wellbeing more thoroughly. New policies and programmes need to be developed to cope better with the health problems of today. Health policy at present is chiefly concerned with the existing system of caring for the sick; it is sectoral in its approach, concentrating most of its resources on cure. Health promotion and illness prevention are neglected despite the fact that the health returns of the traditional health services are diminishing. Of course, behaviour patterns must be changed, but there is also a need to tackle the wider environmental issues that shape individual choices but are beyond the individual's control. In a milieu that is

4

shaped in a health-promoting way, both the desire for and the opportunity to indulge in unhealthy habits would be reduced.

A healthy public policy ought to promote community health through a whole range of public policies, of which traditional health service policies are just one element. It makes health a priority on the public policy agenda, emphasizing positive initiatives rather than restrictive regulations, achieving objectives through rewards rather than penalties, and encouraging self-control, self-management, participation and mutual aid. A healthy public policy has to clarify and highlight the implications for health of the full range of related public policies, including the areas of food, housing, technology, work, recreation and education. Measures of fiscal and social policy need to be stressed, particularly with respect to long-term policies and lasting solutions.

Sometimes the costs to health of self-destructive behaviour are thought to be politically acceptable because, for example, heavy smoking or heavy alcohol consumption are highly profitable. The number of people employed to produce unhealthy goods is substantial; so are the profits and taxes on the production of these goods. However, the economic benefits of alcohol consumption, for example, might be valued less highly if the real costs were taken into account: the loss in total production due to alcohol-related problems, the commitment of health service resources to treating people with alcohol-related problems, the real loss to society from traffic and other accidents in which alcohol is a factor, and expenditure on social services for the prevention and alleviation of alcohol-related problems. Similar arguments hold for tobacco, military goods and the like.

Knowledge of social factors and health has improved considerably during the last century. This can no longer be questioned. Because of the still predominantly medical view of health, however, members of advanced societies suffer from a gap between what they know about social factors in health and what they do about them. We hope that this book will help to overcome this gap.

References

1. **Dubos, R**. *Mirage of health*. New York, Harper & Row, 1959.
2. **McKeown, T**. *The role of medicine*. Oxford, Blackwell, 1979.

5

3.   **Lazarus, R.S. & Folkman, S**. *Stress, appraisal and coping*. New York, Springer, 1984.
4.   **Durkheim, E**. *Suicide*. New York, Free Press, 1951.
5.   **Cassel, J**. The contribution of the social environment to host resistance. *American journal of epidemiology*, **104**: 107–123 (1976).
6.   **Cohen, S. & Syme, S.L**. *Social support and health*. New York, Academic Press, 1985.

Part I

Healthy public policy

Making healthy public policy; developing the science by learning the art: an ecological framework for policy studies[a]

Nancy Milio

During the 1980s increasing attention has been given to the view that a vast array of public policies have great potential for health promotion and that this potential ought to be developed. After briefly discussing the basis for this concept and its policy implications, this chapter turns to a major corequisite for making healthy public policy a political reality: learning how to do it. Where healthy public policy exists, how did it happen? This is a question that calls for a new generation of policy studies, one that is relevant to advocates of healthy public policy within and outside governments. An ecological framework of policy-making is proposed for such studies, delineating the social climate, key players, and strategic action. From it, operational indicators and study methods are suggested, in order to learn some general principles, within a real-world context, of how to develop public policies that are healthful.

Basis for Healthy Public Policy

A turn-of-the-century public health is emerging in many countries, one intent on meeting the complex and interconnected health challenges of humankind to the year 2000 and beyond *(1)*. The new public

[a] Reprinted from *Health promotion,* Vol. 2, No. 3 (1987) by permission of Oxford University Press.

health sees human health in an ecological relationship with all else in our natural and human-made habitats. It is relevant to both high- and low-income countries (2) although its priorities will differ in different nations. This view derives from growing evidence that health and illness are embedded in the household, worksite, school, community and larger environments in which we live and evolve our social and individual, public and private, informal and organized ways of living.

The nature of health

From an ecological perspective, people's health affairs cannot be neatly grouped into diagnoses, symptoms and risk factors to be targeted and eliminated or altered. Health problems, having multiple origins, are themselves interrelated (3–5). The people, for example, who have one major problem are more likely than others to have additional problems (6).[a] The earlier in life people experience illness, the more likely they are to become ill, and more severely ill. This snowballing process continues into old age, for those who survive (7–9). Similarly, disadvantaged groups are likely to be socially vulnerable in more than one way (10,11).

On the more positive side, the groups of people favoured with the lifelong conditions for healthy living carry a robust biological and social capacity into the later decades of life (12–14).

This reveals the cumulative and often multiplicative effects of both lifelong health history and of people's social contexts (15). Further, neither health nor social experience can be understood apart from the other (16–18).

Policy implications

Upon reflection, an ecological view of health leads to an awareness that the many contexts in which people live and the ways that people relate to them are profoundly influenced by the most powerful collective means to shape human living: public policy. Simply put, public policy — the guide to government action — sets the range of possibilities for the choices made by public and private organizations, commercial and voluntary enterprises, and individuals. In virtually every facet of living, the creation and use of goods, services, information and environments are affected by

---

[a] **Rice, D. & LaPlante, M**. *The burden of multiple chronic conditions: past trends and policy implications*. Paper presented at the Annual Meeting of the American Public Health Association, Las Vegas, 1986.

government policies — fiscal, regulatory, service provision, research and education, and procedural.

Public policy then becomes a prime approach to creating the conditions and relations that can nurture health. The new public health thus asserts that all public policies should take into account the health interests of the public. It advocates that policies should make healthful choices easy (less costly in various ways) and damaging choices difficult (high in monetary or other costs) to the chooser, whether a corporate body or individual *(4)*. The recognition of this possibility for public policy has grown and developed in recent years among governments and WHO *(19)*.

To be effective, such an approach must be multisectoral in scope — not confined to the conventional sphere of health policy — and collaborative in strategy, involving not only sectors of national policy, such as employment and income maintenance, agriculture, housing, education and health services, but also other levels of government, and voluntary, economic and community groups *(20,21)*.

The fundamental idea that public policies have important effects on the living conditions and so the health of a nation's people is not new among health professionals *(22,23)*, the international community *(24)*, or to current governments, which provide guarantees of humane living conditions for their people. It is known, for example, that age-specific death rates among poorer people (a measure of physiological aging) are lowest among the poorer sections of the countries that ensure a more equitable distribution of resources and a stable economy *(25)*. What is new today is an effort to make the effects on health of public policy explicit, and where necessary and possible, to alter policies in the direction of health promotion. Recognition of these health effects will allow health criteria to enter public policy discourse in governments, community groups and the media and thereby help develop a social climate favourable to healthful policy decisions. In effect, this will reduce the costs to political leaders of making healthy public policies.

In numerous countries, the move to use public policy explicitly to promote health is being pursued by national legislatures *(5,26)*, ministers *(27,28)*, bureaucracies *(29,30)*,[a] parties *(31,32)*, regional

---

[a] **Kern, A.** *Community health — retrospect and prospect.* Paper presented at the First National Community Health Conference on Social and Environmental Health, Adelaide, Australia, 24–26 September 1986.

and local governments *(1,33,34)*, nongovernmental organizations *(35)*, professional groups *(36)*, community organizations,[a] and the mass media.[b] The means employed include: Sweden's Intersectoral Health Council, in which more than 10 ministries can examine the health effects and implications of their policies, Canada's health policy declaration, to attempt to coordinate intersectoral policy; Norway's comprehensive farm-food-nutrition policy; and Denmark's policy on telematics (new information technology). This includes "electronic village halls" not only providing high-quality communications and information, but also promoting the economic, cultural, and political integration of rural communities by granting them public and collective access to new information technology *(37)*.

An analysis of early experience suggests that among the ingredients necessary to develop a policy strategy for health are high-level political leadership, the designation of institutional responsibility, the design of machinery for collaboration within government and between government and outside groups, and material and intangible support for policy development. The resources needed include not only funds, authority, expertise and time but also new types of information and education for new audiences such as policy-makers, community leaders, and journalists.[c]

Strengthening Prospects for Healthy Public Policy: New Directions in Policy Studies

In the current, embryonic stage of a multisectoral policy approach to health, an important priority is development of new types of information — policy-relevant information (as opposed to data on the lifestyles of individuals) — for politically important audiences such as policy-makers, interested groups and the media. Such information would help advocates of healthy public policy to identify within their own situations points of entry into policy-making processes, sources of support, and strategies to enhance the feasibility of specific health

---

[a] **Milio, N.** *Multisectoral policy and community health.* Paper presented at the First National Community Health Conference on Social and Environmental Health, Adelaide, Australia, 24–26 September 1986.

[b] **Draper, P.** *Reinventing public health.* London, Channel 4 Television, 1986.

[c] **Milio, N.** *Building healthy public policies. Basis for a new public health.* Background paper and presentation at the First International Conference on Health Promotion, Ottawa, Ontario, Canada, 17–21 November 1986.

10

promotion policy options in any given policy sector. Health information must be reframed to address the two basic questions for building healthy public policies *(38)*. The first is substantive. What policy options will make healthy choices easier for society to make in the continuous creation of goods, services and environments? This will require the development of new indicators of health and of the effects on health of current and proposed policies.

The second question is strategic or process-oriented. How can options for healthy public policy be made easier for policy-makers and their supporters to choose? This will require an understanding of policy-making processes — the how of policy — under various conditions. Both questions also mean that a new generation of policy studies is needed, one using nontypical methods of data collection.

New measures
In recent years, efforts have been made to develop new indicators of health, focusing on living conditions and people's relations to their environments and using measures of perceived health and a variety of indices *(39–42)*. Less attention has been given to analysis of the health impact of current or prospective public policies *(43)* with some exceptions *(44,45)*. For example, research is developing on the health consequences of economic policies through their effects on unemployment, inflation and income *(46)*. More is on the horizon through such groups as The Other Economic Summit in Europe and as a result of growing concern over environmental protection. More difficult but as necessary are studies to estimate the probable social and health effects of new domains of policy, such as those related to telematics *(47)*.

Typical health policy studies have almost omitted process-oriented analyses, although this gap in research on policy development *(43,48)*, implementation *(49–51)*, and interorganizational/social change *(52)* has been noted by researchers. The need for this kind of policy-relevant information is also recognized by real-world policy-planners to help move their agendas among constituencies *(53)*[a] and within bureaucracies.[b] Such analyses have

---

[a] **Health Promotion Directorate**. *In-house research*. Ottawa, Health and Welfare Canada, 1986 (unpublished memorandum).

[b] **Rogers, C.** *Community participation in the (Federal) Department of Health*. Paper presented at the First National Community Health Conference on Social and Environmental Health, Adelaide, Australia, 24–26 September 1986.

also been found to be crucial for developing the political skills needed by both insiders (54) and outsiders[a] in policy development to enable them to effectively influence the formal and more visible processes of policy-making (55).

The kinds of process-oriented information that have proven useful to policy planners and others for moving policy forward include an understanding: of the negotiated nature of policy-making; of how to extrapolate the policy implications of data, propose feasible policy options, and judge the social and political responses to issues and proposals; and of who to contact, when, and how (24,54,56–58).[a] The best way to find such policy-relevant information is by observing and analysing the real-world experience of public policy-making.

An Ecological Framework for Policy-Making: A Proposal for Analysts and Activists

To derive lessons in policy-making from actual practice in policy arenas, it is useful to have an explicit conceptual framework, a pair of eyeglasses, to help focus attention on relevant aspects of reality. The perspective taken here, one that perhaps best mirrors the nature of human experience (59,60) and is also appropriate for the new public health, is an ecological view of policy-making.[b] From this vantage point, policy development — initiation, adoption, implementation, evaluation and reformulation — is seen as a continuous, but not necessarily linear, social and political process. Policy substance (content) changes under the influence of both changing social, political and economic conditions (social climate) and the changing perceptions of interested parties. As conditions change, there is a change in the views of such groups on the shape, pace and direction of a policy that best enhances (or least harms) their interests.

It must be remembered that policy is made within a set of broadly shared and implicit expectations derived from historical, socio-political, and organizational experience.

---

[a] **Cross, A.** *Nutritionists in the policymaking process 1969–1977.* Paper presented at the Annual Meeting of the American Public Health Association, Las Vegas, 1986.

[b] **Milio, N.** *Making policy: a mosaic of Australian community health policy development.* (Unpublished paper).

12

Participants

As seen here, the major players are interest groups, broadly defined as any organized groups or parts of groups whose resources, authority, status, influence or survival is affected by a policy. Such groups include political parties; parliamentary committees; ministerial offices and bureaucratic units; commercial enterprises; and voluntary, professional, religious, communications or minority organizations *(61)*. These entities (not the individuals who lead them) are the units of analysis. The analysis focuses on the policy-keeper, the entity that by its own initiative or by mandate holds a specific, articulated policy at any given time, and moves the policy at a pace conditioned by the entity's interests during any phase of policy-making. During the initiation, for example, of Norway's food and nutrition policy, the policy-keeper was a nongovernmental group, the National Nutrition Council. For many years this group advocated the policy before getting the idea on the government agenda. This done, a ministerial office became the policy-keeper, and thus the focal point of interest groups' activities (including those of the National Nutrition Council) as they tried to influence the design of the policy (or, in later phases, its adoption, implementation, evaluation and reformulation) directly or by other routes. The entity identified as policy-keeper may thus change as policy-making progresses.

The key players each separate, in effect, from the larger, aggregate general public. The people comprising the general public — as consumers, taxpayers, voters and audiences — may form opinions but are not likely directly to influence the formulation of specific policies in important ways; thus, their views are seen as part of the climate of policy-making that only rarely has direct effects on specific policy choices *(62)*.

Social climate

The perceived and actual interests and priorities of organized groups, like those of the relatively few political leaders who finally make the decision to adopt a policy (for example, a prime minister and "inner cabinet"), are affected by the broad environmental context that they share and can only partly control. Significant facets of this context — which may either enable or constrain the movement of any given policy — include changes in: population demographics; party alliances and priorities; economic growth, inflation, unemployment or debt; parliamentary and cabinet agendas, procedures or composition; bureaucratic agreements or restructuring; the emergence or dissolution of groups outside of government; priority issues and views of the mass media and public opinion; and natural or techno-logical events. Together, these create a social climate, along with ex-pectations derived from previous experience, that can alter judge-ments about the feasibility of a policy at any point in time.

Generic policy-making questions
These environmental conditions affect how the participants in policy-making will respond to (often implicit) questions of policy-making. These answers are necessary to move a policy from initiation to political reality. The questions include:

— agenda setting, or whether a given public issue is an appropriate problem for public policy;

— problem framing, or determining the definition and scope of the problem;

— priority setting;

— option setting, or finding possible optional solutions, includ-ing goals and strategies;

— criteria selection, or by what criteria options should be chosen;

— policy selection, or who bears the responsibility to decide;

— means choice, or how and by whom the policy should be implemented;

— success indicators, or determining the criteria and sources of evaluation; and

— changing goals or means, or how the policy should be reformulated.

The answers to these questions depend in part on which interested parties have access to the decision-makers and at what point(s) in the process. Issues in job creation, housing, agriculture or telematics, for example, might be defined and shaped into policy solutions in very different ways if health criteria and health advocacy groups (within or outside government) became part of policy deliberations *(24)*.

Players' policy positions
The answers to these questions of policy development also involve often competitive and yet mutually dependent relations among inter-ested parties, and require compromises and other arrangements that

14

necessarily shape, move or deter a given policy *(63,64)*. The major players filter information from factual reality through lenses tinted by their judgements of what is best for the success or survival of their own group (whether a ministerial office or commercial enterprise), although their public statements are often couched in other terms *(65,66)*. Their stated reasons or arguments for their policy stance may be taken as a publicly acceptable justification of their material or political interests. These interests, as indicated by the source(s) of their resources (including their constituencies), offer a better explanation of their policy actions than the public rationale.

Thus, it is important to know both how a policy materially affects interested parties (based on verifiable data and self-reported judgements) and how they frame their verbal support or opposition to it in their responses to the questions involved in its development. Although no group expects to get all that it wants, each usually enters the process with a strong position and has fall-back options that are minimally acceptable *(59)*. It is necessary, in other words, to know groups' material interests and their view of their interests at stake in the policy to understand their preferred and compromise policy positions.

Strategic action
Key players (organized groups) within and outside government develop strategic plans to influence the development of policies that have a high priority according to their perceived interests. The type and effectiveness of these plans depend on such things as the groups' size and other resources, organizational age (affecting experience, contacts and credibility), authority, proximity and dispensability to policy-makers, and their skill in using these assets *(54,67)*.[a] Effective strategic planning often involves: realigning organizational priorities and redeploying resources to develop specific policy preferences and rationales for selected audiences; developing information for advocacy and media strategies; and changing relationships with outside organizations *(68)*. This may mean either establishing or breaking ties with other entities, both allies and potential competitors or opponents *(58)*.

---

[a] **Cross, A.** *Nutritionists in the policymaking process 1969–1977.* Paper presented at the Annual Meeting of the American Public Health Association, Las Vegas, 1986.

Information strategies include developing or using hard, systematically gathered data, or softer, informal word-of-mouth perceptions, and then deploying them either by positive manipulation of symbols or as threats. Information on material disincentives and inducements is, of course, often used.

Whether information is gathered from scientific, social, or political sources, interested parties can use it in two ways. Relatively less active purposes include monitoring, analysing and critiquing policy-making; more directly active efforts are persuading, mediating, or mobilizing others for action.

Strategies may aim at influencing policy-makers indirectly (by going over the head of or around the policy-keeper) by gaining the support of credible public figures or attempting to influence general public opinion and so helping to create a climate favourable to a given point of view. This often involves a mass media strategy by parties at interest, ranging from advertising to staging news events, to gain the attention of the public, of potential supporters within and outside of government, and of editorial writers in the media themselves (69–72).

Roles for the mass media

With the apparent increase in the use of the mass media by politically active groups, the electronic media in particular are rightly viewed as mediating the communications between policy-makers and the attentive or interested sections of the public (73). But the electronic and print media are more than mediators, commentators, and sometimes interested parties in policies concerning communications, information, technology, advertising, or corporate economics (74).

The mass media also, intentionally or not, participate in policy-making through their impact on the nature of public discourse. They contribute to policy-making not only by what they say, but also: by whether they say anything at all (i.e., agenda setting) (75,76); who is allowed to speak (the selection of its news sources) (73,77); how much prominence is given to an issue (priority setting) (78,79); and the "angle" used in covering an issue (problem framing) (80,81). They thus act selectively as channels of communication among key players and would-be participants. Such influence on public opinion and on policy-makers is especially important when other sources of information (from experience or other media) are not readily available to the public or political leaders (82,83).

Thus, any ecological view of policy-making must take account of the mass media as a contributor to the social and political process that links policy-makers with the other interested parties, within and outside of government, and with the remaining section of the public in which opinions may develop and be called into the play of policy-making. Account must also be taken of the function of the media in channelling communication among all these groups.

Summary

Conceptually, within an enabling or restrictive social context or climate, a specific policy issue draws the attention of the groups within and outside government that view a policy change as important to their interests (Fig. 1). Depending on their priorities, the groups deploy their resources to influence the shape, pace, or direction of policy-making in ways that will either enhance or at least not harm their interests. The effectiveness of their efforts depends on their influence, status, resources, and skill relative to competing groups that have different interests. Thus, within an ecological view of policy-making the important environmental conditions form the social climate, and the participants are the interested parties (including the policy-keeper) and their agendas, priorities, resources, and perceptions of timeliness (or whether the general climate in its many facets allows policy movement that will ensure — or not damage — their political, economic or social interests). Important too are the strategies that groups deploy — involving internal organization, information and the mass media, and interorganizational relations — directly or indirectly to influence the shape of a policy. Finally, the extent of involvement of the mass media (including the extent of coverage, prominence, timing, emphasis ("angle"), sources chosen, and commentary, if any) may affect the climate and indirectly influence the perceptions of interested parties about the timeliness of a specific policy and so whether or how they should try to shape it (Table 1).

A Method: Observing the Art

An ecological view of policy-making also suggests the data-gathering methods that are needed to glean usable lessons from political reality in any attempt to analyse the development of a health-related policy in any or all of its phases, from initiation to reformulation.

For analytic purposes, a policy is taken to be the current formal statement (for example, in the form of legislation or a declaration),

17

Fig. 1. The scene and the players in the continuous process
of making policy

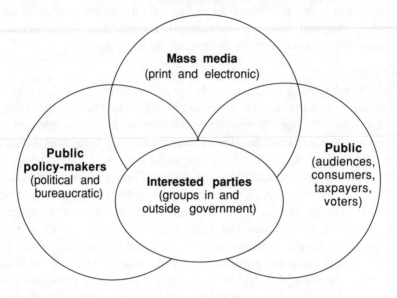

the aim of analysis being to explain why it changes on paper and/or in
process or implementation. Some of the major problems relevant to
learning how to develop healthy public policy are to determine:

— the environmental (political, social, economic, organizational) conditions under which a specific healthy public
policy became feasible;

— the most influential interested parties and the points in policy
development at which they exercised their influence;

— what the interested parties gained and/or lost;

— the strategic actions that succeeded or failed; and

— the consequences of policy-making within and between interested parties, the media, and the general public that may make
healthy public policy more or less feasible in the future.

Gathering policy-relevant information on how to pursue healthy
public policy requires an emphasis on qualitative or soft data, and
methods of data gathering complemented by hard (quantitative) data
whenever possible, rather than relying primarily and typically on data
from either intraorganizational or survey, statistical or economic

18

studies. Qualitative approaches stress relevance, timeliness and use-fulness over rigor and strict accuracy *(84)* and thus are appropriate to the changing circumstances of policy-making and the purposes of people who wish to be more effective participants.

The kinds of data needed to analyse policy-making are implied by the ecological concept. These are mainly information on: the social context or climate available from public documents, opinion polls and the media; the nature and size of the organizations and subunits that are key participants, usually available from their public or in-house reports; the perceptions of these interested parties of their stake in and position on a given policy, in the light of the larger social context as they see it; the strategies they deploy to influence policy development; and their view of the short- and long-term feasibility of a given policy. Such information is best obtained by semistructured interviews *(85)*. In effect, an attempt is made to view the policy-making process from the outside through the documents of organiza-tions and other groups, and from the inside through the eyes of participants.

Tracer studies
Perhaps the most workable approach to such policy studies, given the current rudimentary state of the art, is to identify and trace the development of a specific healthy public policy. The key players must be identified (including the policy-keeper during the phase(s) under study), a cast that will grow (a "snowball sample") through information gained from documents and interviews. Among the techniques that can be employed are historical methods; content analyses, elements of Delphi and scenario approaches; and qualita-tive, systematic analyses of hard and soft data, according to the con-ceptual categories of the ecological model of policy-making.

Description and analyses would include, for example, what participants (organizational units) were involved; how (their positions on the policy questions as the policy developed); what resources and strategies they used; and their success in shaping the policy in their favour. Beyond the effectiveness of the participating interested parties, the impact of the policy and the policy-making process may be evaluated by determining health-related changes. Such changes may occur in: participants' agendas and priorities (whether a participant is a committee, department, business or community group); the definition or scope of public policy problems; the criteria for choosing policy solutions (such as taking health or

Table 1. Suggestive indicators and methods to describe
and analyse the scene and players in the policy-making process

The scene	The changing environment (social climate):	
	Population (age, ethnicity)	Political party agendas, priorities
	Economy (growth, unemployment, inflation, income distribution)	Legislative agendas, priorities, statutes, composition
Policy development phases	*Policy phases (not necessarily linear)*	*Generic questions implicit in policy-making*
and players (interested parties within and outside government)	Initiation	Is issue legitimate for policy? (If so, what is definition and scope of problem? What priority should it have? What are possible solutions (goals, means)? What criteria should guide selection?
	Adoption	Who decides and how (criteria used)?
	Implementation	How and by whom should policy be implemented?
	Evaluation	What are criteria and sources of evaluation?
	Reformulation	How should policy goals/ means be changed?
Research approach	Identify specific *(a)* policy (goals and components (economic, regulatory, direct provision, education/information/ research, participatory guarantees)) and *(b)* phase(s) for study, including points in time	
Major sources of information	Legislative archives; newspapers of record	
Methods	Interviews, modified Delphi and other surveys; content analysis	

political economy and social ecology

Bureaucratic arrangements Extragovernmental groups (new, old, mergers, splits)	Mass media and public opinion natural/ technological crises

Descriptive story (chronology of phases under study; how players answered generic questions; their reasons and actions)	*Analysis and interpretation* (Why is policy in its current form?)
Players: overall agenda, goals, priorities; preferred and fallback position on the policy; initial involvement with policy; own interests at stake gained in policy and feasibility of own success; strategic actions taken (internal; information/media; inter-organizational); organization data on purpose, size, source of funds, age, constituencies, authority, influence (proximity to policy-makers)	Which players had influence? What strategic actions failed and succeeded? Why (in relation to "climate" and competing interests gained or lost)? Did agendas, goals, priorities, policy views, structure, relationships, resources, or influence of players change during policy process? Did media or public opinion change? Which population subgroups gained/lost?
Mass media: extent of policy coverage, timing, prominence, emphasis, sources used,commentary	

Identify parts at interest (including policy-keeper) and major media Gather data on climate, players' views, organizational units (interested parties), media coverage	Analyse and interpret data Consult expert analysis

Major interested parties Organizational and public documents/ data	Primary and secondary data

	Historical, systemic, qualitative, economic, social-epidemiological

21

vulnerable groups into account). Are more or different interested parties involved in consultations on policy? During policy implementation, has the distribution of resources or authority shifted among interested parties? If so, has it shifted in favour of advantaged or disadvantaged groups? Have new formal or informal interorganizational mechanisms or units developed? Have the perceptions of participants, the press or the public changed concerning the value or feasibility of the policy? This might affect its reformulation.

If such process-oriented questions were asked about specific national, regional or local experiences in developing healthy public policies, the answers could improve the science of policy-making. If made part of the skills of policy practitioners through seminars and other means, such answers could help make public policies that promote health easier for policy-makers to choose.

The substantive dimension of a healthy public policy, namely, its effects on people's health, requires attention to direct population measures as well as to changes in the environments and living conditions that nurture health, including changes in access to policy-making processes. Such research findings will indicate whether a policy has actually favoured disadvantaged or advantaged sections of the community.

Conclusion

Once the idea of healthy public policy is accepted, the next step is to put it into practice. Many countries have succeeded in developing policies that benefit health. The current problems for policy analysts are determining not only the nature of these benefits to people's health but also how such policies were enacted. This information, disseminated to people who seek to improve health and wellbeing, can contribute to the prospects for making healthy public policy.

References

1. **Milio, N**. Towards a turn-of-the-century public health: international initiatives and policy support implications. *Environments* (in press).
2. **Patel, M**. An economic evaluation of "health for all". *Health policy and planning*, **1**: 37–47 (1986).

3. **Gardell, B**. Scandinavian research on stress in working life. *International journal of health services*, **12**: 31–41 (1982).

4. **Milio, N**. *Promoting health through public policy*. Philadelphia, F.A. Davis, 1981.

5. *The Swedish health services in the 1990's*. Stockholm, National Board of Health and Welfare, 1985.

6. **Kottke, T**. Disease and risk factor clustering in the U.S.: implications for public health policy. *In*: Office of Disease Prevention and Health Promotion. *Integration of risk factor interventions*. Washington, DC, Department of Health and Human Services, 1986, pp. 1–62.

7. **Jones, H**. A special consideration of the aging process, disease and life expectancy. *Advances in biological and medical physics*, **4**: 281–337 (1956).

8. **Olshansky, S.J. et al**. *The fourth stage of the epidemiologic transition: the age of declining mortality in advanced ages*. Washington, DC, American Public Health Association, 1985.

9. **Schneider, E. & Brody, J**. Aging, natural death, and the compression of morbidity: another view. *New England journal of medicine*, **309**: 854–856 (1983).

10. **Kohler, L. & Martin, J., ed**. *Inequalities in health and health care*. Gothenburg, Nordic School of Public Health, 1985.

11. **Verbrugge, L.M**. Gender and health: an update on hypotheses and evidence. *Journal of health and social behavior*, **26**: 156–182 (1985).

12. **Kaplan, G.A. & Camacho, R**. Perceived health and mortality: a nine-year follow-up of the human population laboratory cohort. *American journal of epidemiology*, **117**: 292–304 (1983).

13. **Rodin, J**. Aging and health: effects of the sense of control. *Science*, **233**: 1271–1276 (1986).

14. **Rosenfeld**, A. *New views of older lives*. Washington, DC, National Institute of Mental Health, 1978.

15. **Smith, R**. Bitterness, shame, emptiness, waste: an introduction to unemployment and health. *British medical journal*, **291**: 1024–1027, 1985.

16. **Dean, K**. Social support and health: pathways to influence. *Health promotion*, **1**(2): 133–150, 1986.

17. **McKinlay, J**. Epidemiological and political determinants of social policies regarding the public health. *Social science and medicine*, **13**(5): 541–558 (1979).

18. **Nizetic, B. et al**. *Scientific approaches to health and health care*. Copenhagen, WHO Regional Office for Europe, 1986.

19. *Targets for health for all*. Copenhagen, WHO Regional Office for Europe, 1985 (European Health for All Series No. 1).

20. Ottawa Charter for Health Promotion. *Health promotion*, **1**(4): iii–v (1986).

21. *Health promotion. Concepts and principles in action. A policy framework*. Copenhagen, WHO Regional Office for Europe, 1986.

22. **Sigerist, H.E**. *The university at the crossroads: addresses and essays*. New York, Henry Schuman, 1946.

23. **Winslow, C.-E.A**. *The evolution and significance of the modern public health campaign*. New Haven, Yale University Press, 1926.

24. **Milio, N**. Promoting health through structural change: analysis of the origins and implementation of Norway's farm-food-nutrition policy. *Social science and medicine*, **15A**: 721–734 (1981).

25. **Brenner, H**. Mortality and the national economy. *Lancet*, **2**: 568–573 (1979).

26. **Norum, K**. Ways and means of influencing nutritional behavior — experiences from the Norwegian nutrition and food policy. *In*: *Influence of modern style of life on food habits of man*. Karger, Basle, 1985, pp. 29–43 (Bibliotheca Nutritio et Dieta, No. 36).

27. *Developing a health promotion policy. The basic considerations*. Dublin, Health Education Bureau, 1986.

28. **Epp, J**. Achieving health for all: a framework for health promotion. *Health promotion*, **1**(4): 413–417 (1986).

29. **Food Committee of 1983**. *Summary report from the Expert Group for Diet and Health*. Uppsala, Expert Group for Diet and Health, 1985.

30. *General plan for the development of health education for 1984–88*. Helsinki, National Board of Health, 1983.

31. **Daneff, T**. *Preventing illness: strategies for a preventive health policy*. London, Social Democratic Party, 1984.

32. *A new vision of health: report of a working group*. London, Labour Party, 1985.

33. *10-year plan for the NHS in Greenwich. Comments from the London Borough of Greenwich*. London, London Borough of Greenwich, 1985.

34. **Social Health Office**. *Discussion paper. Role and functions of the Social Health Office*. Adelaide, South Australian Health Commission, 1986.

35. **Gunji, A**. *An administrative view of the role of private enterprises in health maintenance*. Tokyo, Faculty of Medicine, University of Tokyo, 1986.

36. **Faculty of Community Medicine**. *HFA 2000: charter for action*. London, Royal College of Physicians, 1986.

37. **Qvortrup, L**. *Electronic village halls — teleports for rural village communities*. Odense, Odense University, 1987.

38. **Milio, N**. Creating a healthful future. *Community health studies*, **9**: 270–274 (1985).

39. **Gogstad, A**. The use of social background data in social medicine research. *Scandinavian journal of social medicine*, **14**: 49–50 (1986).

40. **Hunt, S. et al**. *Measuring health*. London, Croom Helm, 1986.

41. **Mossey, J.M. & Shapiro, E**. Self-rated health: a predictor of mortality among the elderly. *American journal of public health*, **72**: 800–808 (1982).

42. **Wilkins, R. & Adams, O**. *Healthfulness of life*. Montreal, Institute for Research on Public Policy, 1983.

43. **Falcone, D**. Health policy analysis: some reflections on the state of the art. *Policy studies journal*, **9(2)**: 188–197 (1980).

44. **Joint Economic Commission**. *Economic change, physical illness, and social deviance*. Washington, DC, US Congress, 1984, pp. 72–110 (Committee Print 98–200).

45. **Office of Technology Assessment**. *Technology and structural unemployment: re-employing displaced adults*. Washington, DC, US Congress, 1986.

46. **Westcott, G. et al**. *Health policy implications of unemployment*. Copenhagen, WHO Regional Office for Europe, 1985.

47. **Milio, N**. Community binding and community building with telematics tools: potential, problems, policies. *In*: Duhl, L., ed. *Urban condition II* (in press).

48. **Hornik, R**. Shedding some light on evaluation's myths. *Development communication report*, **29** (1980).

49. **Altman, D**. A framework for evaluating community-based heart disease prevention programs. *Social science and medicine*, **22**: 479–487 (1986).

50. **Berman, P**. The study of macro- and micro-implementation. *Public policy*, **26**: 157–184 (1978).

51. **Siler-Wells, G**. An implementation model for health system reform. *Social science and medicine*, **24**(10): 821–832 (1987).

52. **Reiss, A., Jr**. Measuring social change. *In*: Smelser, N. & Gerstein, D., ed. *Behavioral and social science. Fifty years of discovery*. Washington, DC, National Academy Press, 1986, pp. 36–72.

53. *Health promotion discussion paper. Followup Communication Plan 14*. Ottawa, Health and Welfare Canada, 1987.

54. **Baum, H**. Policy analysis. Special cognitive style needed. *Administration and society*, **14**: 213–236 (1982).

55. **de Leeuw, E**. *2000. A health odyssey. An inquiry into the planning and design of a regional strategy for health for all by the year 2000 in the European Region of the World Health Organization*. Maastricht, University of Limburg, 1985.

56. **Advisory Commission on Intergovernmental Regulations**. *Citizen participation in the American federal system*. Washington, DC, Government Printing Office, 1980.

57. **Marmor, T. & Dunham, A**. Political science and health services administration. *In*: Marmor, T., ed. *Policy analysis and American medical care*. New York, Cambridge University Press, 1983, pp. 3–41.

58. **Milio, N**. Pressure groups and Australian health policymaking in the 1980s. *Politics*, November: 51–61 (1986).

59. **Morgan, G**. Rethinking corporate strategy: a cybernetic perspective. *Human relations*, **36**: 345–360 (1983).

60. **Vickers, G**. *Human systems are different*. New York, Harper and Row, 1983.

61. **McQuail, D. & Windahl, S**. *Communications models for the study of mass communications*. New York, Harper and Row, 1981.

62. **Lang, G. & Lang, K**. Mass communications and public opinion. *In*: Rosenberg, M. & Turner, R., ed. *Social psychology*. New York, Basic Books, 1981, pp. 654–681.

63. **Barrett, S. & Fudge, C**. *Policy and action*. New York, Methuen and Company, 1981.

64. **Keller, L**. The political economy of public management. An interorganizational network perspective. *Administration and society*, **15**: 455–474 (1984).

65. **Crichton, A**. *Health policy making. Fundamental issues in the U.S., Canada, Great Britain, Australia*. Ann Arbor, MI, Health Administration Press, 1981.

66. **Milward, H**. Interorganizational policy systems and research on public organizations. *Administration and society*, **13**: 457–478 (1982).

67. **Vickers, G**. *Value systems and social process*. Harmondsworth, Penguin, 1970.

68. **Gandy, O**. The information subsidy in health. *In: Beyond agenda setting*. Norwood, NJ, Ablex, 1982.

69. **Freimuth, V. & Van Nevel, J**. Reaching the public: the asbestos awareness campaign. *Journal of communication*, **31**: 155–168 (1981).

70. **Gerbner, G. et al**. Charting the mainstream. TV's contributions to political orientations. *Journal of communication*, **32**: 100–127 (1982).

71. **Strodthoff, G. et al**. Media roles in a social movement. *Journal of communication*, **35**: 134–153 (1985).

72. **Woods, M**. *The influence of community, media, and election factors on fluoridation referenda*. Washington, DC, American Public Health Association, 1985.

73. **Shepherd, R**. Selectivity of sources: reporting the marijuana controversy. *Journal of communication*, **31**(2): 129–137 (1981).

74. **Martenson, R**. *Media competition in the U.S. Research report*. Gothenburg, School of Business Administration, University of Gothenburg, 1985.

75. **Erbring, L. et al**. Front-page news and real-world cues: a new look at agenda-setting by the media. *American journal of political science*, **24**(1) (1980).

76. **Tuchman, G**. *Making news: a study in the construction of reality*. New York, Free Press, 1978.

77. **Gans, H**. *Deciding what's news: a study of CBS Evening News, NBC Nightly News, Newsweek, and Time*. New York, Pantheon, 1979.

78. **Celsing, A**. *Seeing is believing — on the function of the image in TV news' production of reality*. Stockholm, University of Stockholm, 1984.

79. **Turow, J**. Local TV: producing soft news. *Journal of communication*, **33**: 111–123 (1983).

80. **Mackuen, M. & Coombs, S**. *More than news: media power in public affairs*. London, Sage Publications, 1981.

81. **Rubenstein, E. & Brown, J**. *Media, social science and social policy for children*. Norwood, NJ, Ablex, 1985.

82. **Meyerson, J**. *No sense of place: impact of electronic media on social behavior*. New York, Oxford University Press, 1985.

83. **Waldahl, R**. *Communication and political participation*. Oslo, Oslo University Press, 1982.

84. **Patton, M**. *Qualitative evaluation methods*. Beverly Hills, CA, Sage, 1980.

85. **Van Maanen, J**. *Qualitative methodology*. Beverly Hills, CA, Sage, 1983.

2

The relevance of health economics to health promotion

Alan Maynard

The purpose of this chapter is to define and elaborate the role of economics in health promotion. The economic approach to policy choice informs decision-makers about the costs and benefits of alternative courses of action. Such information can help in making decisions, although this can also be evaluated to determine whether the benefits of producing economic information exceed the costs. The economic evaluation of policy options makes explicit in a simple framework the results of competing choices, in a way that facilitates the policy debate and provides an incentive for systematic evaluation of policy options. This framework and the information provided do not necessarily result in efficient policy choices. At worst, it leads to decisions that favour industrial lobbying groups and ignore the potential for improving health, which is very difficult to sustain politically. At best, the economic evaluation of health promotion policies identifies choices that give good value for money and ensures that the scarce resources available are best used to improve health.

The economic evaluation of policy choices is essential to identify cost-effective health promotion policies. For example, does medical advice to stop smoking improve health more than better diets or controlling serum cholesterol levels? The first section of this chapter explores the economic approach to policy choices. This is followed by an examination of the economic theory used to explain the behaviour of producers and consumers. This theory very usefully addresses such questions as which incentives can induce producers or consumers to act more consistently to promote health.

Case studies are presented and empirical results described to illustrate arguments. The appraisal of policy options in health promotion is a multidisciplinary activity. The results of the economic evaluation of alternative forms of health promotion depend on good epidemiology, and can contribute to policy choice in health promotion. Nevertheless, economic techniques are crude, if explicit, and their strengths and weaknesses must be recognized by all students and practitioners of health promotion. It is equally essential for these people and policy-makers to recognize that, without economic evaluation of policy options, choices are poorly informed and likely to use scarce resources inefficiently.

The Economic Approach to Evaluation

Scarcity, choice and efficiency

Economics is the study of how scarce resources are allocated among competing ends. The starting point is recognizing the ubiquitous problem of scarcity. Individual people, households, governments and firms have the same problem: additional resources could purchase many goods and services that benefit these decision-makers but, because of limited budgets, all purchases are not possible and all of these decision-makers have to choose which items are given priority for purchase from finite resources.

Individual people or households can win lotteries; firms can make bumper profits; governments can gain revenue from, for instance, an oil price increase, or can cease to spend on defence; then these decision-makers have more resources to allocate. Nevertheless, the resources available are still finite, demands are still greater than supply and rationing is still necessary.

The problem of rationing health promotion resources is the essence of the economic approach. It can only be resolved by determining how to set priorities for alternative ways of using scarce resources. Of the many ways of spending resources on health promotion, which generate the greatest increase in health at least cost?

Scarcity makes efficiency necessary. Efficiency can be defined as either maximizing improvements in health at least cost or minimizing the cost of improving health by a given amount. Efficiency is a relationship between input (cost) and outcome (improvement in

30

health) and economic evaluation identifies the costs and outcomes of competing ways of spending resources. Once costs and outcomes are identified, a matrix of the competing options can identify the most efficient ways of investing society's scarce resources.

People involved in health promotion who are not interested in efficiency and economic evaluation may act unethically. Failure to evaluate the cost and outcome of a health promotion programme may mean that resources are used inefficiently. The inefficient use of resources means that health promotion programmes are deprived of resources that could produce improvements in the health of citizens. It is unethical to deprive citizens of such benefits, because of inefficiencies not detected by economic evaluation (1).

Economic evaluation in health promotion

Background

There are many ways to improve health. Table 1 is an incomplete list of the inputs that can affect health. For instance, work and leisure environments may significantly affect health. Tobacco (passive smoking) and alcohol (alcohol-induced violence) may damage health and affect the wellbeing of other household members. Which of these inputs gives the greatest improvement in health for each US $1 million invested?

The answer to this question is noticeable by its absence. Most health promotion programmes have not been evaluated. How much is health improved by a 1% reduction in the use of alcohol, tobacco or

Table 1. Health promotion: the production of health

Examples of inputs	Outcome
Income	
Wealth	
Education	
Health care	
Work practices	Improvement
Leisure activities	or deterioration
Household support	in health
Housing	
Nutrition	
Use of addictive substances	

illicit drugs and what is the cost of achieving this? Would the money used for such a programme improve health more if it were spent on free milk for nursery school children, on reducing environmental pollution or on antenatal classes for mothers from low-income households? The list of possible health promotion programmes is very long, but few have been evaluated thoroughly.

The benefits of particular programmes are often asserted rather than identified. For example, *Inequalities in health (2,3)* advocated investment in: child health programmes, day care for children under age 5, screening for hypertension and an enlarged programme of health education. All these proposed investments need careful specification, but even so these priorities are difficult to substantiate by evaluative evidence. These choices are, in fact, based on humane and well intended guesses about the benefits of the programmes. The authors of *Inequalities in health* did not know the relative merits (costs and outcomes) of the competing ways of spending scarce resources on health promotion and health care.

Decision rules
In deciding whether a particular health-promoting activity is to be adopted, two rules should be followed.

1. The activity should be adopted if total benefits exceed total costs. If total costs exceed total benefits, abandon the activity.

2. If the activity (or programme) is adopted:

— if the cost of one more unit (the marginal cost) exceeds the marginal benefit from an increase in activity, reduce the level of activity;

— if marginal benefit is greater than marginal cost, increase the level of activity;

— follow these rules until the marginal cost equals the marginal benefit, which identifies the most efficient level of activity of the programme.

These rules can often produce very useful insight into policy choices. For instance, the debate on screening for cancer of the colon has been elucidated by the economic analysis of Neuhauser & Lewicki *(4)* (Tables 2 and 3). They used marginal analysis to determine the costs of identifying an additional case of cancer of the colon by using successive stool guaiacs (which test for occult blood in

Table 2. Screening for cancer of the colon:
the average cost approach

Number of tests (guaiacs)	Number of cancers found[a]	Total cost (US$)	Average cost per cancer found (US$)
1	65.946 00	77 511	1 175
2	71.442 00	107 690	1 507
3	71.900 00	130 199	1 811
4	71.938 00	148 116	2 059
5	71.941 72	163 141	2 268
6	71.942 00	176 331	2 451

[a] Per 10 000 patients screened.

Source: adapted from Neuhauser & Lewicki (4).

Table 3. Screening for cancer of the colon:
the marginal cost approach

Number of tests (guaiacs)	Incremental increase in cancers found[a]	Marginal cost per cancer found (US$)
1	65.946 00	1 175
2	5.496 00	5 491
3	0.458 00	49 100
4	0.038 00	470 000
5	0.003 72	4 040 000
6	0.000 28	47 000 000

[a] Per 10 000 patients screened.

Source: adapted from Neuhauser & Lewicki (4).

stools). Successful identification of such cancers leads to surgical intervention and enhanced rates of survival.

Nevertheless, Neuhauser & Lewicki did not measure outcome in terms of the duration and quality of survival but in terms of an intermediate outcome, the number of cancers detected. The problem of facing policy-makers was that the screening procedure produced false positives and false negatives and thus repeated testing was necessary to reduce the probability of erroneous conclusions. Neuhauser & Lewicki addressed the costs of identifying a cancer using successive, incremental levels of testing.

As the number of tests is increased from one to six to avoid problems with false positives and false negatives, the average cost of detecting one cancer rises from US $1175 for one test to US $2451 for six tests (Table 2). This modest rise in costs to reduce doubt might seem a small price to pay.

Using a marginal approach (Table 3), however, the cost of detecting an additional cancer using more testing turns out to be very high, rising to over US $47 million in 1968 prices for the sixth guaiac.

What is the efficient level of testing? The answer depends on the productivity of guaiac testing relative to other diagnostic, curative and promotive activities. The cost of the life saved by this test (US $47 million) is high enough that many other lives (the outcome proxy used here) could be saved by allocating funds differently.

There is an efficient level of intervention above which saving lives and mitigating pain and disability misuse resources. All illness cannot be treated, and some people will not be diagnosed or treated or will retain patterns of behaviour (such as smoking) that are inefficient to alter.

Some pressure groups seem to believe that completely eradicating smoking or drinking is an efficient policy. Reducing the use of tobacco and alcohol reduces ill health, but the costs of such policies would probably increase over time, as the behaviour of hard-core users (or addicts) would be increasingly expensive to change. Such resources might produce greater health benefits elsewhere and, unfortunately, it may be more efficient in promoting health to let some smokers and drinkers kill themselves prematurely.

Costing policy options
The primary policy problem in health promotion is identifying efficient policies. Decisions on how to spend scarce resources on competing therapies have to be informed by data on costs and outcomes.

Much costing of health care and health promotion options is incomplete, as it concentrates on the financial (accounting) costs of institutions such as hospitals. Pursuing the policy objective of minimizing costs is easy: the cheapest health promotion policy is to do nothing. Each policy option and choice must be fully explored economically, informed by cost and outcome data for policy alternatives.

Opportunity cost is the cost concept used by economists. What is the value of the alternatives foregone when resources are committed

34

Fig. 1. The evaluation process

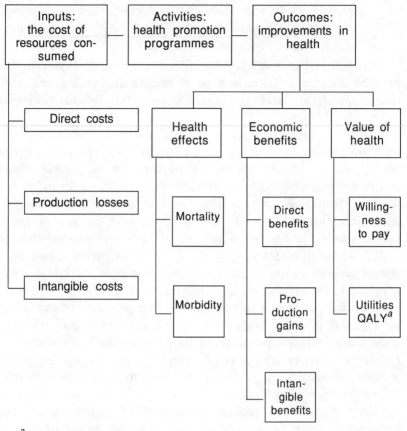

^aQALY: quality-adjusted life-year.
Source: adapted from Torrance *(5)*.

to a particular policy? For instance, the cost of treating diabetes consists of three elements (Fig. 1), direct costs, production losses and intangible costs.

The direct costs comprise the costs of treatment and care:

— costs in hospital and primary care, including materials to test blood sugar and hypodermic needles and drugs needed to maintain insulin levels;

— costs to the household and friends in terms of the time involved in care;

— costs to private and other non-health-care institutions that provide support and care;

— costs to people with diabetes (considerable time may be used to control and treat diabetes; two hours per week is equivalent to 2.5 person-weeks per year of work or leisure foregone).

Production losses affect only diabetics who are employed, but may be substantial because time is needed for testing and self-medicating during working hours and for travel to and waiting at health care facilities.

There are complex methodological problems in valuing working time lost because of illness or gained because of health promotion or health care. In a society that had full employment, the absence of one worker because of diabetes would mean reduced output for individual workers, firms and society. The value of this reduced output is approximated by the average wage of a worker. Thus, if a worker is paid £240 for a 40-hour week, the loss because of two hours' absence is £12. Although no single way of estimating such costs is correct, it is essential not to ignore them. Alternative proxies for this cost are explored in Drummond *(6)* and Drummond et al. *(7)*.

The first problem is the assumption that productivity and wages are linked in this way. Wages may be inflated by monopoly power (a trade union inflating the wage of the lawyer who has diabetes) or reduced by monopsony power (the employer may use buying power to reduce wages below the productivity of the worker and thereby inflate profits by exploitation).

Even if the wage proxies are adjusted for these factors, the opportunity costs of worker absence may be overestimated. If employment is less than full, the employer can hire additional labour at no opportunity cost. The diabetic's input is replaced and the absence caused by illness may have no effect because other labour does the job and maintains the firm's and society's output.

The final problem is that wages put a value on the time the worker spends on diabetes, but what is the value of the time lost by treatment for the nonworking wife, child or retired person with diabetes? Crude economic techniques can solve this problem *(7)*.

The intangible costs to the diabetic are difficult to measure. They may include embarrassment and loss of quality of life (pain and discomfort) at work and at leisure. These costs may be substantial if control is difficult and the diabetic is occasionally found unconscious.

36

All these cost elements are opportunity costs arising from diabetes and various levels of treatment. If the policy issue is the cost of alternative modes of treatment, such as maintenance treatment in hospital or in primary care, the evaluation would estimate the difference in the relative costs of the two treatment modes.

Measuring outcome

These inputs (or costs) are combined in a variety of ways to produce health promotion (or health care) activities such as diabetic screening programmes. How can the benefits or outcome of these activities be measured? Three alternative methods measure: health or medical effects, economic effects and the value of improvements in health (Fig. 1).

The evaluation of medical effects tends to favour mortality and mortality-reducing activities because data on morbidity (illness) are scarce and often not comparable for different programmes. For example, will a programme of exercise reduce morbidity more than a hernia repair? Mortality data, including lives saved or additional years of life produced, tend to be more easily estimated (particularly lives saved), as data on length of survival are not needed and provide a similar unit of measurement for all activities. A life saved by a transplant is the same as a life saved by a programme of smoking cessation.

Nevertheless, the limitations of this measure are obvious. Emphasizing mortality data means that evaluation produces data on programmes that save life but offers little or no insight into the quality of that life. In addition, a life saved at age 25 may be viewed as more valuable than a life saved at age 75, as the former generates 53 life-years and the latter only 3 life-years if life expectancy is 78. Although this problem can be overcome by an additional measure of life-years produced, this again tells decision-makers nothing about the quality of the life-years gained. The additional life-years of the 25-year-old person may be spent in a coma and on a ventilator.

Lives saved or additional life-years produced are used as measures of outcome, but their limitations provide an incentive to search for better proxies of outcome: improvements in health.

Economic evaluation (Fig. 1) involves estimating the costs averted or resources saved as a result of successful health promotion or health care intervention. The direct benefits are the mirror image of the costs: health care costs saved, self-help group time costs, and other institutional costs saved. Production gains are assessed by

37

proxy measures outlined in the discussion of production losses; the intangible benefits and intangible costs are difficult to assess.

Similar to medical evaluation, economic evaluation is severely limited, as it captures very imperfectly the effect of intervention on the length and quality of a person's life. These limitations have catalysed the development of an alternative measurement method, the valuation of improvements in health.

One method of valuing improvements in health is to assign a monetary value to life and injury by using one of three approaches. The first uses legal valuation of life and injury: the damages awarded to accident victims. This is often indirectly and imprecisely related to the human capital approach, which values life in terms of the lifetime earnings of a person. Thus, saving the life of a woman aged 35, if the retirement age is 65, is worth 30 times the estimated annual salary of that woman during the remainder of her working life. This lifetime stream of earnings is discounted to account for time preference.

The human capital approach and therefore the legal approach are ageist and sexist. Lives are not valued after the retirement age. As women have a lower rate of participation in the labour force and receive lower wages than men because of discrimination, their lives are valued lower. Such defects make most economists nowadays very cautious about using the human capital approach. Nevertheless, it is used, despite its limitations, in a potentially naïve and provocative manner.

The third approach to valuing life assesses willingness to pay. People are asked to value a reduction in the probability of death. For instance, assume initially that in a community of 100 citizens the probability is that two (2%) will die from accident or disease in the next year. Then assume that the invention of some health or health care procedure reduces the probability of death in this community to 1%. What value do the 100 citizens place on this reduction? The value of the life saved is equal to the sum of the individual valuations placed on the reduction of the probability of death from 2% to 1%. This approach typically produces high values of life *(8)* and can be criticized in a variety of ways; for example, would people actually pay that amount?

The difficulties associated with calculating and interpreting willingness-to-pay measures have sparked efforts to produce a single composite measure of the effect of health programmes that includes both additional life-years and the quality of these years. The

38

quality-adjusted life-year (QALY) is one year of life in good health, which is assigned a value of 1.0 regardless of who gains the additional year of healthy life. Any period of illness is valued at less than one and thus a health promotion programme that produces an increase in the QALY measure from 0.5 to 0.8 for one year for one person is valued the same as a programme that produces an increase in the QALY measure from 0.6 to 0.9 for another person.

How are the QALY values derived? The first step is to describe the aspects of health that affect the quality of life. Drummond et al. *(7)* classify health states using four dimensions: physical functioning, role functioning, social emotional function and health problems. Rosser et al. use two dimensions, disability and distress (Table 4) *(9)*.

Thus, different measures classify health differently. Each researcher has the same objective: a global measure of the quality of life for all types of health promotion and health care activities. There are many global measures of health status *(10)* and different national research groups are developing and applying these measures.

The classification of health states is only the first stage in creating a measure of the quality of life. The next stage is to obtain valuations for combinations of, for instance, the four dimensions of Torrance *(5)* and the two dimensions of Rosser et al. *(9)*. Different methods can be used to evaluate the combinations of health dimensions in each measure. Torrance uses the time trade-off approach, in which respondents rank alternatives by the amount of time spent on them. Rosser et al. use psychometric techniques to obtain valuations for the combinations of alternative classifications of disability and distress from 70 respondents, and the results are shown in Table 5.

These valuation data can be used to chart changes in health status before and after a health intervention, by asking medical experts to estimate these changes based on experience or by measuring change prospectively in a clinical trial of the intervention. Any trial would ideally use a control and experimental group with substantial follow-up to detect how the health programme affects the quality and duration of life.

Information about any health programme could then be charted (Fig. 2). For instance, a 30-year-old smoker may have a profile of quantity and quality of life like A in Fig. 2 and, in this hypothetical case, die at age 55. An effective smoking cessation programme could create a profile of quantity and quality of life like B: an additional 45 years of life from age 30. The benefit of the smoking cessation

Table 4. Classification of health status

Disability		Distress	
I	No disability	A.	No distress
II	Slight social disability	B.	Mild
III	Severe social disability and/or slight impairment of performance at work Able to do all housework except very heavy tasks	C. D.	Moderate Severe
IV	Choice of work or performance at work very severely limited Able to do light housework only but able to go out shopping		
V	Unable to undertake any paid employment Unable to continue any education Confined to home except for escorted outings and walks and unable to do shopping Able only to perform a few simple tasks		
VI	Confined to chair or to wheelchair or able to move around in the house only with support from an assistant		
VII	Confined to bed		
VIII	Unconscious		

Source: adapted from Rosser et al. *(9)*.

programme is the shaded area in Fig. 2, a composite measure of the quantity (additional life-years) and quality of life gained. This QALY indicator can measure the benefit of all health procedures.

The costs of health procedures can also be measured to determine the cost of producing one QALY using competing procedures. Table 6 presents some estimates of the cost of producing one QALY for alternative ways of spending health resources. Some health promotion activities appear to be very efficient: advice from general practitioners to stop smoking creates a QALY for £167. Similar data from North America are summarized by Torrance *(5)*.

Like all other ways to evaluate outcome, the QALY is crude and imperfect in use. Different researchers use different measures of the quality of life and it is not clear whether the competing measures quantify the same things or whether they might result in different scores if they were used simultaneously, for a given group of people. For instance, it is not clear whether the results of Rosser et al. *(9)* are

40

Table 5. Valuations of combinations of health states (N = 70)

Disability rating	Distress rating			
	A	B	C	D
I	1.000	0.995	0.990	0.967
II	0.990	0.986	0.973	0.932
III	0.980	0.972	0.956	0.912
IV	0.964	0.956	0.942	0.870
VI	0.946	0.935	0.900	0.700
VII	0.677	0.564	0.000	− 1.486
VIII	− 1.028	Not applicable		

Note. Fixed points: healthy = 1; dead = 0. Categories VII - D and VIII - A were rated lower than 0 by respondents. An example might be whether people prefer to be dead or a senile dement with double leg amputation. Some of the respondents rated death higher than these states.

Source: Rosser et al. *(9)*.

replicable for a small group of respondents like those originally used. It is not known whether these results would be different for a large, randomly drawn sample of the population. The advocates of this approach recognize these defects and much current research is attempting to elucidate these difficulties.

Fig. 1 summarizes the alternative ways of measuring outcome. Economists and other evaluators recognize that the economic and willingness-to-pay approaches are incomplete. Because the available morbidity measures are poor, the medical measures are biased in favour of activities that produce additional years of life; quality is not evaluated. Measuring utilities or satisfaction includes length of life and effects on the quality of life. This type of measure could be useful in evaluation.

A final point about evaluation: whose benefits should be included in the analysis? For instance, a programme of respite care for elderly people may benefit them and the people that care for them. Is the benefit of this intervention the sum of the QALY changes for elderly people and care givers? If so, how far should this principle be extended? If a programme to control hypertension reduces mortality and morbidity, the care givers are also allocated QALYs because they do not have to provide as much support. Such issues merit careful consideration regardless of the outcome measure used.

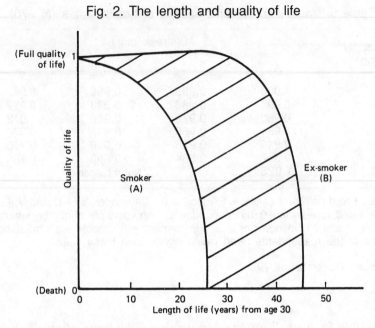

Fig. 2. The length and quality of life

Discounting and sensitivity analysis

The estimates of both costs and outcomes produced by these methods are clearly crude and incomplete. All estimates must therefore be analysed for sensitivity, by systematically varying assumptions by, for instance, 10%, 50% or 100% and determining the effect on the estimates.

Both the cost and outcome measures need to be discounted. The assumption is that it is preferable that benefits be immediate and costs be delayed. To reflect this, benefits and costs that accrue in the future are discounted, perhaps at a rate of 5% per year. Sensitivity analysis can demonstrate the effects of different discount rates on the results. Texts on techniques of economic evaluation *(7)* discuss the need for sensitivity analysis and discounting.

Conclusion

The major advantage of economic evaluation is that it explicitly values the costs and benefits of policy options. Policies are often advocated in good faith but in the absence of evaluative data. Resources may thus be used inefficiently and people may be deprived of procedures that could improve health. Decisions about resource allocation in health promotion need to be informed by cost and outcome data, to avoid such inefficiency.

42

Table 6. The cost of producing one quality-adjusted life-year
(QALY) for competing programmes

Programme	Cost of one QALY (£)
Advice from general practitioners to stop smoking	167
Pacemaker implementation for atrioventricular heart block	700
Hip replacement	750
Valve replacement for aortic stenosis	900
Coronary artery bypass grafting:	
for severe angina with left main vessel disease	1 040
for severe angina with three-vessel disease	1 270
for moderate angina with left main vessel disease	1 330
General practitioner control of hypertension	1 700
General practitioner control of total serum cholesterol	1 700
Coronary artery bypass grafting:	
for severe angina with two-vessel disease	2 280
for moderate angina with three-vessel disease	2 400
for mild angina with left main vessel disease	2 520
Kidney transplant	3 200
Heart transplant	8 000
Hospital haemodialysis	14 000

Source: Williams *(11,12)*.

Another advantage of economic evaluation is that it forces those competing for resources to evaluate their practices. If health promoters and medical professionals know that funding agencies only provide support if evidence is provided on the cost-effectiveness of the proposals, the advocates of specific care and prevention programmes will have to evaluate their practices carefully. Until this happens, policy-makers will ignore the costs and benefits of programmes, and resources will be allocated based on rhetoric rather than on evidence of cost-effectiveness, to the disadvantage of citizens.

Summary
Scarcity is unavoidable and ubiquitous and resources must therefore be used efficiently. Because of scarcity, the way resources are allocated means that some people are allowed to kill themselves by such behaviour as smoking or using drugs, and others are left in pain and

discomfort caused by poor diets, alcohol abuse and inadequate exercise. All health promotion and health care programmes cannot be funded, and choices between alternative ways of using resources should be based on information about the costs and benefits of these alternatives.

Economic evaluation can explicitly provide this information. This process can provide knowledge to inform difficult policy choices and challenge the influence of rhetoric on policy choices in the health sector.

Consumer Behaviour, Producer Behaviour and Health Promotion

Consumer behaviour

Most smokers know that smoking harms their health but they still use tobacco. Why? The answer is important in identifying the variables that can be manipulated to change behaviour. Any policy to change behaviour should be based on evaluative evidence that demonstrates cost-effectiveness.

The consumption of alcohol (measured here in litres of pure alcohol equivalent per person aged ≥ 15 years) has increased by 60% in the United Kingdom in the last 25 years. Why? Can economics explain the effect of price, purchasing power, advertising, health education and other influences on alcohol consumption?

Demand theory asserts that such variables as price, income, the prices of other goods (both close substitutes and other substitutes) and individual tastes and preferences influence individual consumption of a particular commodity (such as beer). If all nonprice variables are constant, the quantity demanded is inversely related to price; if the price falls, consumption increases, and if the price rises, consumption falls.

In the United Kingdom, alcohol prices have fallen while consumption has risen. Consumption rose from 6.0 litres in 1960 to 9.6 litres in 1985, a rise of 60%, while the price indices for spirits, wine and cider rose less than the average price level (Table 7). While consumption has increased, the market shares of the different forms of alcohol (measured in terms of percentage share of consumption of pure alcohol equivalent) have altered radically: the beer market share has declined and that of wine has increased (Tables 7 and 8). One reason for this is the changing relative prices of the different forms of

44

Table 7. Consumption and the price of alcohol in the United Kingdom

Year	Total consumption[a]	Currrent price indices (1963 = 100)			
		Beer	Spirits	Wine and cider	All items
1960	6.0	100.0[b]	100.0[b]	100.0[b]	100.0
1965	6.6	116.6	114.3	111.9	108.7
1970	7.5	148.3	131.9	137.5	135.8
1975	9.3	248.0	189.8	225.7	266.3
1979	10.2	423.3	279.8	330.2	404.7
1980	9.7	515.6	328.2	378.0	471.1
1981	9.4	615.0	373.0	419.1	525.3
1982	9.3	684.5	406.0	456.8	570.2
1983	9.4	746.5	431.4	473.2	600.9
1984	9.6	808.5	465.0	501.2	631.6
1985	9.6	881.4	488.4	525.4	659.1

[a] In litres of pure alcohol equivalent per person aged ≥ 15 years.
[b] Data for 1963.

Source: Maynard & Jones *(13)*.

Table 8. Market shares of alcohol products in the United Kingdom[a]

Year	Market shares (%)			
	Beer	Spirits	Wine	Cider
1960	73	16	6	2
1965	72	16	7	2
1970	72	16	8	3
1975	65	20	10	3
1979	60	23	11	3
1980	60	22	12	3
1981	59	22	13	4
1982	59	21	13	5
1983	58	21	14	5
1984	58	20	16	5
1985	56	22	16	5

[a] As a percentage of the total market in terms of litres of pure alcohol equivalent per person aged ≥ 15 years. All data rounded down.

Source: Maynard & Jones *(13)*.

alcohol (Table 7). Beer has become relatively more expensive as its price has risen faster than the average price level during the last 25 years. This trend makes wine and spirits a relatively cheap way of ingesting alcohol in the United Kingdom.

While this casual empiricism usefully describes market trends, it does not always explain these trends satisfactorily. For instance, the real price of tobacco in the United Kingdom has fallen during the last 25 years; purchasing power has increased but consumption fell from a peak of 132.6 thousand million cigarettes in 1975 to 97.8 thousand million in 1985. If prices fall and incomes increase, other things being equal, an increase in consumption would be expected. This increase has not materialized, reflecting the growing impact of health education on public awareness of the health hazards of tobacco. This public health education has compensated for the economic influences that might have increased the use of tobacco, and such experiences in the United Kingdom and the United States demonstrate that education is potentially effective in promoting health.

Testing the theory

While it is illuminating both to examine the causes of changes in consumption trends and to describe these trends, it is potentially more useful to express these relationships in theories that can be tested empirically and used to predict consumer behaviour.

An example of a simple demand equation that can be estimated in logarithmic values using routine econometric techniques is:

$$Q_D = \alpha_1 + \alpha_2 P + \alpha_3 Y + \alpha_4 E + \alpha_5 A + \mu$$

Q_D = quantity demanded (measured in volume or expenditure terms)

P = price

Y = income

E = health education programmes

A = advertising

α_1 = constant term

α_2 = price elasticity of demand

α_3 = income elasticity of demand

α_4 = health education elasticity of demand

α_5 = advertising elasticity of demand

μ = a dustbin or catch-all variable

The data available and the underlying economic model determine the functional form of this equation. Cross-sectional data that identify smokers and nonsmokers and their characteristics can be explored using models of discrete choice (such as logit and probit). Time-series data can be used to estimate this type of equation. Regardless of the nature of the data and the methods used to estimate the values of the coefficients, it is essential to test for functional form (whether the demand equation is linear as assumed) and for whether the error term has the assumed characteristics. The nature of these tests is specified in econometric textbooks (14).

When the value of the coefficients in this equation is estimated, the results have to be used cautiously. The price elasticity of wine is:

$$\frac{\text{percentage change in consumption of wine}}{\text{percentage change in the price of wine}}$$

Similar definitions apply to the elasticities of income, health education and advertising. If the price elasticity of wine is -1.8, a 10% decrease in the price of wine will increase consumption by 18%.

Such estimates approximate the effects of small changes in price, income, health education and advertising. Thus, the elasticity estimates may predict well for small (10%) changes in these variables, but if the price of wine changes drastically, elasticity estimates will inaccurately forecast the effects on consumption.

Many problems arise in estimating the effects of changes in economic variables on the consumption of such commodities as alcohol, tobacco and food (15,16). Nevertheless, used carefully, these techniques can illuminate policy problems considerably, and they are used extensively by firms to formulate marketing policies.

Some government estimates of elasticities in the United Kingdom are reported in Table 9 (15,17). The predominant form of alcoholic drink, beer, has the lowest price and income elasticities. This result is similar for the predominant products in other countries (for example, wine in Spain and France) and makes predominant products a desirable target for government taxation. Because the elasticity is low, tax increases have little effect on the consumption and considerably increase tax revenue. The price and income elasticities of tobacco for the United Kingdom are small, but higher than many other estimates (15). Most studies find that price increases have little effect on tobacco consumption. These results depend on the data used, time period covered and the form of the equation used. At best,

Table 9. Some estimates of alcohol and tobacco elasticities for the United Kingdom

Product	Price elasticity	Income elasticity
Beer	− 0.20	0.7
Spirits	− 1.39	2.5
Wine	− 1.10	1.8
Tobacco	− 0.50	0.6

Source: H.M. Treasury *(17)* and subsequent revisions.

tobacco tax increases in the United Kingdom can be expected to have only modest effects on consumption, although such increases will generate considerable increases in tax revenue and generate the illusion of an active government antitobacco policy.

The effects of health education are difficult to model. One reason is that the obvious proxies for health education are incomplete. For instance, expenditure on health education excludes the effects of government (for example, the US Surgeon General) or medical (for example, the Royal College of Physicians in the United Kingdom) reports on tobacco. Further, the stock of such knowledge may accumulate and depreciate in uneven ways that are difficult to model. The effect of advertising is also difficult to measure. Should the expenditure of the alcohol or tobacco industry be used as a measure of this effect? What about sports and arts sponsorship by these industries? Should the use of alcohol and tobacco in television programmes and films be regarded as advertising?

The typical estimates for the value of advertising elasticity in the United Kingdom are low (~ 0.1). This may reflect the inadequate estimation techniques, or the tobacco industry could be correct when it claims that advertising does not affect market size but only market share. This claim needs to be investigated using disaggregated studies; although the overall effect of advertising on consumption may be minimal, the responses of particular groups (such as young people, whose preferences may be crucially affected with lifelong effects) may be quite high. As tobacco and alcohol advertising targets young people, it may be inferred that young people are more responsive to advertising than a 0.1 elasticity indicates. As tobacco prematurely kills 100 000 people per year in the United Kingdom, the tobacco industry has to recruit new smokers (an average of 250 per day) to maintain its revenues and profits. Advertising may be crucial in recruiting new, young smokers (7–14 years old).

Economic theory and econometric techniques enable economists to illuminate how consumer demand responds to such crucial variables as price, income and advertising. The results can affect the debate about how to control consumption, although the techniques are crude because of modelling difficulties and the poor data that are available. Nevertheless, even if this analysis identifies the economic levers that will reduce or stabilize consumption, it still offers little insight into the links between consumption and harm.

Consumption and harm
The consumer theory summarized previously indicates the links between policy instruments such as tax increases and the consumption of such commodities as alcohol and tobacco. To measure how such policies affect health, however, it is necessary to determine how changes in consumption affect harm. An increase in the price of alcohol may reduce consumption, but how does this affect morbidity and mortality? Anyone attempting to answer this question has to determine whether to use medical, economic or QALY data.

Some economic analyses have confronted this directly by analysing how policy changes affect accident rates. Saffer & Grossman *(18)* and Grossman & Coate *(19)* econometrically analysed alcohol abuse by young people and mortality from motor vehicle accidents in the United States. They evaluated how an increase in the legal minimum drinking age and increased alcohol taxation affected accident mortality, and concluded that a uniform minimum drinking age of 21 years in the entire United States would reduce mortality among the group aged 18–20 years by 7%. More strikingly, they predicted that offsetting the erosion that has occurred since the 1950s, in the real (adjusted for inflation) level of federal taxation of beer and taxing the alcohol in beer at the same rate as that in spirits would reduce mortality among those aged 18–20 years by 34% and among the group aged 21–24 years by 52%.

Similar work on tobacco by Lewitt et al. *(20)* and Lewitt & Coate *(21)* concluded that teenagers respond more to price changes than adults and that "price has its greatest effect on young males and that it works primarily on the decision to smoke rather than via adjustments in the quantity of cigarettes consumed".

Any study of how health promotion policies affect harmful behaviour or the consumption of harmful commodities has to model the effects of policy on consumption and the harmful effects of consumption. Work in these areas has been very limited and is inhibited by poor data. Nevertheless, exploring such relationships offers both exciting research challenges and potentially very useful insights into the benefits of health promotion policies.

Such benefits would be created at an unknown cost. Econometric analysis can explore the relationships between the consumer and the harmful effects of consumption, but the costs of manipulating these variables are not revealed by this analysis. It may be that an effective policy to reduce road accidents caused by young people would be costly to implement. Benefits cannot be bought regardless of cost, and these analyses can be usefully supplemented by economically evaluating the competing policies.

Producer behaviour and health promotion
Economics offers a variety of approaches to explore the behaviour of producers of alcoholic drinks, tobacco and food.

Structure, conduct and performance
The behaviour of firms and industries can be explored by examining their structure, conduct and performance.

The structure of an industry may cross geopolitical boundaries and is usually related to the range of products it produces and to the firm (the basic unit of production), which is defined by its ownership.

Conduct is the strategies and rules of behaviour adopted by firms. Firms may not always maximize profits (the conventional capitalist paradigm), but may pursue other goals (such as maximizing sales).

Performance is how firms perform on such selected indicators as profitability, employment and growth. Growth is influenced by entry and exit conditions in the industry and by mergers and takeovers. Thus, performance affects the structure of an industry. These categories can be used to analyse the characteristics of industries and firms (13) and the information generated produces valuable insights and inputs for more complex analyses.

Modelling supply-side responses
One of the main responses of industry in the United Kingdom to health promotion policies is to say that they will cause unemployment and disrupt trade. Any health promotion policy that reduced demand for harmful products such as tobacco and alcohol, however, would free money to be used elsewhere in the economy to buy goods and services and create employment and trade. Such changes in demand

may disrupt the structure of the economy as it readjusts, and demand may also shift from domestic products to imports, with adverse effects on the balance of trade.

Some of the effects of particular health promotion policies will be as follows.

- Prices will be increased (via tax increases) to reduce use. How will this affect overall consumer price levels, wage demands and the balance of payments?

- The consumption of harmful products will be reduced. Whose consumption (rich or poor, young or old, male or female) of what goods (beer, wine or spirits) will be changed?

- The production of harmful products will be reduced. What production (domestic or foreign) will be reduced by what amount?

- Employment will be reduced. Where will employment be reduced? How will this reduction be distributed within and between countries? How much will employment be reduced and for how long?

- Profitability will change. Whose profits will be reduced by how much? Whose profits will be increased as demand shifts from alcohol and tobacco to other industries?

- Consumers' responses will change. To what product and service sectors will consumer demand be shifted?

- Producers' responses will change. How will firms and industries respond to changed demand? How will profits be affected and what will be the effects on industrial structure in the sectors that gain or lose?

These effects can be crudely modelled by simulating the effects of alternative assumptions on future behaviour patterns. Such analyses can determine who loses and gains what from health promotion policies.

Public choice
The balance of gainers and gains (consumers and QALYs) and losers and losses (producers and profits) highlights the trade-off between health and wealth in many areas of health promotion. Industrial interests will organize when confronted by health groups whose policies will reduce their markets and profits and therefore transfer

profits and wealth to other producer groups. Policy formation can be explored using public choice theory *(22)*, which analyses how public policy choices are made. This established body of economic theory has not been widely applied to health promotion issues. Nevertheless, the insights that economics provides in other areas makes it a potentially advantageous area in which to invest scarce research resources.

Conclusions

Economic analysis can primarily be used to analyse the costs and benefits of competing health promotion policies. Because of limited resources, all policies cannot be funded, and decision-makers have to choose the projects that are most cost-effective. Mere advocacy of health promotion policies is not enough. As Russell *(23)* has shown, advocating healthy policies can result in the adoption of inefficient policies, and careful evaluation is thus essential. Explicit economic evaluation produces data that illuminate the attributes of competing choices and can facilitate the efficient use of resources. Failure to evaluate may mean that health promotion policies are determined by rhetoric rather than by an explicit factual framework that facilitates choice.

Economic techniques can also demonstrate the effects of policy choice in modelling consumer demand and the supply responses of producers. Conventional economic theory can analyse how changes in price, income and other variables affect the consumption of commodities (such as alcohol, sugar, salt and tobacco) and services (such as leisure activities). This type of analysis can be extended to model the links between consumption or activity and harm to predict, for instance, how increases in alcoholic drink taxes affect motor vehicle accidents.

The behaviour of suppliers can be similarly described and modelled to determine how alternative policies affect profits, sales and employment. These effects may generate opposition to health promotion policies by industries, and this opposition can be studied using established techniques in public choice theory.

All economic techniques have limitations. They need to be applied carefully, and the quantity and quality of the data available influence the results inequitably. The economic approach to policy choice means explicit discussion and analysis of policy options and, when possible, testing theories positively by comparing predictions (such as from elasticity estimates) and outcomes (what occurs). Clearly, economics is only one of several disciplines that can assist in making decisions in health promotion, and economists must work with other policy analysts to produce efficient healthy public policies.

A rigorous interdisciplinary approach to formulating health promotion policies is essential to avoid squandering scarce resources because of casually advocated policies based on a complacent (albeit well meant) approach to allocating resources.

References

1. **Maynard, A**. Economic aspects of health promotion. *Health promotion*, **1**(1): 61–71 (1986).
2. *Inequalities in health*. London, Department of Health and Social Security, 1980.
3. **Townsend, P. & Davidson, N**. *Inequalities in health*. Harmondsworth, Penguin, 1982.
4. **Neuhauser, D. & Lewicki, H**. National health insurance and the six stool guaiacs. *Policy analysis*, **24**: 175–196 (1976).
5. **Torrance, G.W**. Measurement of health state utilities for economic appraisal: a review. *Journal of health economics*, **5**: 1–30 (1986).
6. **Drummond, M.D**. *Principles of economic appraisal in health care*. Oxford, Oxford University Press, 1981.
7. **Drummond, M.D. et al**. *Methods of economic evaluation of health care programmes*. Oxford, Oxford University Press, 1987.
8. **Jones-Lee, M**. *The value of life: an economic analysis*. London, Martin Robertson, 1976.
9. **Rosser, R. et al**. Valuation of quality of life: some psychometric evidence. *In*: Jones-Lee, M.W., ed. *The value of life and safety*. Amsterdam, North Holland, 1982.
10. **Kind, P**. *A review of quality of life measures*. York, Centre for Health Economics, University of York, 1987.
11. **Williams, A**. Economics of coronary artery bypass grafting. *British medical journal*, **291**: 326–329 (1985).
12. **Williams, A**. Screening for risk of CHD: is it a wise use of resources? *In*: Oliver, M. et al., ed. *Screening for risk of coronary heart disease*. New York, Wiley, 1986.

13. **Maynard, A. & Jones,** A. *Economic aspects of addiction control policies*. York, Centre for Health Economics, University of York, 1987.

14. **Johnston, J**. *Econometric methods*, 3rd ed. New York, McGraw-Hill, 1983.

15. **Godfrey, C**. *Factors influencing the consumption of alcohol and tobacco: a review of demand models*. York, Centre for Health Economics, University of York, 1986 (Discussion Paper 17).

16. **Godfrey, C. & Maynard, A**. An economic theory of alcohol consumption and abuse. *In*: Chaudron, D., ed. *Economic, social and political aspects of addiction*. Toronto, Addiction Research Foundation, 1988.

17. **H.M. Treasury**. The change in revenue from an indirect tax change. *Economic trends*, **317**: 97–108 (1980).

18. **Saffer, H. & Grossman, M**. *Endogenous drinking age laws and highway mortality rates of young drivers*. New York, National Bureau of Economic Research, 1986 (Working Paper No. 1982).

19. **Grossman, M. & Coate, D**. *Youth alcohol use and motor vehicle mortality*. New York, National Bureau of Economic Research, 1985.

20. **Lewitt, E.M. et al**. The effects of government regulation on teenage smoking. *Journal of law and economics*, **24**: 545–570 (1981).

21. **Lewitt, E.M. & Coate, D**. The potential for using excise taxes to reduce smoking. *Journal of health economics*, **1**: 121–145 (1982).

22. **Müller, D.C**. *Public choice*. Cambridge, Cambridge University Press, 1979.

23. **Russell, L.B**. *Is prevention better than cure?* Washington, DC, Brookings Institute, 1986.

3

Indicators of health promotion policy: directions for research

Erio Ziglio[a]

The Impact of Public Policy on the Environment and Human Health

Many chapters in this book point out that governments at all levels have public policies that affect health, such as policies on housing, income-maintenance programmes, employment, education, energy, transport, farming and defence. Although health may not be an explicit goal, these policies can have salutary or detrimental effects on people's health *(1,2)*. These policy sectors have a combined greater effect on people's health than traditional health policy conceived of as hospital and medical services *(3,4)*.

Effectively moving towards health promotion therefore necessitates fundamental changes in traditional ways of formulating public policy. These changes should affect both the social and economic facets of public policy. In social policy, planning for health promotion has to deal with poverty, unemployment and other forms of social deprivation and inequalities that are detrimental to health. Thus, non-fragmented policies that comprehensively address such problems need to be implemented as part of a health promotion

[a] The author is very grateful to Dr David McQueen and Dr Claudia Martin of the Research Unit in Health and Behavioural Change, and Dr Mel Bartley of the Department of Social Policy at the University of Edinburgh for the discussions of many of the subjects covered in this chapter.

strategy. In the pursuit of health promotion, social policy must attempt to prevent rather than just mitigate the health-damaging effects of poverty and deprivation (5).

The effects on health of economic development and related decisions in sectors such as farming, energy, transport and defence are also vitally important in conceptualizing health promotion policy. Major pioneering research by Milio (6), Henderson (7) and Valaskakis et al. (8) in North America and Draper et al. (9), Robertson (10), Popay et al. (11), and Barde & Gerelli (12) in Europe (among others) illustrates the risks to health associated with macroeconomic policies in developed countries.

Public policy will increasingly have to deal with the emerging concept of health promotion and its ecological connotation. Since the late 1970s, for example, a number of reports by the Organisation for Economic Co-operation and Development (13–16) have focused on the growing interdependence of the economic and ecological systems. Understanding this interdependence and its implications for public health is obviously central to policies inspired by the concept of health promotion. Thus, fiscal policies in such sectors as agriculture, energy and transport significantly affect the environment and human health. Trade policy influences environmentally relevant products such as chemicals, natural resources and wildlife. Foreign investment policies, private financing practices and bilateral or multilateral aid affect the environment, whether or not they take an ecological viewpoint (16). In exploring these issues, the Brandt Commission (17) advocated that the environmental impact be assessed whenever investment or other development activities may have adverse environmental consequences, either for a country or for the environment of neighbouring countries.

In recent years, public concern about the consequences for health of social and economic development has been monitored by several surveys investigating lay perceptions of ecological and public health issues. A report released by the Commission of the European Communities (18) points out that the 1973, 1976 and 1978 surveys indicated that respondents were highly concerned about pollution and other environmental problems.

In 1982, public opinion on the environment was monitored by an extensive survey of the ten member states (of the European Community) (19). As in earlier surveys, respondents showed substantial concern about ecological issues and about the local and national environment. At the local level, the major concerns were landscape deterioration and noise pollution. The real environmental fears, however, were national or global in scale, such as marine pollution and the dangers of chemical and nuclear waste. This concern and advocacy for policy action was not affected by the regional economic situation of the people interviewed, as results were very similar for high- and low-unemployment areas *(18,19)*. Incidents such as the Seveso disaster in 1976 or, more recently, the Chernobyl catastrophe have further highlighted the danger of ecological deterioration and its effects on human health.

Most atmospheric, land and water pollutants are undoubtedly associated with public policy in general and economic and industrial development in particular. Table 1 gives examples of the effects on people's health and on the environment of some of the major traditional pollutants. Ecological and public health issues are increasingly becoming global. Increased unmonitored industrial procedures lead to the emission of sulphur and nitrogen oxides, effectively illustrating the global nature of ecological issues and the need for national policy action and international cooperation. These emissions can travel long distances and return to land and water surfaces as dry or wet deposits. The deposited compounds acidify soil and water, with deleterious effects on aquatic ecosystems, crops, forests and ultimately public health *(20)*.

The increased use of high-temperature processes such as smelting and fuel combustion in the transport, energy and other industrial sectors has dramatically increased the emissions of some metals. Worldwide human-made atmospheric emissions of lead, cadmium, mercury and arsenic are now 20 to 300 times higher than natural emissions *(16)*. They may affect human health directly or by bioaccumulation. These emissions can cause cancer, kidney and liver damage, and disorders of the nervous system.

In addition to "traditional" pollutants, concern also exists about many "new" pollutants that are not systematically monitored. Some of these are known or feared to cause cancer and degenerative deformities. Although the effect of the new pollutants on human health is uncertain, if governments wait for scientific proof it can often be too late. Research, monitoring strategies, and national and international action towards preventive policies are urgently needed to avoid irreversibly degrading the ecosystem on which human life depends.

Table 1. The effects on health and the environment
of some pollutants

Pollutants	Effects on:	
	health	the environment
Carbon oxides	Carbon monoxide affects the central nervous system	Increased carbon dioxide concentrations in the atmosphere can lead to serious climatic changes
Nitrogen oxides	Nitrogen dioxide affects the respiratory system. Nitrogen monoxide and nitrogen dioxide contribute indirectly to increased susceptibility to infections, pulmonary disease, eye, nose and throat irritation	Nitrogen dioxide and monoxide contribute to acid deposition, damaging aquatic and forest eco-systems
Sulphur oxides	Sulphur dioxide affects lung functioning	Contribute to acid deposition, damaging aquatic and forest ecosystems
Mercury	Central nervous system and kidney disorders	Readily accumulates in the environment with damaging effects on wildlife
Lead	Impairment of haemoglobin synthesis in children and possible neurological problems	Effects on flora
Cadmium	Damage to liver, kidneys, lungs, blood (anaemia) and has possible carcinogenic effects	Has a long half-life, is subject to bio-accumulation, and affects the atmosphere, soil, waters and wildlife

Source: Organisation for Economic Co-operation and Development *(16)* and Commission of the European Communities *(18)*.

Improved collection, interpretation and dissemination of information on the effect of public policy on health and the environment is essential to keep the lay community informed, and it is vital when advocating decision-making practices that incorporate health promotion criteria. It is also urgently necessary to reassess how monitoring systems cover issues and to make them more relevant to policy. They need to monitor the ecological effect of traditional and new pollutants and the effect on health of exposure to combinations of pollutants.

In pursuing healthy public policy, a new generation of more aggressive and comprehensive local, national and international environmental programmes is needed. In searching for indicators of health promotion policy it is therefore very illuminating to analyse the legal, institutional, economic and fiscal means available to encourage and enable public and private bodies to consider health promotion as an integral part of their decision-making. Such analyses are essential in understanding the politics of health promotion and, of course, in building theory.

The Concept of Health Promotion Policy

The ecological view that advocates changes in public policy to favour health promotion has increasingly been supported by WHO reports *(21–23)*. This ecological and public health concern is highlighted by the commitment to health promotion policy expressed in the Ottawa Charter for Health Promotion *(24)*. The Ottawa Charter emphasizes that health promotion policy requires public political commitment by all levels of government to the health of the entire population. The Charter also states that:

> Health promotion policy combines diverse but complementary approaches including legislation, fiscal measures, taxation and organizational change. It is coordinated action that leads to health, income and social policies that foster greater equity.

Target 13 of the strategy for health for all by the year 2000 of the European Region of WHO *(25)* recommends that Member States ensure appropriate mechanisms for providing intersectoral support and resources for promoting public health. Thus, one of the challenges facing health promotion policy is emphasizing health criteria in developing public policy. Dealing with this challenge effectively requires identifying and facilitating the processes by which health promotion can be placed on the agenda of public policy sectors at various levels of policy-making.

59

Health promotion is a process that is said to be co-produced.[a] Health promotion cannot be equated solely with government policies. The circumstances and environments within which people live are the result of government action and of social relations and processes involving a broad range of institutions, groups and individuals. Governments are more likely to act when organized groups generate political pressure for reforms. This clearly has implications for community participation in creating political support for health promotion and in developing health-promoting policies.

Given the diverse structures of policy-making in different socio-economic and cultural settings, policy measures and processes vary widely from country to country. Different political, economic and sociocultural circumstances may greatly influence a country's development of a health promotion policy and its content and scope. Each country has a potential for making public policy more consistent with health promotion criteria (22,23).[b] As health is very dependent on culture and values, this diversity is appropriate as long as there is a commitment to evaluate the impact of policy and to learn from the health promotion approach chosen. Global and inflexible prescriptive statements are inappropriate for a clear and constructive discussion of health promotion policy, including both strategies and health promotion indicators.

Health promotion policy may be the greatest opportunity for public health in the future; it may also pose the toughest conceptual, political and programmatic challenges (26). A substantial investment in research is needed to understand better the conditions favouring or impeding the formulation and implementation of health promotion policy. This research is needed because ambiguities often lie beneath rhetorical commitments to improving health. Government documents and policy statements often pay lip-service to public health, but they rarely clarify how intersectoral decision-making can facilitate the introduction of health promotion criteria, or the kind of policy-making processes and mechanisms to resolve conflicts that bring about changes in health-related public policies (5).

---

[a] *Vienna dialogue on health policy and health promotion — towards a new conception of public health*. Copenhagen, WHO Regional Office for Europe, 1987 (unpublished document ICP/HSR 623).

[b] See also Chapter 1.

60

The search for indicators of health promotion policy represents an opportunity to analyse policy and to build theory. Indicators of health promotion policy need to be developed: for example, indicators of intersectoral decision-making at the macro level. This is only one of the key areas in which indicators need to be developed. Process and outcome indicators of community action in health promotion must also be developed to monitor experiences and to build theory. The development of such indicators may be difficult in health promotion, as theory and methods are still incomplete. The data necessary to develop valid and sensitive indicators of intersectoral decision-making are discussed here to specify the type of information on which such indicators should be based.

Developing and Interpreting Policy Indicators

Policy indicators can provide information on several phases of policy-making, from the preformulation stage through various implementation stages to policy termination. Thus, policy indicators aim to fulfil such tasks as: describing the social organizations and institutions that make policy, describing policy-making processes and outcomes, indicating policy directions, and illustrating past, present and future trends. Appropriate policy indicators should provide guidance to decision-makers, including consumers, health professionals, planners and legislators (27).

The development of health promotion policy indicators presents two immediate problems. The term policy is interpreted in diverse ways, which can convey different meanings according to context. A single standardized definition of health promotion policy cannot be universally relevant, and general definitions imply a conceptual vagueness that may make putting concepts into operation arbitrary or even impossible. Of course, when health promotion is implicit in or a side-effect of public policy, it is very difficult to draw boundaries and operationalize policy stages in terms of indicators of health promotion policy.

The second problem is the danger of overemphasizing measurement as a reductionist exercise. Indicators, like other forms of operationalized information, may give a simplified and misleading representation of reality, particularly when measurement is blindly pursued without reference to competing theories and explanations.

61

Every explicit or implicit health promotion policy has unique features, owing to its location and time of occurrence. Uniqueness, however, militates against the ability to generalize indicators and measurement in general. This is a particularly serious problem in interpreting indicators of process and outcome in comparative policy analyses. Policy-making processes that work effectively in one given context may prove inapplicable elsewhere. Moreover, government decisions may have different meanings in different policy-making contexts. For example, the interpretation of government decisions related to health promotion should take into account that the probability of a decision becoming embodied in legislation, or receiving other forms of authorization, varies according to the legislative and political structure of different countries. The reason for such complexity is not the policies, nor a recalcitrant or perverse reality, but naïve efforts to impose reductionist generalizations upon the many shapes that reality may take (28). In developing and interpreting indicators of policy, this complexity needs to be respected rather than denied or overlooked by a priori formulations. It is thus undesirable to make prescriptive and inflexible statements about the form that health promotion policy should take and to construct indicators accordingly.

Indicators of policy formulation (desired output) and indicators of policy implementation (actual output) must be distinguished. If policy is seen just as output, health promotion policy would be measured in terms of what government actually delivers, as opposed to what has been promised or authorized through legislation (29). Nevertheless it is often very difficult to decide and operationalize in the form of indicators, what the final output of health promotion policy is. Intermediate output, such as the funds allocated to health promotion activities and the number of trained staff and health promotion programmes, can at best contribute to the desired output and should not be confused with the output itself. For example, a formal authorization of resource allocation for health promotion programmes could be measured by several indicators, ranging from financial indicators or resource allocation to personnel motivation and cooperation. These indicators are mainly oriented towards input rather than towards output and process, indicating what is put into the system rather than the result of invested resources.

Policy outcome is the effect of the activities of governments, or other policy agencies. Indicators of outcome alone are insufficient because they say nothing about the process by which a particular outcome has been achieved. There is rarely a straight-line relationship between a single policy and a clear-cut result. Hogwood & Gunn *(29)* point out that several organizations frequently operate in the same policy area and affect the same targets, thus producing interaction effects. Hence, the impact of policy may not necessarily reflect the sum of the purposes of the organizations trying to promote health, or the intentions of the original decision-makers.

Thus, the complexity of the policy-making process must also be analysed. This can be a lengthy and difficult case-study analysis or process evaluation and does not always result in concise and simple indicators. Nevertheless, case studies can usefully guide policy analysis, particularly when based on a clear theoretical framework.

Empirical research on health promotion policy can both describe and evaluate the policy measures adopted. Descriptive analysis focuses on such elements as the nature of the policy chosen, the degree of involvement of local residents in certain issues, the categorization of the policy objectives and the magnitude of cooperation between professionals and organizations. These analyses should not be difficult.

The key question in evaluation is which theoretical framework and empirical evidence enables researchers to hypothesize about how policy affects health promotion. This question is relevant both in interpreting indicators of outcome and in searching for indicators of process.

In developing indicators related to health promotion policy, questions should be addressed. For example, what indicators could measure the outcome of a given policy in terms of health promotion? What processes might influence health promotion policy-making and how could they be operationalized in indicators? Moreover, evaluation is often complicated by the multiple objectives of health promotion policy. For example, many community-based health promotion projects have broad objectives and effects that may be diffuse, hard to define and difficult to convert into precise operationalized indicators. Traditional baseline measures, controlled trials or epidemiological research would largely be inadequate. Significant indicators of process cannot be easily quantified. Researchers usually choose variables that can be quantified. Researchers analysing health promotion policy, however, must consider the meaning, values, aspirations and motives that the participants attach to the project being investigated, all of which are less able to be meaningfully quantified *(28)*.

This situation poses remarkably intertwined theoretical and methodological problems for developing indicators of health promotion policy. To have meaning, indicators must be grounded in a strong theoretical framework. Such a framework is still underdeveloped in the emerging concept of health promotion policy. This should warn of the danger of overloading the information contained in any indicator. The overemphasis placed on social indicators in the formulation and evaluation of policy in the last two decades illustrates just this danger. In the 1960s and 1970s, social scientists, planners and policy-makers involved in public policy formulation at various levels of government put increasing faith into developing a system of social indicators that attempts to measure salient aspects of the quality of life and to monitor societal change (30). Although the social indicator movement was particularly strong in the United States, it had considerable impact in many European countries, too (31). As Land (32) points out, perhaps the most publicized definition of social indicators was given in *Toward a social report (33)*:

> A social indicator . . . may be defined to be a statistic of direct normative interest which facilitates concise, comprehensive and balanced judgements about the conditions of major aspects of society. It is in all cases a direct measure of welfare and is subject to the interpretation that, if changes are in the "right" direction, while other things remain equal, things have gotten better, or people are "better off".

The rationale for developing social indicators was heavily influenced by the use of economic indicators and the emphasis placed on quantitative operationalized information. All too often, however, social indicators — presented as averages, proportions, rates or indices — have been taken uncritically to convey more information than is merited by the actual data (32,34–36). In explaining the danger of overloading the information derived from social indicators, Sheldon & Freeman (36) argue that social indicators cannot be used to develop a system of social accounts because "there is no social theory capable of defining the variables of a social system and the interrelations between them, and such a system is an essential prerequisite to the development of a system of social accounts" (see also 30). Thus, although indicators can be useful in planning activities, one must be cautious, especially in evaluating policy or building theory.

The difficulties in generating and interpreting indicators of health promotion policy suggest caution towards the whole question of

64

measurement. Indicators should make sense out of phenomena that are not familiar, but the interpretation of these indicators should result from a validated theory. As theory-building in health promotion is still primitive, indicators of policy or other operationalized information may produce more questions than answers, particularly at this early stage. This should not be considered detrimental to understanding and analysing health promotion policy, but such questions should be openly acknowledged and, when possible, addressed.

The rush to a reductionist type of measurement may denigrate indicators that have a subjective component. Yet an appropriate strategy in developing indicators may emphasize the development of valid and reliable subjectively based indicators of health promotion policy (37,38). Indeed, subjectively based indicators may be congruent with the underlying subjective ethos of health promotion policy. In the end, well developed subjectively based indicators may be more sensitive and, thus, attuned to the apparent vagaries of culturally biased health promotion strategies in different countries. A good example of the importance of subjectively based indicators of health promotion policy is the approach to health promotion chosen by the New Zealand Maori Women's Welfare League (39). Dyall (40) points out that:

> Although the Maori population, and particularly Maori women, have amongst the highest rates of lung cancer and heart disease in the world, these are not our health priorities at present. Instead, we are concerned about rebuilding and strengthening our culture. The biggest health problem facing Maori people is cultural alienation. To be healthy, young people need to feel proud of who they are . . . Maori people are now rebuilding those institutions which provide the foundation for good health. From our perspective, these are: language, strengthening family and tribal links, rebuilding Maori meeting places (marae), regaining ownership of land and water resources and transmission of cultural values and beliefs.

Indicators of Intersectoral Decision-making

Some countries have already set up intersectoral decision-making mechanisms for health promotion. For example, the Swedish Parliament established an advisory Intersectoral Health Council in 1985. The Council comprises senior personnel from ministries such as Health and Social Affairs, Labour, Housing and Physical Planning, Agriculture, Transport and Communication, and Finance. The

Council provides an organizational focus to strengthen the links between different public policy sectors and health promotion objectives *(41)*.

The Norwegian national nutrition and food policy, formulated in the mid-1970s, also attempted to promote health using intersectoral decision-making *(42–44)*. The Norwegian Government set up an interministerial coordinating body to promote cooperation in implementing this policy by ensuring that nutritional considerations are given sufficient attention in the work of various ministries. Thus, intersectoral decision-making is designed to facilitate policy decisions related to food and nutrition and make their ultimate implementation smoother.

The feasibility and desirability of devising intersectoral decision-making mechanisms at a national level vary from country to country. In Canada, in the late 1970s, there was an attempt to promote a national food strategy based on intersectoral decision-making *(45)*. This attempt was short-lived because some government departments and vested interest groups resisted. The author has analysed the reasons for the failure of the 1977 food strategy for Canada *(46,47)*. By and large, intersectoral decision-making is more feasible in certain European countries (particularly in Scandinavia) than, for example, in North America. This does not mean that Canada and the United States cannot find appropriate policy-making devices (often bypassing central government control) to promote health effectively. For example, the United States has a history of minimal central government intervention in human activities. This reduces the desirability of adopting intersectoral decision-making at a macro level *(6,26)*. This tendency stems from assuming individual freedom of choice and from the political faith that the free-market economy maximizes individual and social welfare *(48)*. Tilson *(26)* reviews the role of the various levels of government in the United States in health-promotion-related activities.

To understand health promotion policy, it is necessary, but not sufficient, to have nominal indicators, descriptive statements that indicate whether intersectoral decision-making operates, or whether a given policy exists. For instance, a nominal indicator would pick up the existence or absence of: legislation to protect the public from the production, distribution, promotion and use of harmful goods; appropriate channels that allow public participation in shaping health promotion policy; policy measures that specifically have health promotion as a fundamental goal; and established organizational mechanisms for intersectoral decision-making. In conceptual terms, nominal indicators provide only a superficial attempt to analyse policy and an unsophisticated, sometimes misleading, representation of the real situation. Normal indicators do not convey information on the ways policies are implemented and only prove to be of marginal use in interpreting policy change over time.

Indicators need to go beyond description to be sensitive enough to distinguish between the formal aspect of intersectoral decision-making (which can be very impressive on paper) and what happens in practice. If indicators lack this sensitivity they will not be able to detect the cases in which intersectoral decision-making is merely a routine bureaucratic procedure without efficacy or application. In order to ensure that indicators are sensitive, a set of indicators is necessary that at least covers areas such as the decision-making process and the outcome of intersectoral decision-making.

Of course, in assessing the role of health promotion in a given country, the impact on health of policies not explicitly formulated as health promotion policy, or policy decisions as outcomes of non-intersectoral decision-making (such as housing, pricing, unemployment, defence, energy, income and social security) must also be monitored. Based on this, a system of indicators measuring the implications for health of public policy is necessary, to enable public participation in health promotion policy-making.

Indicators of processes of intersectoral decision-making
The appropriate method of policy analysis and the task of finding policy indicators vary according to the policy-making context within which health promotion issues are perceived and the decision-making process within which they are handled. The type of information to be gathered in developing these indicators has varying salience according to the features of the decision-making process within which policy-making operates. At least three styles of decision-making can be identified: rational–deductive, incremental and mixed-scanning. Elsewhere, the author has analysed these different decision-making processes as applied to health promotion policy *(49)*.

If health promotion policy is inspired by a rational–deductive style of decision-making, the policy tends to be structured in terms of a strategy. A series of sequential steps is worked out to obtain a specific health promotion objective. The basic features of

67

rational–deductive decision-making have been illustrated by many authors *(50,51)*. Wiseman *(52)* points out that this approach:

> ... involves the policy-maker in identifying the goals or objectives that should govern the choice of solutions to the problem, and in undertaking a comprehensive review of all possible alternatives and their consequences. On this basis, a solution is chosen as a master plan for maximizing the objectives chosen.

This approach emphasizes its apparent rationality, the logical sequence of steps and the objective evaluation of the policy alternatives. Despite varying fortunes over the years, the popularity of the rationalist process of policy-making is reflected in the introduction of research units in government departments to monitor the effects of public policies and reliance on: systems analysis, operational research, the planning–programming–budgeting system, the programme evaluation and review technique and cost–benefit and cost-effectiveness studies *(53)*. The supporters of incrementalism have argued, however, that adopting rational–deductive decision-making is naïve, as it seeks to objectify political variables, such as the policy-making process itself *(54)*.

In a rational–deductive decision-making process, indicators should be built on the types of information illustrated in Table 2. This information is essential to assess how effectively the rather rigid, positivistic, rational–deductive decision-making is developing health promotion policy. Countries adopting this style of decision-making have (or are assumed to have) homogeneity among policy-makers. A policy tends to be viewed as an essentially static product *(51)*. Hence, indicators should be sensitive enough to pick up the distinctions made between ends and means, values and decisions, and policy outcomes and processes at different stages of policy development *(55, 56)*. Moreover, they should be sensitive to the very assertions of rationality on which decisions are made and justified. Indicators of rationality would be very useful in comparative work or in attempting to translate a particular policy from one country to another. In fact, there is no consensus that rationality represents a universal concept.

The idea behind any health promotion policy that is inspired by an incremental style of decision-making is to arrive at policy decisions by muddling through, resulting in only marginal change. This style of decision-making requires that:

68

— rather than attempting a comprehensive evaluation of all the policy alternatives, the decision-maker focuses only on those that differ incrementally from the existing ones;

— for each policy alternative, only a restricted number of important consequences are evaluated; and

— the problem confronting the decision-maker is continually re-defined to make it more manageable *(57–60)*.

Table 2. Rational–deductive style of decision-making.
Examples of information and analyses
needed in developing process indicators

1. Health promotion goals and objectives that have governed the selected policy

2. Decision power of the actors involved in the decision-making process (for example, policy-makers, organized groups, voluntary organizations)

3. Evaluation criteria used in ruling out possible policy alternatives

4. Implementation schedule for short-term and long-term policy

5. Policy evaluation criteria and feedback mechanisms

6. Channels and processes for modifying policy as a result of 5

The final set of priorities and decisions is obtained by a political process in which pressure exerted by different interest groups plays the most important part in decision-making *(49)*. This style of decision-making is common in most western industrialized countries.

As muddling through is the result of give-and-take among many interests, it is vital to have indicators composed of quantitative and qualitative information on the nature and dynamics of the interaction of such vested interests (Table 3). Mutual adjustment among various interest groups often reflects their different power and lobbying activities. Indicators constructed using the types of information outlined in Table 3 should then be sensitive enough to show whether the policy chosen copes only with remedial or marginal change. Further, indicators should help in assessing whether the manner in which incrementalism interprets a policy is a barrier to the innovation and change so badly needed in health promotion policy *(61,62)*.

Table 3. Incremental style of decision-making. Examples
of information and analyses needed in developing
process indicators

---

1. Interests involved in the area of health promotion policy and magnitude of competing goals and objectives

2. Number, composition and power of vested interest groups, lobbying and policy advocacy groups and agencies

3. Interaction, processes and bargaining involved in 2

4. Compromise, outcome and short-term marginal change as a result of 3

5. Assessment of 4 in relation to innovation and change implied by health promotion objectives

---

Finally, countries may become increasingly interested in experimenting with a mixed-scanning process of intersectoral decision-making that attempts to incorporate both rationalistic and incrementalist principles. In a mixed-scanning process, a policy is not seen simply as a rigid goal-oriented mechanism. Political considerations and different interest groups are also included as variables in the decision-making process *(63)*; a key task is distinguishing between fundamental decisions (such as a policy shift towards health promotion) and incremental decisions. Etzioni *(64)* points out that:

> Fundamental decisions are made by exploring the main alternatives the actor sees in view of his conception of his goals, but, unlike what rationalism would indicate, details and specifications are omitted so that an overview is feasible ... Incremental decisions are made but within the context set by fundamental decisions and fundamental reviews.

Mixed-scanning affords wide scope for incremental decisions, but within the context set by fundamental decisions taken in a relatively rational or synoptic mode *(29,51)*. Wiseman *(52,65,66)* of the Scottish Institute for Operational Research is one of the few researchers who deliberately uses a mixed-scanning process of decision-making. Wiseman developed a mixed-scanning process to filter issues so that those requiring an analytical (rather than administrative) approach could be selected for detailed planning attention *(52)*.

Four types of criteria were identified to concretize this selection process:

— the size of the issue (resources committed, project need);

— the nature of the issue (the range of choices about future courses of action, the complexity of the problem);

— the future implications of the issue (type of innovation involved, implications for future resources, retaining flexibility of future action, significance of the outcome); and

— the political setting of the issue (level of urgency, consistency in decision-making, strategic relevance, and nature and purposes of pressure for change).

The collection and analysis of information as suggested in Table 4 would allow an evaluation of whether mixed-scanning decision-making is turning out, in practice, to be as cumbersome as rational–deductive processes, or just as lethargic in implementing substantial policy changes as incrementalist processes.

Table 4. Mixed-scanning style of decision-making. Examples of information and analyses needed in developing process indicators

1. Policy statements of health promotion as a fundamental goal or objective
2. Process through which 1 has emerged (for example, the role and interaction of policy actors involved)
3. Criteria used in selecting health-promotion-related issues for further analysis
4. Degree of scanning used in 2 and 3 and its impact on actual decision-making
5. Analysis of how different interests affect 2, 3 and 4

Indicators of the intersectoral decision-making process should portray what happens and what does not happen in intersectoral policy-making. They should encompass not simply the decisions that have been made but also:

— the major interactions between the policy-making actors;

— the process by which decisions have been made;

— the combinations of causes and effects that appear to be at work in the policy chosen;

— the options that have been ruled out;

— the process by which the policy is implemented, modified or terminated.

Although the term policy implies a purposive course of action, purposes are very often defined retrospectively. Purposes defined retrospectively may imply greater strategic justification than one might actually have inferred by analysing earlier stages of the policy-making process. To avoid misrepresentation of reality, indicators of the decision-making process should therefore be able to identify the situations where purposes and objectives are formulated retrospectively in an attempt to rationalize past actions, rather than prospectively as a deliberate effort to attain specific goals (29).

To address this issue, it would be appropriate to monitor longitudinally policy-makers' intentions at the various stages of policy development. It has been argued, however, that as the analysis proceeds it is often difficult to reconcile observed decision behaviour with stated intentions (29). This is also one of the reasons why nominal indicators of intersectoral decision-making lack sensitivity and provide only general descriptive information if they are not supported by more sophisticated data and analysis.

Indicators of outcomes in intersectoral decision-making

Outcome is defined here as the result, or end-product, of the intersectoral decision-making process in terms of decisions made. Indicators in this area can attempt to categorize decisions and policy actions according to their salient features (67–69). Decisions are usually categorized as:

— routine, where there is consensus on the desired goal and how to achieve it; and the technology, staffing and other resources necessary to achieve the goal exist; or

— creative, where there is no agreed method of dealing with the problem; this lack of certainty may be related to incomplete knowledge of causation, lack of an appropriate solution strategy, or uncertainty about the political and technical desirability of potential policy options; decision-makers rely on subjective forecasting and intuition, usually accompanied by a search for flexibility in reframing strategies chosen in the pursuit of innovation and change; or

— negotiated, where there are differences in norms, values and interests within opposing interest groups in the policy-making process that confront each other over ends and means; the outcome of this process is usually a negotiated decision reflecting power struggles within policy-making.

In areas related to health promotion, preventive measures such as immunization programmes are possible routine decisions. Inter-sectoral decision-making on environmental issues is more likely to arrive at negotiated outcomes. In developed countries, policy measures dealing with pollution of soil, water and air and with contamination by irradiation and toxic wastes are good examples of such negotiated outcomes (70,71). The categorization of a decision-making outcome as creative poses more problems of interpretation. First, the difference between negotiated and creative outcomes is often unclear. Second, the dynamic nature of creative outcomes, and their link with strategy and long-term commitments, cannot easily be operationalized by indicators.

Nevertheless, creative decision-making outcomes can be vital in developing health promotion policy. For example, to obtain participation by non-health sectors, intersectoral decision-making has to take account of the interests and concerns of a wide range of policy sectors. For intersectoral decision-making, the question is not just what other sectors can do to promote health, but also what health promotion policy can do to support non-health interests. Many policy sectors overlook the impact on health of policy decisions, and even where this is understood, health is not necessarily the main concern in policy formulation. Thus, from a pragmatic point of view, in inter-sectoral decision-making it may be strategically sound to present issues in such a way that an immediate negative response by non-health policy sectors is avoided.

On the one hand, intersectoral decision-making tends to avoid presenting issues in a black-and-white manner, which allows policy-makers more scope for manoeuvre. On the other hand, the built-in tendency to reach compromise and to mediate divergent interests may mean that the decision outcome loses credibility. Further, inter-sectoral cooperation has other political and bureaucratic boundaries that may severely affect decision-making outcomes. For example, politicians' and bureaucrats' decision-making behaviour is generally motivated by competition to acquire power over decisions, rather than a desire for power-sharing (49).

This built-in trade-off component of intersectoral decision-making can affect decision outcomes in a variety of ways. For example, difficulties may emerge in devising decision criteria that have meaning and relevance for all the policy sectors involved. These difficulties may be reflected in decision-making outcomes in the form of negotiated decisions and/or contingency actions. Such difficulties may seriously affect the desirability and feasibility of implementing particular policy measures characterizing different approaches to health promotion.

Another way of classifying decision-making outcomes is to focus on the policy measures that are adopted to achieve health promotion objectives *(17,72)*. Health promotion policy measures can be classified into three broad categories:

— educational, providing advice, information and even specific training to change individuals' attitudes and behaviour;

— regulatory, mainly legislative measures (sanctions, for example) to prevent undesirable actions or regulate the production, distribution and consumption of goods;

— facilitative, including educational and regulatory measures, but also incorporating fiscal measures (or other incentives or disincentives) to direct action towards desired goals (making healthy choices easy).

These policy measures can be considered as proxy indicators of the rationale behind the approach to health promotion policy chosen by a particular country. In fact, diverse approaches towards health promotion policy are characterized by differing emphasis on the desirability of particular decision outcomes. In general, two divergent approaches inspire health promotion policy *(72)*. The first is the individual-oriented approach, in which the policy measures used are primarily educational. Intersectoral decision-making is usually ruled out (or confined to a very marginal role), as health promotion is seen mainly as the responsibility of the individual. Nevertheless, this approach could also represent the intersectoral decision-making outcomes when non-educational policy measures are considered politically undesirable or technically unfeasible.

The rationale of educational policy measures is to inform people about diseases and their prevention, to motivate people to change their health-damaging behaviour through persuasion, and to help individuals to gain the skills necessary to minimize health risks.

74

Many health education programmes and campaigns in the areas of smoking, drinking, nutrition, drug abuse and sexually transmitted diseases are based on this rationale.

The predominance of individualistic approaches to health promotion in most developed countries is not surprising. According to Draper,[a] it suits the interests of most interested parties in the health field. It accommodates the medical model of health and disease prevention that has been predominant for decades, and it allows governments to commit themselves to health promotion without confronting the complex political questions implied by more structural policy measures.

The structuralist approach to health promotion has a societal and environmental orientation *(47)*. For example, the Norwegian nutrition and food policy attempted to use regulatory and facilitative policy measures, in addition to educational ones *(43,47)*.[b,c] The desirability of structuralist approaches to health promotion over individual-oriented ones has been reinforced by the Ottawa Charter for Health Promotion *(24)*. In this approach, educational, regulatory and facilitative measures are available, and intersectoral decision-making is essential for implementation.

Sensitive indicators should be able to pick up the trade-off between health and other considerations when intersectoral policy-making mechanisms are established. Qualitative and quantitative information could be gathered on the desirability and feasibility of the decision taken and of the options that have been rejected. This type of information can be distilled by collecting decision-makers' subjective assessments on the desirability and feasibility of possible resolutions of various policy issues. To this end, such techniques as interviewing, Delphi and cross-impact analysis could be useful to collect data. Analysing documents related to different stages of policy development can also provide relevant information.

---

[a] **Draper, R.** *Healthy public policy and individual behavioural change: a modern dialectic.* Paper presented at the First International Conference on Health Promotion, Ottawa, Ontario, Canada, 17–21 November 1986.

[b] **Helsing, E.** *The Norwegian nutrition policy: research programme on measures for its implementation*: report on a seminar. Copenhagen, WHO Regional Office for Europe, 1986 (unpublished document).

[c] **Norwegian National Nutrition Council.** *Intersectoral action for nutrition and health: Norwegian policy.* Paper presented at the Workshop on Intersectoral Action for Health, Trivandrum, India, 22–26 November 1982.

Table 5 gives some examples of the information necessary to interpret decision-making outcomes, classified in terms of the category of decisions (for example, routine, creative, negotiated) and in terms of the policy measures adopted (for example, educational, regulatory and facilitative). This information is relevant not only for descriptive and retrospective analysis, but also for evaluating the desirability and feasibility of prescriptive policy recommendations. Policy options characterized by high levels of desirability and feasibility are obviously likely to be resolved quickly. Thus, policy options rated by policy-makers as being very desirable and very feasible can easily be taken within intersectoral decision-making. Options that are either desirable but very unfeasible, or vice versa, necessitate further analysis and cannot be resolved quickly.

Information on the level of agreement or disagreement among policy-makers in rating desirability and feasibility, and the justification for their ratings, is very relevant in forecasting the probability that a specific policy event will occur (that is, the probability of resolving a given policy issue or implementing a set of facilitating policy measures).

Finally, indicators of the outcome of intersectoral decision-making should also specify whether the decision taken is the result of, or brings about, particular types of policy action. Indeed, for many kinds of policy, a decision is qualified by the action resulting from it (49,73). Decisions can bring about actions ranging from interim to contingency action.

Interim action is taken before the cause of a problem has been found and before corrective action becomes possible. Interim action is taken to maintain a policy. It gives time to complete specification and analysis of the health-promotion-related policy problem.

Adaptive action is taken after the cause of a particular problem is identified and after it is acknowledged that the problem cannot be influenced or controlled by a given policy or organization. Adaptive action copes with the effects of the problem and, when possible, minimizes or eliminates such effects.

Preventive action attempts to remove the cause of a problem or attempts to reduce the probability that the cause will occur. Since problems related to health promotion may have many possible causes, several preventive courses of action may therefore be considered in intersectoral decision-making. Preventive action can only be taken when the cause is known and political will to remove this cause exists.

Table 5. Qualitative and quantitative information on decision-makers' assessment of the desirability and feasibility of taking a policy decision

Rating scale for decision desirability

Very desirable:	a policy decision will have positive effect and little or no negative effect; social benefits far outweigh social costs; the decision is justifiable on its own merits.
Desirable:	a decision will have positive effect with minimum negative effect; social benefits are greater than social costs; the decision is justifiable in conjunction with other items.
Undesirable:	a decision will have negative effect; social costs greater than social benefits; it may only be justifiable in conjunction with another highly desirable item.
Very undesirable:	a decision is judged to have a major negative effect; social costs far outweigh any social benefits; not justifiable.
Definitely feasible:	a policy decision can easily be implemented; no further research and development required; the necessary resources (financial, staffing, etc.) are available at present; no major political obstacles; acceptable to the general public.
Possibly feasible:	some indication that the policy decision can be implemented; some research and development still required; available resources have to be supplemented; some minor political obstacles and/or further considerations may have to be given to public reaction, although some indication exists that this may be acceptable.
Possibly unfeasible:	some indication that the policy decision cannot be implemented; major research and development needed; large-scale increase in resources needed; major political obstacles and/or not acceptable to a large proportion of the general public.
Definitely unfeasible:	implementation of a policy decision is unrealistic; unprecedented allocation of resources would be needed; politically unacceptable and/or unacceptable to the general public.

Contingency action usually occurs when the stakes are very high and when failure at one point of the plan is likely to jeopardize the whole operation. Preventive action to remove the cause of a problem or significantly reduce its probability cannot be relied on.

In intersectoral decision-making, decision outcomes are often a compromise between the ideal and what can be achieved politically and technically. Although preventive actions are most desirable in health promotion policy, policy-makers and planners are often compelled to pursue contingency actions. Thus, longitudinal monitoring of intersectoral decision-making could indicate eventual shifts in outcomes. Moreover, indicators of decisions and actions taken, as suggested above, should allow more thorough analysis of the outcome components of the policy under investigation. Indicators of decision-making outcome should always be interpreted in conjunction with indicators of the decision-making process. This procedure should minimize the risk of reductionism and of making inappropriate generalizations.

Conclusion

This chapter has explored some major methodological and theoretical issues concerning indicators of intersectoral decision-making. In developing such indicators, both qualitative and quantitative information should be combined, thus avoiding naïve reductionist approaches. Some of the most pressing issues in the future development of health promotion policy indicators thus involve basic research questions of theory and method. Policy indicators should provide more than simple pictures of information on policy development. The dynamics of the policy-making process and interpretation of decision-making outcomes need to be addressed in developing policy indicators.

The key elements of process in reaching policy decisions cannot be articulated in static, nondynamic indicators that are inherently descriptive. Process and outcome indicators need to incorporate the varying cultural components that influence health promotion policies in different countries. Specific indicators that take account of the variety of decision-making processes need to be emphasized. This may result in the need for subjective indicators, in addition to objective indicators. Process and outcome indicators need to be specifically tied to the variety of expectations raised by policies to promote health. In particular, process indicators must be directly associated with the dialectic of policy-making, whereas outcome indicators must be able to demonstrate that the outcomes are, in fact, the result of specific decision-making related to health promotion policy.

References

1. **Martin, C. et al**. Housing conditions and ill health. *British medical journal*, **294**: 1125–1127 (1987).
2. **Townsend, P. & Davidson, N**. *Inequalities in health*. Harmondsworth, Penguin, 1982.
3. **Hancock, T. & Perkins, F**. The mandala of health: a conceptual model and teaching tool. *Health education*, **24**(1): 8–10 (1985).
4. **McKeown, T**. *The role of medicine: dream, mirage or nemesis?* London, Nuffield Provincial Hospitals Trust, 1976.
5. **Research Unit in Health and Behavioural Change**. *Changing the public health*. Edinburgh, University of Edinburgh, 1989.
6. **Milio, N**. *Promoting health through public policy*. Philadelphia, PA, F.A. Davis, 1981.
7. **Henderson, H**. *The politics of solar age*. New York, Anchor Press, 1981.
8. **Valaskakis, K. et al**. *The conserver society: a workable alternative for the future*. New York, Harper & Row, 1979.
9. **Draper, P. et al**. Health and wealth. *Royal Society of Health journal*, **97**(3): 121–126 (1977).
10. **Robertson, J**. *The sane alternative: signposts on a self-fulfilling future*. London, Villiers Publication, 1978.
11. **Popay, J. et al**. The impact of industrialization on world health. *In*: Feather, F., ed. *Through the '80s: thinking globally, acting locally*. Washington, DC, World Future Society, 1980.
12. **Barde, J.-P. & Gerelli, E**. *Economia e politica dell'ambiente* [The economics and politics of the environment]. Bologna, il Mulino, 1980.
13. *Macroeconomic evaluation of environmental programmes*. Paris, Organisation for Economic Co-operation and Development, 1978.
14. *The environment: challenges for the '80s*. Proceedings of a special session of the OECD Environmental Committee. Paris, Organisation for Economic Co-operation and Development, 1981.
15. *Environment and economics*. Paris, Organisation for Economic Co-operation and Development, 1984.
16. *The state of the environment*. Paris, Organisation for Economic Co-operation and Development, 1985.

17. **Brandt Commission**. *Common crisis north-south: coopera-tion for world recovery*. London, Pan Books, 1983.
18. **Commission of the European Communities**. *The state of the environment in the European Community 1986*. Luxembourg, Office for Official Publications of the European Communities, 1987.
19. *The European and the environment*. Brussels, Commission of the European Communities, 1983.
20. *Proceedings of the 1982 Stockholm Conference on Acidifica-tion of the Environment*. Stockholm, Ministry of Agriculture, 1982.
21. Health promotion: a discussion on the concept and principles. *Health promotion*, **1**(1): 73–76 (1986).
22. A framework for health promotion policy: a discussion document. *Health promotion*, **1**(3): 335–340 (1986).
23. *Intersectoral action for health: the role of intersectoral coop-eration in national strategies for health for all*. Geneva, World Health Organization, 1986.
24. Ottawa Charter for Health Promotion. *Health promotion*, **1**(4): iii–v (1986).
25. *Targets for health for all*. Copenhagen, WHO Regional Office for Europe, 1985 (European Health for All Series No. 1).
26. **Tilson, H.H**. Governmental legislative policies to control and direct the promotion of health. *In*: Holland, W.W. et al., ed. *Oxford textbook of public health: history, determinants, scope and strategies*. Oxford, Oxford University Press, 1984, Vol. 1.
27. **Bice, T.W**. Comments on health indicators: methodological perceptions. *In*: Elison, J. & Siegmann, A.E., ed. *Socio-medical health indicators*. New York, Baywood Publishing, 1977.
28. **McLaughlin, R.T**. Four levels of disagreement about inter-national development. *Futures research quarterly*, **2**(2): 33–53 (1986).
29. **Hogwood, B.W. & Gunn, L.A**. *Policy analysis for the real world*. Oxford, Oxford University Press, 1984.
30. **Brooks, R.M**. Social planning and societal monitoring. *In*: Wilcox, L.D. et al., ed. *Social indicators and societal monitor-ing*. Amsterdam, Elsevier Scientific Publishing, 1972.
31. **Zapf, W**. Systems of social indicators: current approaches and problems. *International social science journal*, **27**(3): 479–498 (1975).

32. **Land, K.C.** On the definition of social indicators. *The American sociologist*, November: 322–325 (1971).

33. **US Department of Health, Education and Welfare.** *Toward a social report.* Washington, DC, US Government Printing Office, 1969.

34. **Carley, M.** Tools for policy-making: indicators of impact assessment. *In:* Bulmer, M., ed. *Social science and social policy.* London, Allen & Unwin, 1986.

35. **Land, K.C.** Theories, models and indicators of social change. *International social science journal*, **27**(1): 7–37 (1975).

36. **Sheldon, E.B. & Freeman, H.E.** Notes on social indicators: promises and potential. *Policy sciences*, **1**: 97–111 (1970).

37. **Hunt, S.** *Subjective health indicators for health promotion research.* Edinburgh, Research Unit in Health and Behavioural Change, 1987 (Working Paper No. 18).

38. **Hunt, S.** Subjective health indicators and health promotion. *Health promotion*, **3**(1): 23–34 (1988).

39. **Murchie, E.** *Rapuora: health and Maori women.* Wellington, New Zealand Maori Women's Welfare League, 1984.

40. **Dyall, L.** The Tangata Whenua: Maori people and their health. *Radical community medicine*, Winter: 9–13 (1986/1987).

41. **Eklund, B. & Petterssen, B.** Health promotion policy in Sweden: means and methods in intersectoral action. *Health promotion*, **2**(2): 174–194 (1987).

42. **Milio, N.** Promoting health through structural change: analysis of the origins and implementation of Norway's farm-food-nutrition policy. *Social science and medicine*, **15A**: 721–734 (1981).

43. *On Norwegian nutrition and food policy.* Oslo, Ministry of Agriculture, 1976 (Report No. 32 to the Storting).

44. *On the follow-up of Norwegian nutrition policy.* Oslo, Ministry of Social Affairs, 1982 (Report No. 11 to the Storting).

45. **Departments of Agriculture and Consumer and Corporate Affairs.** *A food strategy for Canada.* Ottawa, Department of Agriculture Publications, 1977.

46. **Ziglio, E.** *Uncertainty and innovation in health policy: the Canadian and Norwegian approaches to health promotion.* Edinburgh, Department of Social Administration, University of Edinburgh, 1985.

47. **Ziglio, E.** "Uncertainty" in health promotion: nutrition policy in two countries. *Health promotion*, **1**(3): 257–268 (1986).

48. **Johnson, R**. *The ethical aspects of government intervention into individual behaviour*. Ottawa, Department of National Health and Welfare Publications, 1976 (Staff papers, long-range health planning).

49. **Ziglio, E**. *Policy-making and planning in conditions of uncertainty: the case of health promotion policy.* Edinburgh, Research Unit in Health and Behavioural Change, 1987 (Working Paper No. 7).

50. **Meyerson, M. & Banfield, E.C**. *Politics, planning and the public interest*. London, Collier, 1955.

51. **Robertson, A**. Approcci alla presa delle decisioni nel settore sanitario [Decision-making approaches in the health field]. *In*: Niero, M. et al., ed. *Politice di welfare state e modelli decisionali* [Policies of a welfare state and decision-making models]. Milan, Unicopli, 1983.

52. **Wiseman, C**. Selection of major planning issues. *Policy sciences*, **9**: 71–86 (1978).

53. **Robertson, A. & Gandi, J**. Policy, practice and research: an overview. *In*: Gandi, J. et al., ed. *Improving social intervention*. London, Croom Helm, 1983.

54. **Braybrooke, D. & Lindblom, C.E**. *A strategy of decision: policy evaluation as a social process*. New York, Free Press, 1963.

55. **Hyderbrant, R**. Administration and social change. *Public administration review*, **24**(3): 163–165 (1964).

56. **Smith, G. & May, D**. The artificial debate between rationalist and incrementalist models of decision-making. *Policy and politics*, **8**(2): 147–161 (1980).

57. **Lindblom, C.E**. The science of muddling-through. *Public administration review*, **19**: 79–88 (1959).

58. **Lindblom, C.E**. Context for change and strategy: a reply. *Public administration review*, **24**: 157–158 (1964).

59. **Lindblom, C.E**. *The intelligence of democracy*. New York, Free Press, 1965.

60. **Lindblom, C.E**. *The policy making process*. Englewood Cliffs, NJ, Prentice-Hall, 1968.

61. **Dror, Y**. Muddling through: science or inertia? *Public administration review*, **24**: 153–157 (1964).

62. **Wildavsky, A**. *The art and craft of policy analysis*. London, Macmillan, 1980.

63. **Etzioni, A**. Mixed-scanning: a third approach to decision-making. *Public administration review*, **27**: 385–392 (1967).

64. **Etzioni, A**. *Modern organization*. Englewood Cliffs, NJ, Prentice-Hall, 1964.

65. **Lind, G. & Wiseman, C**. *Setting health priorities — experiences and opportunities*. Edinburgh, Scottish Institute for Operational Research, Tavistock Institute of Human Relations, 1978.

66. **Wiseman, C**. Strategic planning in the Scottish health service: a mixed-scanning approach. *Long range planning*, **12**: 103–113 (1979).

67. **Delbecq, A.L**. The management of decision-making within the firm — three types of decision-making. *Academy management journal*, December: 323–339 (1967).

68. **Harrison, E.F**. *The managerial decision-making process*. Boston, Houghton Mifflin, 1975.

69. **Thompson, J.D**. *Organization in action*. New York, McGraw-Hill, 1967.

70. **Bernstein, J.Z. & Freedman, M**. United States governmental control of environmental health hazards. *In*: Holland, W.W. et al., ed. *Oxford textbook of public health: history, determinants, scope and strategies*. Oxford, Oxford University Press, 1984, Vol. 1.

71. **Castleman, B.I. & Navarro, V**. International mobility of hazardous products, industries and wastes. *In*: Breslow, L. et al., ed. *Annual review of public health*. Palo Alto, CA, Annual Reviews, 1987, Vol. 8.

72. **Ringen, K**. The new ferment in national health policies: the case of Norway's nutrition and food policy. *Social science and medicine*, **13**(1): 33–41 (1979).

73. **Kepner, C.H. & Tregoe, B.B**. *The rational manager*. New York, McGraw-Hill, 1965.

4

Conceptualizing and measuring health

Horst Noack[a]

There seems to be widespread consensus that indicators and measures of several dimensions of health, and of changes towards positive health, constitute an important tool for developing and implementing health policies that emphasize health promotion. Major conceptual and methodological contributions to the measurement of health and the development of health indicators and health information systems have been made in the fields of health statistics, social indicators and assessment of the quality of life.

Most developed countries have routinely produced statistical reports on mortality and other disease-related data for at least 100 years. During recent decades, new health information systems have been built in many countries that include population-based information on morbidity, disability, the use of health services, cardiovascular risk factors, lifestyle and self-perceived health. Many countries regularly conduct health surveys or microcensuses to collect these data.

Since the 1960s interest has been growing in social reporting and social accounting. The so-called social indicators movement has created a new research field, built a social theory of the quality of life, and developed and applied indicators of the quality of life as an important methodological tool *(1)*. The quality of life is a broad

---

[a] The author wishes to thank Monika Iseli-Felder for technical assistance.

concept that includes feelings people express in such areas as standard of living, income, housing, neighbourhood, job and health.

More recently, several scales for measuring the health-related quality of life and the dimensions of health have been built and applied in research on health services and in clinical epidemiology. Most of them were designed to assess the effect of chronic disease on everyday life and to evaluate changes in quality of life caused by major surgery, organ transplants, preventive clinical trials and rehabilitation *(2,3)*.

While traditional health indicators and measures focus on ill health or disease, indicators of the quality of life and health scales tend to be more comprehensive and to cover aspects of positive health and wellbeing.

This chapter reviews the state of the art of measuring health in the context of the rapid growth of health promotion and health research. Concepts and meanings of health are reviewed that have emerged in the social and behavioural sciences, epidemiology and public health. Based on some of the key concepts, a general conceptual framework for health research and health measurement is proposed and discussed. Using this framework, selected measures and indicators of health are reviewed in relation to health assessment, health promotion and evaluation. Finally, some of the unresolved issues are briefly discussed and conclusions drawn about possible new directions in measuring health.

Concepts of Health

Scientific interest in general wellbeing and in good or positive health seems to be a recent development. Compared with the literature on illness and disease, surprisingly few social science and epidemiological studies have treated general and positive health.

Some sociological studies using an anthropological or ethnographic approach have investigated the social and cultural meanings of health and derived health categories from qualitative interviews. In one of the first investigations in Europe, Herzlich *(4)* asked 80 men and women in France, half middle class and half professionals, for their views on health and illness. Three main categories were derived: health-in-a-vacuum (being), reserve of health (having) and health as an equilibrium (doing):

> Health-in-a-vacuum is simply the absence of illness. Health is strictly speaking not something positive, it's simply not being ill. The fact of

86

not having a body, so to speak, if it doesn't bother you in any way, health is basically an absence, it isn't anything positive, it's rather a negative thing.

... the reserve of health expresses an organic-biological characteristic as such... It may be good, less good or poor, and may also vary according to the kind of life the individual leads; one may build up one's reserve of health or break into it. This capital asset of vitality and defence may increase or dissipate... [It] does not consist only of resistance to illness, it also appears as the "substructure" of the other types of health.

Equilibrium ... , both in its presence and in its absence, represents an autonomous experience; one feels that one has equilibrium or that one has lost it... [It comprises] physical well-being, plenty of physical resources, absence of fatigue, psychological well-being and evenness of temper, freedom of movement and effectiveness in action, good relation with other people... [Nevertheless] there is no such thing as perfect health, it's much more a matter of being able to keep a balanced life... To be slightly ill, for example, to have a tendency to bronchitis isn't to be in bad health... I am in good health when I am in equilibrium, when I feel myself capable of doing what I want.

In a sample of about 4000 people in France undergoing a health examination, d'Houtaud & Field (5) found that the responses to an open-ended questionnaire about health were clearly associated with socioeconomic class. The higher, nonmanual classes perceived health more in personalized, positive and expressive ways, and the lower, manual classes perceived health in negative, socialized and instrumental ways. A sociological study of a sample of about 600 people in Switzerland (6) found a similar pattern. For the middle and upper social classes health tended to be a value in itself, whereas working-class people tended to conceptualize health in terms of its instrumental value for productive functions, in particular work.

In the structural–functionalist perspective of sociology, health has been defined as prerequisite for social status and economic achievement, or as the capacity to perform social tasks and roles adequately (7). Within this framework, social psychiatry and social epidemiology have studied social adjustment as an important dimension of social health. The main emphasis is on individual functioning in different accepted social roles, such as occupation, marriage and family, and in the community (8). Social functioning (conforming to social roles) has also been viewed in terms of personal equilibrium or success in satisfying one's own needs and others', and reducing tensions (9).

Social support has emerged as a powerful concept in social epidemiological and psychosocial studies. It predicts differences in mortality and in the incidence of disease and serves as a buffer for stressful experiences *(10,11)*. Social support is the availability of people on whom a person can rely and who value him or her as a person. A general distinction is made between social support and the social network, which is the family members, close friends, neighbours or acquaintances that provide support *(9,12,13)*. An adequate social network and sufficient social support indicate social integration.

As already indicated, the quality of life has been studied extensively in social indicators research and social measurement, both in national and cross-national projects. This concept has also recently been introduced into health services research. The quality of life has two aspects: the adequacy of material and social circumstances, and people's feelings about and evaluations of these circumstances *(9)*. For example, in a comprehensive study involving samples of over 5000 adults in the United States, Andrews & Withey *(14)* investigated global aspects of wellbeing such as life as a whole, and specific feelings such as concerns about health, work, marriage and income. Feelings were expressed according to such criteria as happy, satisfying, rewarding, or worried. The authors studied in detail how specific perceptions of wellbeing related to one another, how they combined, how they changed over time and varied between social, cultural and geographical groups.

Psychological studies of health have focused mainly on mental, physical and overall wellbeing and functioning. Although the quality of life and wellbeing conceptually overlap, measures of psychological wellbeing tend to tap two components: affective wellbeing (feeling states) and cognitive or mental functioning *(9)*. In an early study of affective wellbeing conducted in the United States using a sample of 2000 people *(15)*, positive and negative affect were found to be unrelated, and a composite measure of the relative balance of the two affective states was associated with several social and demographic factors. A study of over 12 000 people in Canada *(16)* did not confirm the independence of positive and negative affect, and affect balance was not considered adequate to summarize the data. A study of almost 1000 adults in Australia *(17)*, however, found that wellbeing and illbeing were independent and the balance of wellbeing and illbeing was found to be a valid concept. Other frequently measured

88

concepts of the affective state are such negative feelings as anger, anxiety and depression and such positive feelings as happiness, satisfaction and joy.

The other component of psychological wellbeing, cognitive functioning, summarizes concepts such as alertness, attention, memory and orientation in space and time. More recent sociopsychological and sociological studies have emphasized the importance of such specific aspects of the self-concept as sense of coherence and perceived control over life and life circumstances *(12,18–21)*. Physical wellbeing and functioning include the ability to perform everyday activities, the integrity of the body and overall physical condition. General wellbeing and general functioning comprise perceived overall health and expected future health *(9,22)*.

Epidemiology has focused primarily on ill health, although the literal meaning of the Greek root (knowledge across people) does not imply this somewhat limited commitment. Mortality data are clearly the most reliable and widely used epidemiological data. Instead of using them in negative terms, the alternative positive concepts of survivorship and life expectancy have sometimes been applied. They may have certain advantages, such as in studies of social inequality or social differences in health *(23)*. There are several different ways to present statistics of death, sickness and disability, such as indicators of life expectancy at certain ages, life expectancy free of disability, and years of life gained. These measures can be used to evaluate improvements in the health of populations *(24)*. Further, epidemiologists and clinical scientists have applied and used many indicators of: physical health (physical growth and velocity of growth *(25)*), health risk (body mass index and cardiovascular risk factors) and psychological and social health (subjective wellbeing, social functioning, life satisfaction).

Several of the social science and epidemiological health concepts have become key concepts in major programmes of WHO. Thus, *Targets for health for all (26)*, adopted by the Member States of the European Region, advocates action to:

— *ensure equity in health*, by reducing the present gap in health status between countries and groups within countries;

— *add life to years*, by ensuring the full development and use of people's integral or residual physical and mental capacity to derive full benefit from and to cope with life in a healthy way;

— *add health to life,* by reducing disease and disability;

— *add years to life*, by reducing premature deaths, and thereby increasing life expectancy.

Based on a discussion document on the concept and principles of health promotion *(27)*, the Ottawa Charter for Health Promotion *(28)* defines health in connection with the promotion of health:

> Health promotion is the process of enabling people to increase control over, and to improve, their health. To reach a state of complete physical, mental and social well-being, an individual or group must be able to identify and to realize aspirations, to satisfy needs, and to change or cope with the environment. Health is, therefore, seen as a resource for everyday life, not the objective of living. Health is a positive concept emphasizing social and personal resources, as well as physical capacities. Therefore, health promotion is not just the responsibility of the health sector, but goes beyond healthy life-styles to well-being.

Health refers to a dynamic quality of being, acting and interacting, and it is both individually and socially valued. Health therefore has subjective and objective dimensions (objective in the sense of intersubjectivity or social consensus). Further, health can be viewed both as a global quality (overall or holistic health) and as a set of specific qualities (physical, psychological and social wellbeing and functioning).

The specific processes of being versus acting and interacting suggest that the time dimension is an important aspect of health. Health reflects an experience and a process of equilibrium or balance that people tend to perceive as wellbeing and adequate functioning. Health means command over resources, a constellation of certain capacities and opportunities, or a potential.

A Conceptual Framework for Measuring Health

For researchers, the biggest difficulty in defining and measuring health is the conceptual pluralism that characterizes many socially and culturally defined terms. Depending on the particular focus of the scientific or practical discourse about health, each concept of health emphasizes specific aspects and leaves out others. An adequate conceptual or theoretical framework is needed to identify and define health concepts that fit the aims and strategies of health promotion. Such a framework would be of particular help in selecting and

90

operationally defining reliable and valid health indicators and health measures.

In this section a general framework is outlined to serve this purpose. It draws on and extends a previously suggested framework *(29)* and seems to follow a proposal made by Bergner *(30)* to define health potential as a dimension of health status. This framework is based on several underlying considerations. First, the health of an individual is phenomenologically and conceptually different from the health of a social group or population. A distinction therefore needs to be made between the health of individuals and of populations. Second, health represents a meaningful, positively or negatively valued state of an active individual that can be viewed as a dynamic open system consisting of biological, psychological and social processes. Third, health refers to a set of physical, psychological and social resources that may also be valued positively or negatively. Fourth, health-related actions and resources are located in time in two ways: within the life cycle of the individual and within the history of a social group or population.

The conceptual framework for health measurement first distinguishes between the health of individuals and the health of population groups or populations. Based on three time frames (past, present and future), the framework posits three different categories of health: health history, health balance and health potential.

Health history is the quality of health experiences and the pattern of health-related actions and interactions in the past. For example, an individual health history may express whether the level of physical and social functioning has been stable, improving or declining. The health history of a population group may indicate the proportion of fully active (nondisabled) people over a given period of time.

Health balance is a dynamic equilibrium of both positively and negatively valued experiences and actions *(29)*. Individual health balance designates both an equilibrium in a person's present internal (physiological and psychological) state and processes, and an equilibrium in individual interaction (symbolic or physical exchange, communication and action) with the physical and social environments. These dynamic equilibria tend to be experienced as physical, psychological and social wellbeing and functioning. At the level of a population, health balance may, for example, indicate a high level of wellbeing, satisfactory and productive social interactions and minimal social disruption because of ill health.

Health potential is the capacity of an individual, social group or population to maintain an acceptable level of health balance and to re-establish it when it is lost *(29)*. For individuals, health potential designates adequate social, psychological and physical health resources and the ability to use them. Examples are good social relations, a positive self-concept, adequate health knowledge and skills, and good physical condition, indicated by such factors as physical fitness, immunological resistance and absence of illness. For a population, health potential is indicated by such factors as an adequate level and distribution of income and social welfare, healthy lifestyles among all population groups (characterized by a balance between health-enhancing and health-damaging behaviour) and a high life expectancy free of suffering and disability.

The proposed framework (Table 1) combines the two health levels (individual and population) and the three time-related health categories (health history, health balance and health potential). The resulting six cells define more specific health concepts.

The main purpose of this framework is to clarify the kind of health indicators or measures that are needed for a specific purpose. For example, describing the health problems and health needs of a particular population group requires measures of health balance. To predict future health, measures of health potential may be more suitable. In principle, both health balance and health potential can be explained by indicators of the health history of a given population group. To assess health improvements, changes in health potential or in health balance may be of interest.

The conceptual and theoretical basis of measuring health is not yet well developed and a number of thorny issues persist. They can only be resolved in an ongoing process of health research and dialogues between researchers, practitioners and policy-makers *(31,32)*.

Aspects of health can be viewed holistically and from certain specific perspectives. Either or both perspectives may be valid in a particular practical or research context. For example, physical, mental and social functioning can be expected to be associated with a person's level of general wellbeing, but physical functioning gener-ally depends on specific physical capacities.

Most health issues have an objective and a subjective dimension and both may be important. For example, one aspect of health is how well people are able to climb stairs (objective); another is how

Table 1. A conceptual framework for measuring health

Time	Concept	Level	
		Individual	Population
Past	Health history	Health balance in personal life Positive health career (growing health balance) Negative health career (declining health balance)	Stable and high level of wellbeing over time Increasing level of well-being over time Decreasing level of well-being over time
Present	Health balance	General wellbeing and functioning Social functioning and social support Psychological wellbeing and functioning Physical wellbeing and functioning	High prevalence of general wellbeing Social integration and mutual support High prevalence of psychological wellbeing High prevalence of physical wellbeing
Future	Health potential	Overall personal health resources Strong supportive social relations Strong, positive self-concept Life and coping skills Level of somatic risk factors Level of physical fitness	Equity of access to general health resources Life expectancy free of suffering and disability Survival and quality of life of chronically ill people Frequency of self-help activities Overall level of positive lifestyle

Note. The entries are only examples that are neither representative nor exhaustive.

relevant this is to them and how well they feel while doing it (subjective).

Most health issues tend to be located between some negative and some positive ends on the illness–health or the disease–health continuum *(19)*. Within this framework, measuring health may serve two purposes: locating an individual or social group on this continuum, or measuring changes along the health continuum. In measuring changes the meaning or quality of the previous level of health of an individual or group is crucial to understand the quality of change. For example, recovery from serious illness has a quality different from successful coping with psychosocial distress. Health change may not simply be reducible to the difference between two points on a particular health scale but may be a unique phenomenon in itself.

Many concepts of health are specific to age and gender. For example, the meaning of physical fitness tends to change during the life cycle from childhood through adolescence, adulthood and old age, and it can differ somewhat for men and women. This has important implications for defining adequate concepts and standards of health, and for comparing different age and sex groups.

The meaning of health depends on social and cultural context. As mentioned earlier, there are well known differences in health concepts between groups of low and high social status. There are obviously no context-free concepts and standards of health. This has serious consequences for defining health standards and for comparing the health of different populations or population groups.

Measuring Health

Methodological issues

Measurement is defined as the process of applying a standard instrument (or scale) to objects or events. Numbers are assigned to the objects or events according to rules specified by the instrument. Health refers to many diverse physical, psychological and social phenomena. Obviously, to develop scales or other instruments to measure health, suitable methods must be applied and reasonable standards defined.

As in psychological and social measurement, the basic principle in measuring health is to assemble indicators that are assumed to represent the concept to be measured (9,33). Indicators are either specific observations or experiences that occur in a defined situation, or responses to standardized questions (items). A value is assigned to each indicator. For example, Andrews & Withey (14) have used a delighted-terrible scale to assess self-ratings of quality of life and life satisfaction, including satisfaction with health (Fig. 1).

These authors have also tested a nonverbal measure, a faces scale, which can be used with children and other people who have difficulty reading (Fig. 2). In these single-item measures, respondents' ratings directly express the value on the health scale ranging from 1 to 7.

Most health scales consist of a number of items with several response categories. Response categories usually range from two (for example, 1 = no, 2 = yes) to numbers as big as ten (for example,

94

Fig. 1. A scale to assess self-ratings of quality of life and life satisfaction

Respondents were instructed:

Please indicate the feelings you have now — taking into account what has happened in the last year and what you expect in the near future . . . How do you feel about your health?

Source: Andrews & Withey *(14)*.

Fig. 2. A nonverbal scale to assess self-ratings of quality of life and life satisfaction

Here are some faces expressing various feelings . . . Which face comes closest to expressing how you feel about your health?

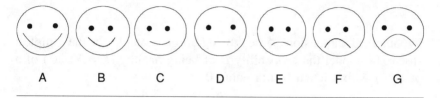

| A | B | C | D | E | F | G |

Source: Andrews & Withey *(14)*.

1 = not at all, 2 = no more than usual, 3 = rather more than usual, 4 = much more than usual). The Nottingham Health Profile measures perceived departures from normal functioning, including physical morbidity, pain, social isolation, emotional reactions and energy level (Fig. 3).

There are two fundamentally different methods to calculate an overall score or to estimate a scale value. According to the linear model of classical test theory, the total score Y_j of the jth respondent is generally defined as a weighted sum of the item scores X_{ij} where W_i is the weight of the ith item:

$$Y_j = \sum_{i=1}^{n} W_i X_{ij}$$

Modern measurement theory applies stochastic models to estimate an individual's position on a postulated latent trait, such as a

95

Fig. 3. Excerpt from the physical ability section of the Nottingham Health Profile

Listed below are some problems people can have in their daily life. Please read each one carefully. If it is *true* for you put a tick (   ) in the box under Yes. If it is *not true*, put a tick (   ) under No. If you are not sure whether to answer yes or no to a problem, ask yourself whether it is true for you in general.

	Yes	No
I find it hard to stand for long (e.g. at the kitchen sink, waiting for a bus)	☐	☐
I can walk about only indoors	☐	☐
I find it hard to bend	☐	☐
I have trouble getting up and down stairs or steps	☐	☐
I find it hard to reach for things.	☐	☐

hypothetical dimension of health *(34)*. For example, in the simplest stochastic model the probability P of being healthy ($X = \text{Yes}/\theta_j$) of a person j with a latent health value θ_j is:

$$P\ (X = \text{Yes}/\theta_j)\ =\ \frac{\exp\ (\theta_j - b_i)}{1 + \exp\ (\theta_j - b_i)}$$

where b_j is a parameter indicating the point on the health continuum where item j discriminates most between respondents. Efficient mathematical procedures are available to estimate the health values θ_j and the item parameters b_i. Without going into detail, if stochastic models fit the data, they have appreciable advantages over the classical measurement model. Thus, the estimated health values θ_j are largely independent of the sample of people and items included in the study, and the health scale has mathematical properties that allow calculation of the change scores for individuals *(35)*.

Measures of two or more dimensions of health can be presented either as a profile of specific values or as a composite score or index. An index is a combination of two or more component measures. Constructing indices raises the difficult issue of weighting the individual components. Weighting may be determined arbitrarily by experts or estimated from empirical data. Composite measures present a further problem of interpretation. For example, a given score can result from several combinations of different components and therefore have several meanings.

The conclusions that can be drawn from a measure depend on the mathematical properties of the scale it produces. Measurement theory distinguishes between four types of scale *(9)*. The nominal (or categorical) scale uses numbers arbitrarily as category labels (for example, 1 = male and 2 = female). The only inference that can be drawn from two measures A and B is that either A = B or A ≠ B. The ordinal scale uses numbers to express an increasing qualitative order of an attribute of interest (1 = very dissatisfied, 2 = fairly dissatisfied and 5 = very satisfied). This scale allows the inference A > B > C; distances between the categories have no meaning. The interval scale assigns values to items with a natural or otherwise meaningful distance between them (such as temperature in degrees Celsius). This may be expressed as $A - B = C - D$. The ratio scale defines ratios between scale values so that a particular value can be said to be so many times more than another value, or $A = B \times C$ (for example, mortality rate and blood pressure). The improvement over the interval scale is that the ratio scale includes a meaningful zero point.

The mathematical properties of a scale affect statistical methods. In a strict sense, adding and subtracting scores and calculating averages are allowed only for interval and ratio scales. Nevertheless, without an adequate measurement model and a substantive theory of a health dimension, it is virtually impossible to determine the properties of a given scale. Ordinal measures are very often treated as if they were interval measures, a violation of principles that does not usually seem to introduce serious bias. Psychological and social measurement have their roots in psychophysics, which was established over 100 years ago *(36)*. Today an elaborated body of measurement theory *(34,37)* can be applied to health measurement.

The subjective bias inherent in psychological judgement seems to be more serious than the bias caused by using inappropriate statistical models. Health ratings combine objective components such as degree of disability and subjective components such as the tendency of respondents to hide or to exaggerate the problem, or to express what is seen as socially desirable. Subjective response tendencies may, of course, vary over time. To control bias and ensure the quality of measurement, it is important to demonstrate the reliability and validity of a scale. Reliability expresses the degree to which measurement scores are free of error and can be replicated. Validity expresses the degree to which a measurement measures what it is claimed to measure. Reliability and validity need to be demonstrated in well designed studies, which makes the development of high-quality health measures time-consuming and costly *(9,33)*.

Measuring the health of individuals

In clinical, social science and epidemiological research, health has almost always been viewed as an individual attribute. Both other reported health information (data recorded by physicians, psychologists, nurses and family members) and, increasingly, self-reported health information (subjective data) have been used in this research. In this section, some of the more recent literature on health measurement will be reviewed. Growing interest in measuring health, with a particular focus on general and positive health, is indicated by several publications:

— *Measurement in health promotion and protection*, published by WHO and the International Epidemiological Association *(38)*;

— *Measuring health: a guide to rating scales and questionnaires (9)*;

— two issues of the *Journal of chronic diseases* covering two conferences, the Portugal Conference measuring quality of life and functional status in clinical and epidemiological research *(2)* and the Conference on Advances in Health Assessment *(3)*.

To organize this diverse field, the categories of health history, health balance and health potential illustrated in Table 1 will be used. The examples of measurements and scales selected are not meant to be representative but merely illustrative.

Health history of individuals
Since ancient times the personal history of health has been an important element of clinical diagnosis and decision-making, but this seems to have lost its attraction because of progress in biomedicine. With the emergence of a new type of holistic general practice or family medicine, a renaissance of historical medicine has been identified *(39)*. This development appears to be paralleled by growing interest in psychosomatic medicine and psychosocial health and in the study of careers of health and illness: for example, the careers of patients recovering from chronic diseases or of very old healthy

98

people. It is plausible that health careers are quite unique and that specific patterns of health history will help to explain health balance and health potential.

This perspective is novel and only a few systematic efforts to measure health history have been reported. For example, in the RAND Corporation health insurance experiment in the United States, perceptions of past health problems (number of health problems, disability and utilization of services) were summarized in the General Health Rating Index, an instrument developed as a principal outcome measure *(40)*. Researchers of some cohort studies, as well as physicians, employers and bureaucracies, often collect data on: several physical measures (weight, blood pressure and blood count), behavioural measures (diet, smoking and engagement in social and physical activities), and clinical symptoms and diseases. Such information could be used to describe individual health careers and to define measures of health history.

Health balance of individuals
Many indicators of the present health of individuals do not reflect just one health dimension but the global health situation, which consists of a balance between positive and negative aspects of wellbeing and functioning. The dynamic concept of health balance is therefore preferable to the more static concept of health status. Thus, objective physical measures such as body mass index, diastolic and systolic blood pressure, heart rate, serum cholesterol, body temperature and immunological status indicate a specific balance between different homeostatic subsystems of the human body *(29)*. Several such measures could be combined into a more global index of physiological balance; for example, measures of heart rate, blood pressure and aerobic capacity could comprise an index of somatic cardio-vascular health balance.

The Alameda County study *(10)* combined reported frequency and/or quantity of cigarettes and alcohol consumed, regular meals eaten, snacking, hours of sleep per night and amount of overweight into an index of health practices, a measure that independently predicted mortality and prevalence of self-reported health problems at the nine-year follow-up. The same principle can be used to build indices or to define profiles of lifestyle balance; for example, by combining indicators of health-enhancing and health-damaging behaviour, or by constructing indices of preventive health behaviour *(41)*.

Most indices of health balance are based on self-reported measures of specific health dimensions. McDowell & Newell *(9)* have described 50 scales of functional disability and handicap, psychological wellbeing, social health, the quality of life and life satisfaction, pain measurement and general health measurements, selected on the basis of reported reliability and validity. Patrick & Erickson *(42)* and Andrews & Robinson *(43)* have reviewed the most frequently used scales of health-related quality of life and given examples of health scales frequently used in the United States.

Several health scales (Table 2) illustrate the dimensions covered in subjective measures of health balance. Except for the dimensions of physical limitations, days in bed and anxiety or depression, the scales in Table 2 tend to tap the positive end of the illness-health continuum, the wellbeing range *(22)*. Some of these scales can therefore be used for individuals or groups in moderately good health. It is an open question whether health scales that discriminate between individuals in the upper range of the health continuum can be developed. Hunt *(58)* sees serious conceptual and methodological obstacles to building indicators of positive health because of the paucity of language that expresses positive health experiences and because of difficult problems of reliability.

Health potential of individuals
Individual health potential is related to individual health resources. Health potential differs, however, in that it includes the specific capacity, skills and opportunities to use physical, mental and psycho-social resources to maintain or reach a certain level of health balance. Opportunities are the social, economic and ecological conditions necessary to maintain and promote health. Health potential is clearly a functional term and can therefore be defined only in terms of a specific purpose or end.

One example of an individual's physical health potential is resistance to certain viruses or bacteria. This can theoretically be tested objectively by specific immunological reactions to standardized exposure to these microorganisms. Another example is physical performance capacity under certain conditions, such as maximal aerobic power measured by a bicycle ergometer or treadmill test, or physical fitness measured by a 12-minute running test *(59)*.

Generalization of the notion of immunological resistance to the psychosocial world has led to the concept of psychosocial resistance.

Antonovsky *(19)* describes a whole range of hypothetical generalized resistance resources in proposing a salutogenetic model including material resources, knowledge and intellect, ego identity, coping strategy, social support and ties, commitment, continuance, cohesion and control, cultural stability, magic and religion, philosophy and art, a stable set of answers to important questions in life, and a preventive health orientation. In a specific context several of these resources may determine an individual's health potential.

The salutogenetic model postulates a specific determinant of health, the sense of coherence, defined as *(19)*:

> a global orientation that expresses the extent to which one has a pervasive, enduring though dynamic feeling of confidence that one's internal and external environments are predictable and that there is a high probability that things will work out as well as can reasonably be expected.

Based on subsequent refinement and operationalization, this construct was differentiated into three components: comprehensibility, manageability and meaningfulness. A 29-item scale has been submitted to extensive field tests in several countries *(20,21)*. If the construct turns out to predict health, a reliable and valid measure of health potential will be available.

Measuring the health of populations
Measures of the health of populations can be derived from health measures of individuals by aggregating data, or they can be defined as unique characteristics of populations and data collected from such sources as families, communities and other social institutions. This section covers mainly the former type of health measurement by applying health history, health balance and health potential to social groups and populations.

Health history of populations
Demographers and epidemiologists have described the past health of populations in terms of patterns of mortality and life expectancy. The data reveal interesting trends. For example, in countries that have such data, the difference between standardized mortality rates for men and for women has remained about the same over the last 100 years, despite a substantial decline in overall mortality *(60,61)*. The gradient of life expectancy in selected European countries today is about the same as it was 100 years ago. Thus, the relative order of life expectancy of countries could have been predicted from the data

101

Table 2. Selected scales measuring dimensions of health balance

Dimensions	Definition	Abbreviated items	References
General health			
Perceived health	Self-rating of health at present	In general, is health excellent, good, fair or poor?	NCHS (44)
		Health is excellent	Davies & Ware (45)
		Energy, pep, vitality	Dupuy (46)
		Been feeling bad lately	Davies & Ware (45)
Social health			
Interpersonal contacts	Frequency of visits with friends and relatives	Number of friends visited	Donald & Ware (47)
		Going out less often to visit people	Bergner et al. (48)
Social resources	Quantity and quality of social ties, network	Number of close friends, people to talk with	Donald & Ware (47)
Role functioning	Freedom from limitations in performance of usual role activities (such as work, housework, school) because of poor health	Limited in kind or amount of major role activity	NCHS (44)
		Working shorter hours	Bergner et al. (48)
		Health causes problems at work	Hunt et al. (49)
		Unable to work because of health	Stewart et al. (50)
Mental health			
Anxiety or depression	Feelings of anxiety nervousness, tenseness, depression, moodiness or downheartedness	Depressed or very unhappy	Bradburn (15)
		Bothered by nervousness or nerves	Dupuy (46,51)
Psychological wellbeing	Frequency and intensity of general positive affect	Happy, pleased, satisfied with life	Dupuy (46,51)
		Wake up expecting an interesting day	Costello & Comrey (52)
		Feel cheerful, lighthearted	Veit & Ware (53)

Table 2 (continued)

Dimensions	Definition	Abbreviated items	References
Behavioural and emotional control	Control of behaviour, thoughts and feelings during specified period	Feel emotionally stable	Dupuy (46
		Lose control of behaviour, thoughts, feelings	Veit & Ware (53)
		Laugh or cry suddenly	Bergner et al. (48)
Cognitive functioning	Orientation to time and place, memory, attention span and alertness	Feel confused, forget a lot, make more mistakes than usual	Bergner et al. (48)
Physical health			
Physical limitations	Limitations in performance of self-care, mobility and physical activities	Needs help with bathing, dressing	Katz et al. (54)
		In bed, chair, couch for most of the day	Kaplan et al. (55)
		Does not walk at all	Bergner et al. (48)
Physical abilities	Ability to perform everyday activities	Able to walk uphill, upstairs	Hulka & Cassel(56)
		Able to participate in sports, strenuous activities	Stewart et al. (50)
Days in bed	Confinement to bed because of health problems	During past 30 days, number of days in bed all or most of the day	NCHS (44)
Physical wellbeing	Personal evaluation of physical condition	Rating of physical shape or condition	Dupuy (51) Chambers et al.(57)

Source: Ware (22), pp. 476–477.

collected 100 years ago (24). In general, mortality rates and life expectancies are not sensitive enough to measure important changes in health in developed countries.

Other objective indicators of the health history of populations or population groups have been collected over relatively short periods of time. Examples are physical measurements, such as body mass;

somatic cardiovascular risk factors, such as blood pressure and serum cholesterol; and health-related behaviour such as number of cigarettes smoked per day and number of consultations with physicians for preventive reasons per year. A knowledge of time trends in these indicators helps to evaluate health policies and to predict the future health of the population. It is, however, more difficult to measure and evaluate time trends in subjective health and perceived morbidity. For example, perceived wellbeing measured regularly in population surveys has declined in recent decades, while life expectancy has increased *(42)*. Since wellbeing is socially and culturally defined, changes in sociocultural values and expectations affect subjective ratings of health. The data may, however, be interpreted as indicating a shift in general health perspective or perceived quality of life.

Health balance of populations
The health situation of a population or a large population group is complex and dynamic. Within any population there is constant individual mobility between groups with excellent, good, fair and poor health balance. Single snapshots of the overall health situation, taken using a general health survey of a population sample during a given time period, cannot provide more than a relatively crude and static picture. Such snapshots tend to show that even adults in good or excellent health frequently report symptoms and minor health problems, in most cases self-limiting. Positive health does not seem to be as positive as might be expected *(62)*.

Objective population measures of health balance are rare. An example is the prevalence of health conditions that can be identified by objective criteria such as chronic diseases, disability or confinement to bed. Since health balance means general physical, psychological and social wellbeing and functioning, it can only be described and measured using subjective judgements, ratings or group consensus. Many countries conduct population surveys to assess perceived health, the health-related quality of life and lifestyle factors. Although a survey is a powerful way to collect information on the health balance of both populations and population groups (such as groups of defined age, sex or socioeconomic status), it also has definite limitations. For example, to assess and evaluate changes in population groups, carefully selected cohorts must be studied over some period of time.

104

Health potential of populations

Although health potential is a relatively new concept, several other traditional measures can indicate health potential. Perhaps the best known examples are life expectancy at birth or at specific ages, and life expectancy free of disability (well-years) *(24)*. These indicators can also measure change. Thus, improvement in a population's health potential could be measured in terms of well-years gained. Nevertheless, such measures would be quite insensitive to more specific changes in health potential.

Life expectancy (or mortality rate) is associated with sex and social class *(61,63)* and part of this association can be explained by differences in lifestyle factors related to social support and health. Thus, social class, social support, lifestyle and more specific practices of self-help, coping with psychosocial and health problems, and preventive behaviour are possible social indicators of health potential. Further measures can be derived from person-specific indicators such as self-esteem, sense of coherence *(19,21)* and perceived control of the intended outcomes of actions *(12)*.

Current Issues and Possible New Directions in Measuring Health

Health measurement is a diverse and rapidly developing field. It is therefore not surprising that many theoretical, methodological and practical issues have arisen that must be taken seriously if further progress is to be made.

The concept of health and measures of health is very wide in scope and multidimensional. Whenever measures of health are needed, questions have to be answered. What section of the continuum between poor and good health should the concept cover? Which is more appropriate, different measures of good and of bad health, or a single measure including both the positive and negative ends of the continuum? What indicators of physical disability are needed in health promotion and what indicators of the quality of life are needed in clinical work? How many and which dimensions of health are relevant? Should they be defined in terms of health balance, health potential or both? These questions can only be answered in a particular applied context.

The application of measures of health differs considerably, and frequently a specific instrument is required for each specific purpose *(62,64)*. Are these measure intended to test a theory about health, or will they be used in a practical context such as assessing the health needs or health problems of a population, monitoring health trends in a general population or evaluating a health promotion programme? The measuring instruments to be used for any of these purposes must, of course, be either selected or constructed. Constructing an instrument normally implies transforming general or global concepts to more specific components that can be operationalized. Both the selection and construction of instruments are greatly facilitated if they are guided by a suitable health theory.

Appropriate health theories are lacking. Most measures of health have been developed empirically for a particular research project or for some practical reason. Theoretical considerations, if they exist, have seldom been explicitly stated. If the purpose of measuring health is to test a theory, it is important to ask what the theory covers. For example, is it a theory about differences between social groups in terms of the meaning of health and health-related aspects of life-styles? Does a theory postulate differential changes in perceived wellbeing and symptoms caused by clinical intervention or a health promotion programme? If the purpose is related to policy or practice, the predictions the theory makes about the links between health-related resources and health outcomes may be important.

In developing measuring instruments, several difficult methodological problems must be solved. Their reliability and validity must be demonstrated and data must be compiled and presented in a meaningful way. Several questions need to be answered. How does one sample indicators or items that represent the health concept to be measured? What is a suitable theory and what are meaningful criteria for judging the validity of measures of health? How should validity be tested? How reliable should an instrument be in measuring, for example, group differences in certain dimensions of health and change in health? Should multifactorial health information be presented in terms of profiles or in terms of composite measures, such as a global index of health? How should the different components of such an index be weighted?

The difficulty with these issues is that they can only be resolved in a given context and with a specified purpose or objective in mind, such as health research, clinical practice and health promotion. In

106

selecting or developing instruments to apply in these contexts the requirements in terms of content, conceptual scope, reliability and validity will often not be complementary but competitive *(64)*.

Research on health is an interdisciplinary field addressing many difficult questions. In health sociology and psychology important questions derive from stress theories such as the social demands–control model *(65)*. One such question is how the interraction of specific patterns of psychosocial demands (in the family, the workplace and other institutions) and the capacity to control them affect both risk to health and health. In epidemiology consensus appears to be growing that health is an appropriate subject of research, separate from disease. There are serious difficulties in developing comprehensive health indices that assemble and weight disparate data appropriately *(66)*. One particular challenge will be to expand the traditional epidemiology of disease into a more comprehensive epidemiology of health to use in planning health programmes *(67)*.

Both in clinical practice and health policy, people are asking what the expected health outcomes are and whether they are an improvement over some previous stage. Thus, in clinical health promotion programmes, many specific health measures are needed to assess relevant aspects of the quality of life and, in particular, significant changes in the quality of life *(2,3)*. To evaluate community and institution-based health promotion programmes, it is necessary to translate health targets or objectives into measurable constructs and to develop, test and apply reliable and valid instruments.

Improving the state of the art in measuring health requires a systematic dialogue between decision-makers and researchers *(32)*. There are signs that such a dialogue is developing.

References

1. **Carley, M**. *Social measurement and social indicators. Issues of policy and theory*. London, Allen & Unwin, 1983.
2. **Katz, S**. The Portugal Conference: measuring quality of life and functional status in clinical and epidemiological research. *Journal of chronic diseases*, **40**(6): 459–650 (1987).
3. Proceedings of the Advances in Health Assessment Conference. *Journal of chronic diseases*, **40**(Suppl. No. 1): 1–191 (1987).

4. **Herzlich, C**. *Health and illness*. London, Academic Press, 1973.

5. **d'Houtaud, A. & Field, M.G**. The image of health: variations in perception by social class in a French population. *Sociology of health and illness*, **6**(1): 30–60 (1984).

6. **Buchmann, M. et al**. *Der Umgang mit Gesundheit und Krankheit im Alltag*. Berne, Verlag Paul Haupt, 1985.

7. **Parsons, T**. Definition of health and illness in the light of American values and social structure. *In*: Parsons, T., ed. *Social structure and personalities*. New York, Free Press, 1964.

8. **John, K. et al**. Assessment of psychosocial status: measures of subjective wellbeing, social adjustment and psychiatric symptoms. *In*: Abelin, T. et al., ed. *Measurement in health promotion and protection*. Copenhagen, WHO Regional Office for Europe, 1987 (WHO Regional Publications, European Series, No. 22), pp. 133–150.

9. **McDowell, I. & Newell, C**. *Measuring health: a guide to rating scales and questionnaires*. New York, Oxford University Press, 1987.

10. **Berkman, L.F. & Breslow, L**. *Health and ways of living*. New York, Oxford University Press, 1983.

11. **Cohen, S. & Syme, S.L., ed**. *Social support and health*. New York, Academic Press, 1985.

12. **Hibbard, J.H**. Social ties and health status: an examination of moderating factors. *Health education quarterly*, **12**(1): 23–34 (1985).

13. **Payne, J.M. & Jones, J.G**. Measurement and methodological issues in social support. *In*: Kasel, S.V. & Cooper, C.L., ed. *Stress and health: issues in research methodology*. Chichester, Wiley, 1987, pp. 167–205.

14. **Andrews, F.M. & Withey, S.B**. *Social indicators of well-being. Americans' perception of life quality*. New York, Plenum Press, 1976.

15. **Bradburn, N.M**. *The structure of psychological well-being*. Chicago, Aldine, 1969.

16. **McDowell, I. & Praught, E**. On the measurement of happiness. *American journal of epidemiology*, **116**(6): 949–958 (1982).

17. **Heady, B. et al**. Well-being and ill-being: different dimensions? *Social indicators research*, **14**: 115–139 (1983).

18. **Abbey, A. & Andrews, F.M.** Modelling the psychological determinants of life quality. *Social indicators research*, **16**: 1–34 (1985).

19. **Antonovsky, A.** *Health, stress and coping: new perspectives on mental and physical well-being.* San Francisco, Jossey-Bass, 1979.

20. **Antonovsky, A.** The sense of coherence as a determinant of health. *In*: Matazzaro, J.D. et al., ed. *Behavioural health: a handbook of health enhancement and disease prevention.* New York, Wiley, 1984, pp. 114–129.

21. **Antonovsky, A.** *Unravelling the mystery of health: how people manage stress and stay well.* San Francisco, Jossey-Bass, 1987.

22. **Ware, J.E., Jr.** Standards for validating health measures: definition and content. *Journal of chronic diseases*, **40**(6): 473–480 (1987).

23. **Hansluwka, H.E.** Measuring the health of populations, indicators and interpretations. *Social science and medicine*, **20**: 1207–1224 (1985).

24. **Schach, E.** Alternative ways of presenting statistics on sickness, disability and death. *In*: Abelin, T. et al., ed. *Measurement in health promotion and protection.* Copenhagen, WHO Regional Office for Europe, 1987 (WHO Regional Publications, European Series, No. 22), pp. 213–231

25. **Falkner, F.** Measures of human growth. *In*: Abelin, T. et al., ed. *Measurement in health promotion and protection.* Copenhagen, WHO Regional Office for Europe, 1987 (WHO Regional Publications, European Series, No. 22), pp. 109–122.

26. *Targets for health for all.* Copenhagen, WHO Regional Office for Europe, 1985 (European Health for All Series No. 1).

27. Health promotion: a discussion document on the concept and principles. *Health promotion*, **1**(1): 73–76 (1986).

28. Ottawa Charter for Health Promotion. *Health promotion*, **1**(4): iii–v (1986).

29. **Noack, H.** Concepts of health and health promotion. *In*: Abelin, T. et al., ed. *Measurement in health promotion and protection.* Copenhagen, WHO Regional Office for Europe, 1987 (WHO Regional Publications, European Series, No. 22), pp. 5–28.

30. **Bergner, M**. Measurement of health status. *Medical care*, **23**: 696–704 (1985).
31. **McQueen, D. & Noack, H**. Health promotion indicators: current status, issues and problems. *Health promotion*, **3**(1): 117–125 (1988).
32. **Noack, H. & McQueen, D**. Towards health promotion indicators. *Health promotion*, **3**(1): 73–78 (1988).
33. **Noack, H. & Abelin, T**. Conceptual and methodological aspects of measurement in health and health promotion. *In*: Abelin, T. et al., ed. *Measurement in health promotion and protection*. Copenhagen, WHO Regional Office for Europe, 1987 (WHO Regional Publications, European Series, No. 22), pp. 89–102.
34. **Lord, F.M. & Novick, M.R**. *Statistical theories of mental test scores*. Reading, MA, Addison-Wesley, 1968.
35. **Noack, H**. *Application of latent trait models to the act mathematics usage test*. Doctoral dissertation, Ames, IA, Iowa State University, 1973.
36. **Luce, R.D. & Galanter, E.** Discrimination. *In*: Luce, R.D. et al., ed. *Handbook of mathematical psychology*. New York, Wiley, 1963, pp. 191–244.
37. **Lazarsfield, P.E. & Henry, N.W**. *Latent structure analysis*. New York, Houghton-Mifflin, 1968.
38. **Abelin, T. et al., ed**. *Measurement in health promotion and protection*. Copenhagen, WHO Regional Office for Europe, 1987 (WHO Regional Publications, European Series, No. 22).
39. **Armstrong, D**. *Political anatomy of the body*. Cambridge, Cambridge University Press, 1983.
40. **Ware, J.E., Jr**. Scales for measuring general health perceptions. *Health services research*, **11**: 396–415 (1976).
41. **Bucher, H. & Gutzwiller, F**. Evaluating an indicator of preventive health behaviour derived from a national study. *Health promotion*, **3**(1): 67–72 (1988).
42. **Patrick, D.L. & Erickson, P**. What constitutes quality of life? Concepts and dimensions. *Journal of clinical nutrition*, **7**(2): 53-63 (1988).
43. **Andrews, F.M. & Robinson, J.P**. Measures of subjective well-being. *In*: Robinson, J.P. et al., ed. *The measurement of social attitudes*, 2nd ed. Orlando, FL, Academic Press, 1990.

44. **National Conference on Health Statistics**. *Health*. Washington, DC, US Department of Health and Human Services, 1981.

45. **Davies, A.R. & Ware, J.E., Jr**. *Measuring health perceptions in the health insurance experiment*. Santa Monica, CA, RAND Corporation, 1981 (R-2711-HHS).

46. **Dupuy, H.J**. The psychological general well-being (PGWB) index. *In*: Wenger, N.K. et al., ed. *Assessment of quality of life in clinical trials of cardiovascular therapies*. New York, Le Jacq, 1984, pp. 170–183.

47. **Donald, C.A. & Ware J.E., Jr**. The measurement of social support. *In*: Greenley, J.R., ed. *Research in community mental health*. Greenwich, CT, JAI Press, 1984, pp. 325–370.

48. **Bergner, M. et al**. The sickness impact profile: validation of a health status measure. *Medical care*, **14**: 57–67 (1976).

49. **Hunt, S.M. et al**. The Nottingham health profile: subjective health status and medical consultations. *Social science and medicine*, **15A**: 221–229 (1981).

50. **Stewart, A.L. et al**. Advances in the measurement of functional status: construction of aggregate indexes. *Medical care*, **19**: 473–488 (1981).

51. **Dupuy, H.J**. The psychological section of the current health and nutrition examination survey. *Proceedings of the Public Health Conference on Records and Statistics meeting jointly with the National Conference on Health Statistics*. Washington, DC, National Conference on Health Statistics, 1972.

52. **Costello, C.G. & Comrey, A.L**. Scales for measuring depression and anxiety. *Journal of psychology*, **66**: 303–313 (1967).

53. **Veit, C.T. & Ware, J.E., Jr**. The structure of psychological distress and well-being in general populations. *Journal of consulting and clinical psychology*, **51**: 730–742 (1983).

54. **Katz, S. et al**. Studies of illness in the aged. *Journal of the American Medical Association*, **185**: 94–99 (1963).

55. **Kaplan, R.M. et al**. Health status: types of validity and the index of well-being. *Health services research*, **11**: 478–507 (1976).

56. **Hulka, B.S. & Cassel, J.C**. The AAFP-UNC study of the organization, utilization and assessment of primary medical care. *American journal of public health*, **63**: 494–501 (1973).

57. **Chambers, L.W. et al**. The McMaster health index question-naire as a measure of quality of life for patients with rheumatoid disease. *Journal of rheumatology*, **9**: 780–784 (1982).

58. **Hunt, S.M**. Subjective health indicators and health promotion. *Health promotion*, **3**(1): 23–34 (1988).

59. **Lange Andersen, K. & Rutenfranz, J**. Physiological indices of physical performance capacity. *In*: Abelin, T. et al., ed. *Measurement in health promotion and protection*. Copenhagen, WHO Regional Office for Europe, 1987 (WHO Regional Publications, European Series, No. 22), pp. 123–132.

60. **McKeown, T**. *The role of medicine: dream, mirage or nemesis?* London, Nuffield Provincial Hospitals Trust, 1976.

61. **Verbrugge, L.M**. Gender and health: an update of hypotheses and evidence. *Journal of health and social behaviour*, **26**: 156–182 (1985).

62. **Bice, T.W**. Comments on health indicators: methodological prospectives. *In*: Elinson, J. & Siegmann, A.E., ed. *Socio-medical health indicators*. Farmingdale, NY, Baywood Publishing, 1976, pp. 185–196.

63. **Townsend, P. & Davidson, N**. *Inequalities in health*. Harmondsworth, Penguin, 1982.

64. **Kirshner, B. & Guyatt, G**. A methodological framework for assessing health indices. *Journal of chronic diseases*, **1**: 27–36 (1985).

65. **Baker, D.B**. The study of stress at work. *Annual review of public health*, **6**: 367–381 (1985).

66. **Stallones, R.A**. Epidemiological studies of health: a commentary on the Framingham studies. *Journal of chronic diseases*, **40**(Suppl. No. 1): 177–180.

67. **Brown, V.A**. Towards an epidemiology of health: a basis for planning community health programmes. *Health policy*, **4**: 331–340 (1985).

Part II

Social and behavioural factors in health promotion

5

Socioeconomic status and disease

Michael G. Marmot, Manolis Kogevinas
& Mary Ann Elston

Social Class and Epidemiology

Epidemiological studies tend to include the category of social class or socioeconomic status as regularly but with as little thought as the category of sex. The large social differences in mortality in many societies make analysis by social class crucial, but the largely unthinking use of social class is unfortunate. It may not only contribute little to but actually retard the understanding of the factors affecting health and disease.

This review explains why we look at social class, what social class is and its meaning. Using data mostly from England & Wales, trends are examined over time. Data from England & Wales are used not only because they are easily available but, for better or worse, because there is a long tradition of analysis by social class in these data. Given that in England & Wales, as in many countries, division into social class is based on occupation, we ask whether the relationship between social class and disease is similar for men and women. The generality of findings by social class in different cultures is then examined. Patterns of mortality from specific diseases are not always the same as mortality from all causes. The reasons for the remarkably widespread and persistent social differences in health and disease are not clear. Different explanations are considered.

Why look at social class?

In England & Wales social class has traditionally been based on the Registrar-General's classification of occupations: at first five and now six classes. This classification includes the level of skills, responsibility and prestige of each occupation. This loose aggregation of diverse occupations has been widely criticized; it is unclear, its definition and measurement are imprecise and its relation to sociological concepts of class is uncertain. This system persists in epidemiological studies because during infancy, childhood, maternity, middle age and old age, there are clear social differences in mortality and morbidity and in health behaviour. People lowest on the social scale have an adverse health profile (Tables 1 and 2).

There are at least three overlapping reasons to examine social class: theory, research strategy and public health action.

Theory

The social forces affecting health are expressed in class terms. This division into classes encompasses economic, political and cultural differences, all of which may affect health. Differences in health and in prevalence of disease by social class at least indicate the importance of the social environment. The tradition of medicine focuses on individuals: individual differences in biological characteristics, in disease, in lifestyle and in choices about health. Medicine implies that where disease is not genetically determined it is determined by individual exposure. This is not necessarily incorrect, but it is incomplete. Data indicate that, regardless of individual differences, broad social forces determine states of health and disease (Tables 1 and 2). Although the decision to smoke may ultimately be individual, men in the lowest social class are three times as likely to smoke as men in the highest social class.

Societies have characteristic rates of disease, although the people affected by disease may change (4). More recently, Rose (5) has elaborated this theme, suggesting that the determinants of disease rates of populations may be quite different from the determinants of which individuals develop disease within a population. For populations, social and environmental influences must be examined; within populations, genetic differences and individual differences in lifestyle may be important.

Analysis by social class can potentially explain how the organization of society affects health and disease.

114

Table 1. Birthweight and mortality in England & Wales by social class

	Social class[a]					
	I	II	IIIN	IIIM	IV	V
Birthweight[b,c]						
Percentage of babies ≤ 2500 g (1980)	5.3	5.3	5.8	6.6	7.3	8.1
Mortality[b,d]						
Perinatal mortality per 1000[c] (1978–1979)	11.2	12.0	13.3	14.7	16.9	19.4
Standardized mortality ratio[c] (aged 1–14 years, 1970–1972)						
males	74	79	95	98	112	162
females	89	84	93	93	120	156
Standardized maternal mortality ratio[e] (1970–1972)	79	63	86	99	147	144
All-cause standardized mortality ratio (aged 15–64 years, 1970–1972)						
males	77	81	99	106	114	137
married females[e]	82	87	92	115	119	135
single females[f]	110	79	92	108	114	138
Standardized mortality ratio from coronary heart disease (males, aged 15–64 years, 1970–1972)	88	91	114	107	108	111
Proportional mortality ratio from diseases of the respiratory system (males, aged 65–74 years	60	74	82	105	108	123

[a] Registrar–General's social class categories: I — professional, etc.; II — intermediate; IIIN — skilled occupations (nonmanual); IIIM — skilled occupations (manual); IV — partly skilled; V — unskilled.

[b] Source of data: Marmot & Morris (1).

[c] Social class according to father's occupation.

[d] Mortality cause classified according to Office of Population Censuses and Surveys (2).

[e] Social class according to husband's occupation.

[f] The number of women in this category was very small.

Table 2. Morbidity and health behaviour in Great Britain
by socioeconomic group

	Sex	Socioeconomic group[a]					
		1	2	3	4	5	6
Morbidity[b] (aged 45–64 years)							
Percentage reporting	M	35	31	41	42	47	52
longstanding illness	F	32	36	40	41	49	46
Average number of days							
of restricted activity	M	4	14	30	31	27	38
per person per year	F	22	23	28	27	33	39
Health behaviour [b,c] (adults)							
Prevalence of cigarette							
smoking,	M	17	29	30	40	45	49
1984 (%)	F	15	29	28	37	37	36
Participation in active							
outdoor sports,	M	42		34	23	17	15
1977 (%)	F	30		27	17	14	11

[a] Socioeconomic group: 1 — professional; 2 — employers and managers; 3 — intermediate and junior nonmanual; 4 — skilled manual and own account nonprofessional; 5 — semiskilled manual and personal service; 6 — unskilled manual.

[b] Source of data: Office of Population Censuses and Surveys (3).

[c] Source of data: Marmot & Morris (1).

Research strategy

One of the main strategies of the epidemiologist investigating disease etiology is to find substantial variations in disease prevalence and hunt out the possible reasons. In England & Wales, as in many other countries, variations in disease rates by social class are striking and may indeed hold clues to etiology. Studying these variations may contribute to understanding the causes of disease and the possible links between social class and the risk of disease.

Public health action

In the developed countries, eliminating social inequalities in health is an urgent task for public health and health promotion. This is one of the regional targets set for the WHO European Region in the strategy for health for all by the year 2000 (6). As detailed later, there are no grounds for complacency. General improvements in health and declining mortality do not affect all classes equally. As mortality rates fall, social inequalities often widen.

Explaining differences by social class by finding intermediaries is only part of the answer. For example, the higher mortality rates in social classes IV and V are probably related to a higher prevalence of smoking (Table 1). Such knowledge is of little use in public health, unless it is understood why the antismoking message has been readily adopted by classes I and II and not by IV and V.

The use of social class
To be simplistic, let us characterize some viewpoints. The definition of social class is crucial for people interested theoretically or politically in the link between social structure and the forces that affect health. The apparently nontheoretical way that epidemiologists aggregate individuals into arbitrary groups for statistical analysis seems to deny all meaning to an analysis of social class (7). From this perspective, it is incorrect to attempt to relate differences by social class in rates of disease to individual differences in lifestyle, as this focuses downstream from the group level to the individual level, implying that the focus for action to improve health should be the individual. This is neither politically desirable nor likely to be effective. For example, the goal of intervention should not be to change smoking or diet behaviour, but the class divisions in society — the focus should be upstream.

From a quite different perspective (viewpoint 2), the aim of an analysis by social class is to explain away social class. This viewpoint implies that if, for example, differences in infant mortality by social class could be explained by differences in maternal nutrition, infections and smoking, and lack of antenatal care, social class would no longer be important. It merely identifies groups at differential risk and has no more meaning than calendar year or area of residence.

Whether or not one takes the overtly political view, focusing upstream (viewpoint 1), using social class as a mere marker certainly misses something crucial. Effecting changes in lifestyle at an individual level is extremely difficult. Dropping social class from the analysis seriously reduces the possibility of change. If concrete factors are responsible for a worse outcome of pregnancy in mothers of social class IV and V, the task must be to find out why these risk factors show social segregation. For some people (viewpoint 1), health becomes one part of a political struggle to remove social divisions.

We have a third viewpoint: regardless of political views, it is appropriate to focus on the chain of causation: social forces lead to differences in lifestyle and exposure, which lead to differences in health. It is appropriate to focus on the intermediaries between social class and disease without ignoring the social causation.

Measuring social class is then important not only for its theoretical interest (how it might relate to the concepts of Marx and Weber, for example) but because it might explain the forces at work. This can be illustrated by national data in England & Wales on mortality by social class from the Office of Population Censuses and Surveys (OPCS) longitudinal study that follows a 1% sample of the national population identified in the 1971 census *(8)*. All-cause mortality is related to housing tenure and to access to cars (Fig. 1): people who own their houses and have greater access to cars have lower mortality than people who do not (about one quarter of the population neither own their house nor have access to a car). Within each social class (based on occupation) owner-occupiers have lower mortality than renters (Table 3). One interpretation is that income, as reflected by occupational class, and wealth, as reflected by housing tenure and access to cars, are independent predictors of mortality.

The challenge is to determine whether these predictors are causally related to mortality and, if so, how the links in the causal chain can be broken. If differences in income and wealth were reduced, would social inequalities in mortality be correspondingly reduced, or are there other causes such as prestige, self-esteem, education or occupation? Epidemiological analysis can potentially provide answers.

Social Class and Trends in Mortality over Time

All-cause mortality
Differences by social class in the mortality statistics from England & Wales persist over time (Fig. 2). The data come from the 1921–1923 *Decennial supplement on occupational mortality* and subsequent supplements in 1930–1932, 1949–1953, 1959–1963 and 1970–1972. Age-adjusted mortality rates have declined in all classes, but the differences between classes remain.

Blaxter *(9)* has commented that when mortality rates fall, class differentials tend to widen. She attributes this to a time lag in innovation. When environmental, lifestyle and health care conditions improve, higher classes tend to be affected first and the others more slowly. It is difficult to chart changes over time in the differences by

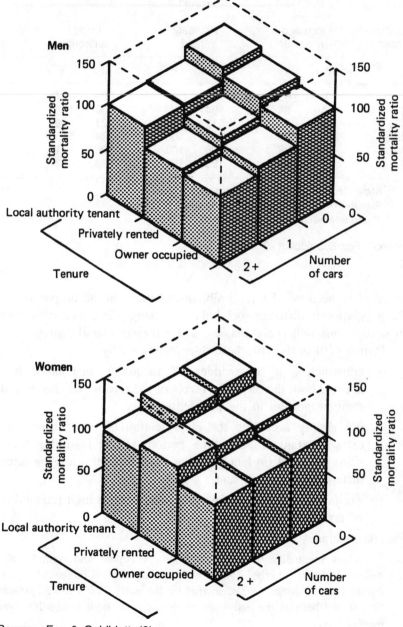

Fig. 1. Standardized mortality ratios of men and women
aged 15–64 years, in England & Wales,
by tenure and access to cars, 1971–1975

Source: Fox & Goldblatt *(8)*.

119

Table 3. Standardized mortality ratios for men and married women[a] aged 15−64 years at death, by housing tenure and social class[b] in England & Wales, 1971−1975

| Social class | Housing tenure | | | | | |
| | Occupied by owner | | Privately rented | | Local authority | |
	M	F	M	F	M	F
I	79	65	93	81	99	57[c]
II	74	84	104	96	99	142
IIIN	79	69	112	94	121	99
IIIM	83	88	99	106	104	115
IV	83	93	100	105	106	111
V	98	108	126	161	123	13

[a] Social class based on husband's social class.
[b] Registrar-General's social class categories as in Table 1.
[c] Based on fewer than 5 deaths expected.

Source: Fox & Goldblatt *(8)*.

social class because of three problems: changes in the proportion of the population in different social classes, changes in the classification of occupations into social classes, and errors in classification.

Pamuk *(10)* deals with these three problems by:

— constructing a slope index of inequality that takes into account both the mortality levels of the five social classes and their proportion in the population;

— not simply accepting the classification of occupations into classes extant at each time period, but reclassifying them using standard (in fact, this was done three times using three different standards); and

— excluding occupations for which there was a high probability of error in classification.

Pamuk concludes that:

. . . class inequality in mortality among occupied and retired adult males declined in the 1920s and . . . inequalities increased again during the 1950s and 1960s, so that by the early 1970s it was greater than it had been in the early part of the century, both in absolute and relative terms.

120

Fig. 2. Mortality from all causes (per 100 000 per year) in social classes I to V, in England & Wales, 1931--1971

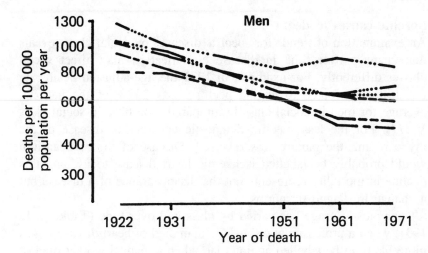

Men

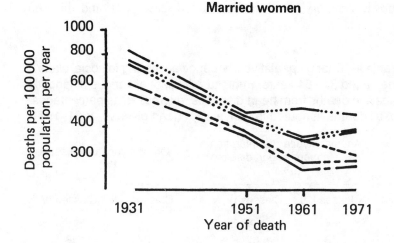

Married women

Source: **Koskinen, S**. *Time trends in cause–specific mortality by occupational class in England and Wales*. Paper presented at XX General Conference of the International Union for Social Studies of Population, Florence, 1985.

121

For married women, who were categorized by their husbands' social class, there was a similar increase in inequality from the 1950s to the 1970s. The comparison with the period before 1940 is less clear.

Specific causes of death

An examination of trends for specific diseases by social class reveals that changes over time in disease classification may affect social classes differently. For example, in 1931 the age-adjusted death rate for deaths attributed to angina pectoris was 237% of the national average for men in social class I, compared with 67% in social class V *(11)*. For the less specific diagnostic category of disease of the myocardium, the picture was reversed. Disease of the myocardium would probably be labelled ischaemic heart disease today, and this decline in mortality represents not the disappearance of a disease but a change in diagnostic norms.

Diagnostic usage has varied by class and over time (Table 4). In 1931, when a professional or businessman died of heart disease it was more likely to be labelled angina than when a manual worker died of the same condition. By 1971, for all classes, the predominant heart disease diagnosis was ischaemic heart disease or coronary heart disease. To chart trends over time it is useful to employ a broader diagnostic category, nonvalvular heart disease *(12)*, and this shows

Table 4. Changing relative frequency according to social class[a] (men aged 35–64 years, England & Wales) of various diagnostic labels in deaths from heart diseases, expressed as percentages of all deaths attributed to nonvalvular heart disease, 1931–1971

Year	Angina, myocardial infarction and ischaemic heart disease (%)		Other myocardial diseases (%)	
	Classes I, II	Classes IV, V	Classes I, II	Classes IV, V
1931	25	13	69	87
1951	73	62	27	38
1961	87	84	13	16
1971	92	90	8	11

[a] Registrar-General's social class categories as in Table 1.

Source: Rose & Marmot *(11)*.

that, for men aged 35–64, heart disease mortality increased more rapidly in social classes IV and V than in I and II, and the curves crossed between 1950 and 1960 (Fig. 3).

To examine the effect of the recent decline in mortality from coronary heart disease in England & Wales on differences by social class, data were compared from two successive *Decennial supplements,* 1970–1972 and 1979–1983 *(13).* This minimized the problems of changes in the coding of disease but, because of apparent changes in errors in the coding of social class, nonmanual and manual classes were compared. For all causes, lung cancer, coronary heart disease and cerebrovascular disease, the nonmanual advantage increased from 1970 to 1980 (Fig. 4 and 5) in accordance with Blaxter's observation *(9).*

Fig. 3. Mortality from nonvalvular heart disease (per million per year) in men and married women aged 35–64 years in England & Wales, 1931–1971, comparing social classes I and II with IV and V

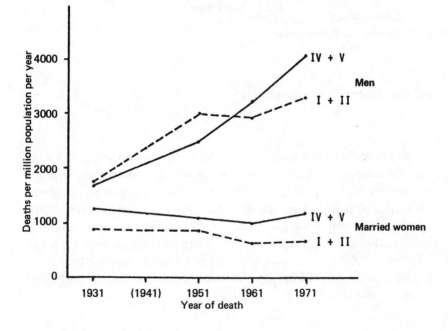

Source: Marmot et al. *(12).*

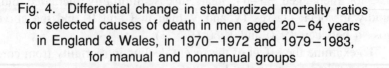

Fig. 4. Differential change in standardized mortality ratios
for selected causes of death in men aged 20–64 years
in England & Wales, in 1970–1972 and 1979–1983,
for manual and nonmanual groups

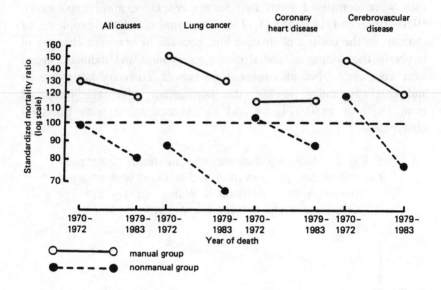

Source: Marmot & McDowell *(13)*.

Koskinen[a] examined data up to 1970–72 and showed that, for all specific causes of death except malignant melanoma, the relative position of higher classes has either remained constant or improved. This general pattern puts the data on coronary heart disease in perspective. General etiological factors must affect a wide range of specific diseases. Nevertheless, the change in distribution by social class of coronary heart disease from class I predominance to class V predominance may have specific etiological reasons: in particular, smoking and diet *(12)*.

---

[a] **Koskinen, S.** *Time trends in cause-specific mortality by occupational class in England and Wales.* Paper presented at XX General Conference of the International Union for Social Studies of Population, Florence, 1985.

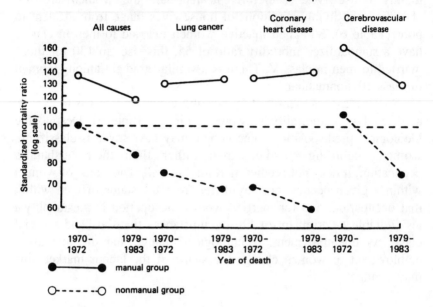

Fig. 5. Differential change in standardized mortality ratios for selected causes of death in married women[a] aged 20–54 years in England & Wales, in 1970–1972 and 1979–1983, for manual and nonmanual groups

[a] Classified according to husband's occupation.

Source: Marmot & McDowell *(13)*

Social Class and Sex

The question of what is being measured by social class is brought sharply into focus when one considers whether the same measures should be applied to both men and women. In England & Wales, data on social class have traditionally classified married women according to their husband's social class. This assumes that: most women are not active in the labour force; social class represents more than the characteristics of the occupations on which it is based; social class is a guide to income, wealth, education, culture and general conditions of life; and the social position of married women is better summarized by their husband's occupational class than by their own.

The OPCS longitudinal study *(8)* provides the opportunity to examine these assumptions. When women are classified into social classes according to their own occupation, the manual classes have

125

higher mortality than the nonmanual classes but there is no gradient within these two groups (Table 5). Nearly half the women who die are officially described as unoccupied or inactive. These are, of course, mainly housewives. Therefore, nearly half the women are not classified; the living conditions of housewives range from affluent to poor (Table 6). So-called inactive women married to men in class I have a standardized mortality ratio of 55; this rises to 130 for those married to men in class V. There is a similar gradient among women in class III nonmanual.

Social class, as measured by housing tenure and access to cars, is associated with mortality in women (Fig. 1, Table 6). Despite the ideological predisposition some people may have towards classifying women according to their own rather than their husband's occupation, it does not predict mortality as well. The status of women within a given occupation may differ from the status of men within that occupation, and for married women occupation is presumably a less reliable determinant of life circumstances than husband's social class. As unemployment, technological change and the increasing employment of women change the shape of the labour market, this may change.

Table 5. Mortality of women aged 15–59 years by social class[a] based on own occupation in England & Wales, 1971–1975

Social class	Deaths observed	Standardized mortality ratio
I, II	118	79
IIIN	232	79
IIIM	78	91
IV, V	291	89
Unoccupied[b]	747	119
Total[c]	1550[c]	100

[a] Registrar-General's social class categories as in Table 1.

[b] Mainly housewives.

[c] Also includes members of the armed forces and inadequately described people.

Source: Fox & Goldblatt *(8).*

Table 6. Mortality of married women aged 15–74 years by own and by husband's social class[a] in England & Wales, 1971–1975

| Husband's social class | Women's own social class | | | |
| | Class IIIN | | Inactive[b] | |
	Deaths observed	Standardized mortality ratio[c]	Deaths observed	Standardized mortality ratio[c]
I	9	72	50	55
II	51	88	315	89
IIIN	47	94	147	79
IIIM	74	98	572	101
IV	42	119	308	102
V	11	117	187	13

[a] Registrar-General's social class categories as in Table 1.

[b] Mainly housewives.

[c] Expected deaths based on death rates for all married women in the study.

Source: Fox & Goldblatt *(8)*.

Social Class and Mortality in Different Cultures

General effects

England & Wales is the logical place to examine the relationship between social class and health and disease, not simply because of the class divisions in British society, but because there are 70 years of data on the subject. Do the concept of social class and its measurement translate across cultures?

It appears that they do. Mortality varies by class, in a way similar to England & Wales, in the United States *(14)*, Denmark and Norway *(15)*, Finland *(16)*, France *(17)*, New Zealand *(18)* and Japan *(19)*.

Despite a lack of definition, social class is very useful in predicting differences in mortality in developed countries. There are few data available to test the association in developing countries, but data on emigrants from developing countries are useful. Mortality patterns for migrants are influenced both by the pattern prevailing in the country of origin and by that in the new country. Thus, for immigrants to England & Wales from the Indian subcontinent, from the Caribbean and from Commonwealth countries in Africa, the major

127

burden of disease is not tropical and infectious diseases but chronic diseases — cardiovascular diseases and cancer. The pattern of total mortality by social class therefore represents the social distribution of these diseases (Fig. 6).

The pattern for England & Wales is the familiar pattern of lower mortality among higher classes. Immigrants from Ireland and Poland have a similar pattern, although with each social class immigrants from Ireland have a higher mortality ratio than the overall average for England & Wales. Clearly, the conventional measurement of social class does not capture all the influences on the mortality of Irish immigrants, either because the measurement is deficient or because the influences on mortality are not all associated with current social class. They may, for example, be related to: experiences prior to migration, the selection of who migrates, the experience of migration and settling, or a social and cultural environment different from others in the same social class.

The pattern of mortality by social class is quite different for immigrants from the Indian subcontinent, the Caribbean and Africa. Indeed, for the immigrants from the Caribbean and Africa, mortality is higher than average at both extremes of the social scale.

A similar picture is seen in New Zealand Maoris, in contrast to the non-Maori pattern, which is similar to that for non-immigrants in England & Wales *(18)*. The pattern of chronic disease by social class in these traditional cultures, and cultures in or originating in developing countries, seems to be different from the pattern of the cultures in developed countries.

Specific diseases

The different relationships between social class and mortality for immigrants to England & Wales from the Caribbean, Africa and the Indian subcontinent are primarily explained by the pattern of circulatory disease.

In England & Wales the pattern of mortality by social class from circulatory disease follows that of all-cause mortality (Table 1), but this is not always the case. At a time in England & Wales when mortality from circulatory disease was rising, the rise presumably began first in social classes I and II and only later in IV and V. Thus, at a time when all-cause mortality was higher in classes IV and V, mortality from circulatory diseases was higher in classes I and II (Fig. 3). When the mortality rate from circulatory disease levelled off and began to fall (Fig. 4 and 5) it fell first in classes I and II.

128

These data support the apparent paradox that, although coronary heart disease is often considered a disease of affluence that is apparently more common in developed than developing countries, in developed countries it is now more common among the less affluent *(21)*. The social class patterns suggest that, as coronary heart disease becomes epidemic, it first affects the wealthier groups in society, perhaps by a combination of excessive fat in the diet, lack of exercise, smoking and stress. Later these lifestyle patterns diffuse throughout society to other groups, causing an increase in the prevalence of coronary heart disease. Change in lifestyle in a healthier direction (adaptation) then occurs first in classes I and II and, in England & Wales at least, it has not yet occurred in manual workers (Fig. 4 and 5). This pattern has also been observed for peptic ulcer *(22)*.

If this model is correct, as heart disease emerges as a major cause of death in developing countries, it will probably first affect higher classes and city residents. If the data for immigrants reflect the pattern of mortality in the country of origin, they support this model. Among immigrants to England & Wales from the Caribbean and Africa, mortality from circulatory diseases is higher for nonmanual than for manual classes *(20)*. The picture is less clear for immigrants from the Indian subcontinent.

Although the inverse relationship between social class and mortality is consistent in developed countries, the factors related to mortality from specific diseases may not be consistently related to social class across cultures, or across time periods. If the prevalence of a disease is related to innovations in lifestyle, the social distribution of prevalence depends on the social distribution of these lifestyles.

Leclerc *(17)* compared mortality differences by social class in France and Great Britain. The largest differences in France were for mortality from alcoholic cirrhosis and accidents, and in Great Britain for respiratory diseases and cancer (there are large differences for tuberculosis by social class in both countries). These diseases precisely characterize the overall mortality pattern in these countries. Great Britain differs most from other countries in high mortality from chronic respiratory disease and lung cancer, and France stands out because of high death rates from cirrhosis and accidents. It seems that the diseases most sensitive to the effects of environment and culture show the largest gradients by social class.

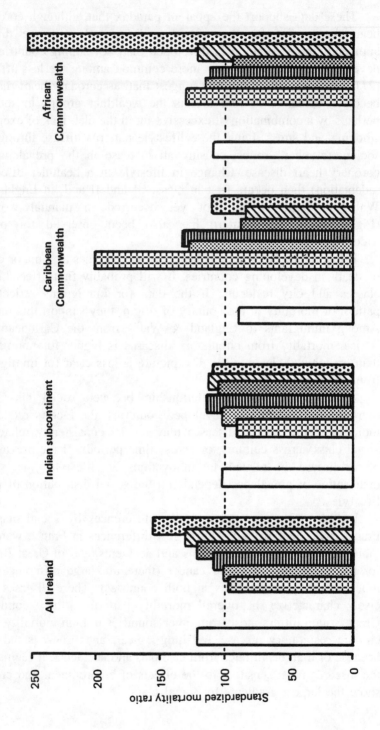

Fig. 6. Standardized mortality ratios for male immigrants to England & Wales aged 15–64 years, by country of birth and social class, 1970–1972

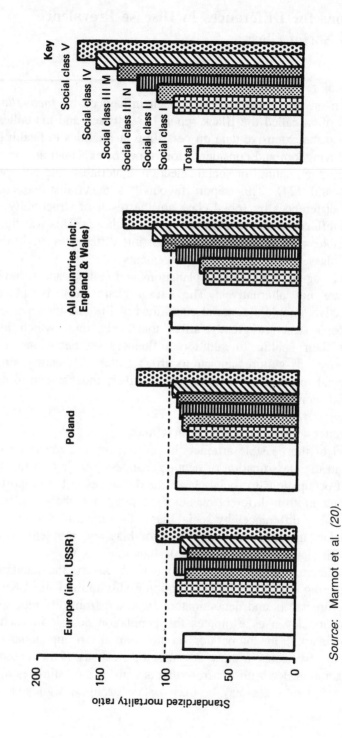

Source: Marmot et al. *(20).*

Reasons for Differences in Disease Prevalence by Social Class

Types of explanation

Opinion on this issue has been much influenced by *Inequalities in health*, often called the Black report *(23)*. Black and his colleagues reviewed the extensive data on persisting inequalities in health in the United Kingdom and considered four types of explanation: measurement artefact, natural or social selection, materialist, and cultural and behavioural *(24)*. This report favoured a materialist explanation: health differences by social class are the result of structurally determined influences on the members of social classes. This was the most reasonable way to account for persisting differences in health by social class despite general improvements.

Once again, materialist explanations and cultural and behavioural ones are not alternatives. The causal chain must be placed in perspective. People's material conditions of life and their position in the social structure greatly affect their behaviour, which in turn affects their health. In addition, influences on behaviour, loosely categorized as culture, appear to affect patterns of eating, drinking and social relationships and may be relatively independent of current material conditions.

Differences by social class as artefacts

Several of the possible artefacts have been mentioned: social differences in the classification of deaths, changes over time in the allocation of occupations to social classes, and changes in the proportion of the population in different classes. These are not likely explanations of mortality differences by social class. Two possible further sources of artefact are numerator–denominator bias and problems with the Registrar-General's social class designations (I–V).

Numerator–denominator bias potentially affects the standard way of gathering data on social class and mortality in the United Kingdom *(25)*. Numerators and denominators are taken from different sources. The national census estimates the population at risk in each class (denominators); the numerators come from the occupational coding of death certificates in the years around the census. If the recording of occupation at death differs from that at census, the estimates of death rates by social class may be biased. The strongest argument against this hypothesis comes from the OPCS longitudinal study *(8)*. By linking deaths as they occurred to a 1% sample of the 1971 census, a strong inverse relationship between social class and mortality was found, particularly in recent years.

Similarly, other longitudinal studies in Great Britain avoid numerator–denominator bias by linking deaths during follow-up to individuals identified at the baseline. The Whitehall study of civil servants working in London examined mortality rates over a ten-year period among men aged 20–64 years who were classified, at entry to the study, according to grade of employment (Fig. 7). There was a steep inverse association: men in the lowest grade (others — messengers, doorkeepers, etc.) had a threefold higher mortality rate than men in the highest grade (administrators).

The Whitehall study also deals with the Registrar-General's social classes (I–V). This classification has been strongly criticized *(7)*. The heterogeneity of occupations grouped into a single class certainly leaves room for differing interpretations. The Whitehall study avoids some of these problems by concentrating on one sector in which there is little heterogeneity within occupational grades and clear social divisions between grades. This more precise social classification may account for the steeper gradient of mortality by grade of employment of civil servants than in the national mortality rates by social class *(27)*, disproving an artefact explanation.

Social mobility or effect of early environment

It has been assumed that social class determines health. An alternative interpretation is that health determines social class *(28)*. This could occur if people who are less healthy are more likely to experience downward social mobility or less likely to be upwardly mobile. Stern *(28)* showed that such differential social mobility based on health status could, theoretically, account for the observed differences in mortality by social class. But does it?

Wilkinson *(29)* argues that, although some selection into social classes does occur because of health status, there is too little to have any major effect on social differences in health. Downward social mobility occurs for specific conditions such as schizophrenia. If social mobility had an appreciable impact on mortality differentials, one would expect social class recorded at or immediately before death to be more strongly related to mortality rates than class recorded years previously. Data from the OPCS longitudinal study showed the

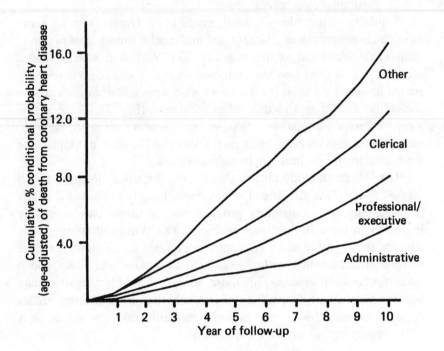

Fig. 7. All-cause mortality by grade of employment in male British civil servants aged 40–64 years

Source: Marmot et al. *(26).*

opposite to be true. Following a sample of men from 1971 to 1981, Fox et al. *(30)* found that mortality differentials in the first five years after identification in the 1971 census were narrower than in the years 1976 to 1981: the longer the gap between recording of occupation and death, the wider the social differences in mortality. Fox et al. postulate that, at census, some sick people were not assigned to a social class and were designated unoccupied. If this affected classes IV and V more than others, it would lead to a flattened social gradient.

Social mobility in adult life probably has a small effect, but what about mobility from childhood to adulthood? Selective social mobility could occur in two ways. Ill health could be a barrier to upward mobility (or cause downward mobility) or, more indirectly, factors that are related to health in adult life could also predict upward social mobility. There is scanty evidence either way for the direct effect of health on social mobility. Data from a longitudinal study of births in Great Britain from one week in March 1946 show that serious illness in childhood is related to a lower achieved social class as an adult, but Wilkinson *(31)* calculates that the proportions affected are sufficiently small that only 1.5% of people who became seriously ill in their early twenties have suffered downward mobility as a result of previous childhood illness. It is not clear whether more minor illness in childhood could play a role.

Illsley *(32)* examined women's reproductive performance (perinatal mortality rates) and argued that children brought up in a poor environment reflect that environment in later life. One possible explanation is that poor health in childhood may lead to lower achieved social class in adulthood, but the effect might be more indirect. Illsley *(33)* showed earlier that women who are upwardly mobile (comparing their husband's class with their father's) are taller than women who marry within their class. Data from studies of civil servants (Table 7) show, similarly, that for men from class IV and V families (father's occupation), height is related to the level achieved in the civil service. This is of interest because shorter men have higher

Table 7. Mean height of male civil servants according to current employment grade and father's social class

Social class of father[a]	Own employment grade				
	Adminis-trators	Professional and Executive	Clerical	Other	Total
	Height N (cm)	Height N (cm)	Height N (cm)	Height N (cm)	Height N (cm)
I, II	178.5 95	176.2 58	171.7 36	172.3 12	176.2 201
IIIN	178.4 32	175.5 20	175.7 11	176.5 8	176.9 71
IIIM	178.8 37	175.0 59	174.6 37	174.2 25	175.7 158
IV, V	176.7 9	174.8 25	174.3 11	170.0 16	173.8 61
Total	178.4 175	175.5 164	173.4 98	173.5 64	175.8 501[b]

[a] Registrar-General's social class categories as in Table 1.

[b] Includes 10 men whose fathers' occupations were not known.

Source: Marmot *(27)*.

mortality rates, independent of grade of employment *(26)*. This does not necessarily mean that health determines educational and occupational performance and hence social class in adulthood, but that social environment in childhood affects achieved adult height, life chances and ultimately mortality rates in adult life.

The effect of childhood social conditions has been further demonstrated by two geographic analyses, one in Norway *(34)* and one in England & Wales *(35)*, that find cohort rates of mortality from coronary heart disease in adulthood to be correlated with that cohort's infant mortality rate 50–60 years previously. Although the prevalence of coronary heart disease may therefore be affected by social environment in childhood, this does not preclude a role for the social conditions prevailing in adulthood. In a multivariate analysis of the Whitehall study, short height and low employment grade were independently related to mortality rates from coronary heart disease *(26)*.

It is unlikely that social differences in health in later life can be explained simply by selection into class because of health. It is likely, however, that in addition to the influences acting in adulthood, the social circumstances present in childhood have a continuing effect on disease rates in adulthood.

Links between social class and mortality
The following phenomena need to be explained:

— social inequalities in mortality have persisted or increased while overall mortality rates have decreased; although the forces leading to premature death have abated and changed, social differences remain;

— countries with different mortality patterns (different distribution of causes of death) such as France, Japan and the United Kingdom all show an inverse association between social class and mortality;

— the relationship between social class and mortality is remarkably general; the Whitehall study of civil servants shows that grade of employment is associated with each specific cause of death, as well as causes grouped by their association with smoking (Table 8).

It is therefore likely that there are a variety of possible intermediaries between social class and mortality. They may differ over time, across cultures and by disease category. The common feature is social class or relative position in a social hierarchy. Although the search for specific links may lead to benefits to public health, changing any one factor is unlikely to eliminate differences in health between classes, if general differences in social class persist.

General explanations

One possible general link between low social class and mortality is low income (29). Low income means poorer housing, poorer diet, fewer social amenities and worse working conditions. In the Alameda County Human Population Laboratory in California, over 18 years of follow-up, people with inadequate family incomes had 2.1 times higher risk of death than people with adequate incomes.[a] After adjustment for age, sex, race, smoking, alcohol consumption, sleep habits, leisure-time physical activity, body mass index and presence of high blood pressure, heart trouble, chest pain, diabetes or cancer, the risk was still 1.6 times greater for people with inadequate incomes.

Low income is correlated with low employment status, and these data are analogous to those from the Whitehall study. Low employment grade was associated with obesity, smoking, less leisure-time physical activity, more baseline illness, higher blood pressure and shorter height. Controlling for all of these accounted for no more than 40% of the grade difference in mortality from coronary heart disease (26,36).

Low income is also associated with poorer social environment. In Alameda County, residence in a poverty-stricken area was associated with a 30% higher mortality rate, independent of individual income or behavioural risk factors such as those listed above.

In the United Kingdom, as in many developed countries, increasing unemployment is now a factor. Unemployment in the OPCS longitudinal study (37) was associated with a 20% higher mortality rate, independent of class. It is unclear whether this effect is caused by increased poverty or by other factors (1).

Psychosocial explanations

It is questionable whether psychosocial explanations should be considered general explanations or specific factors. The search for specific factors to explain differences by social class has only been

---

[a] **Kaplan, G.A.** *Twenty years of health in Alameda Country: the Human Population Laboratory analyses.* Paper presented at the Annual Meeting of the Society for Prospective Medicine, San Francisco, 1985.

Table 8. Age-adjusted mortality and number of deaths for ten years by civil service grade and cause of death

Cause of death (ICD code)[a]	Ten-year mortality percentage (number of deaths)			
	Adminis-trators	Profes-sional and executive	Clerical	Other
Lung cancer (162.1)	0.35 (3)	0.73 (79)	1.47 (53)	2.33 (59)
Other cancer (140-239 excluding 162.1)	1.26 (12)	1.70 (195)	2.16 (73)	2.23 (46)
Coronary heart disease (410-414)	2.16 (17)	3.58 (399)	4.90 (160)	6.59 (128)
Cerebrovascular disease (430-438)	0.13 (1)	0.49 (51)	0.64 (23)	0.58 (14)
Other cardiovascular (404, 420-429, 440-458)	0.40 (4)	0.54 (58)	0.72 (24)	0.85 (24)
Chronic bronchitis (491-492)	0.00 (0)	0.06 (8)	0.43 (15)	0.65 (13)
Other respiratory (460-490, 493-519)	0.21 (2)	0.22 (24)	0.52 (18)	0.87 (15)
Gastrointestinal disease (520-577)	0.00 (0)	0.13 (15)	0.20 (7)	0.45 (15)
Genitourinary disease (580-607)	0.09 (1)	0.09 (10)	0.07 (2)	0.24 (6)
Accident and violence (800-949, 960-978)	0.00 (0)	0.13 (17)	0.17 (5)	0.20 (3)
Suicide (950-959, 980-989)	0.11 (1)	0.14 (18)	0.15 (4)	0.25 (4)
Other deaths	0.00 (0)	0.16 (18)	0.26 (9)	0.40 (6)
Causes not related to smoking[c]				
Cancer	0.86 (9)	1.24 (145)	1.53 (50)	1.57 (33)
Non-cancer	1.00 (10)	1.94 (216)	2.76 (93)	4.19 (82)
All causes	4.73 (41)	8.00 (892)	11.67 (393)	15.64 (326)

[a] ICD = International Classification of Diseases.

[b] Calculated from logistic equation adjusting for age.

[c] All causes, less 140 −141, 143−149, 150, 157, 160−163, 188−189, 200, 202, 410− 414, 491, 492.

Source: Lynge *(15)*

Relative mortality[b]				Chi-square test for trend (1 degree of freedom)	Cause of death (ICD code)[a]
Adminis-trators	Profes-sional and executive	Clerical	Other		
0.5	1.0	2.2	3.6	54.62	Lung cancer (162.1)
0.8	1.0	1.4	1.4	7.08	Other cancer (140-239 excluding 162.1)
0.6	1.0	1.4	1.7	38.24	Coronary heart disease (410-414)
0.3	1.0	1.4	1.2	1.70	Cerebrovascular disease (430-438)
0.9	1.0	1.4	2.0	6.95	Other cardiovascular (404, 420-429, 440-458)
0.0	1.0	6.0	7.3	21.01	Chronic bronchitis (491-492)
1.1	1.0	2.6	3.1	11.99	Other respiratory (460-490, 493-519)
0.0	1.0	1.6	2.8	6.26	Gastrointestinal disease (520-577)
1.3	1.0	0.7	3.1	2.46	Genitourinary disease (580-607)
0.0	1.0	1.4	1.5	1.36	Accident and violence (800-949, 960-978)
0.7	1.0	1.0	1.9	0.97	Suicide (950-959, 980-989
0.0	1.0	1.9	2.0	4.18	Other deaths
					Causes not related to smoking[c]
0.8	1.0	1.3	1.4	4.70	Cancer
0.6	1.0	1.5	2.0	31.83	Non-cancer
0.6	1.0	1.6	2.1	144.05	All causes

partially successful. For example, the Whitehall and Alameda County studies showed that there are mortality differences by class independent of known and measured risk factors. Lower classes may be generally more susceptible to disease *(38)* and this may be related to psychosocial factors. Cassel *(39)* proposed that the social environment may contribute to resistance to disease. It is easier for some people to accept the role of psychosocial factors in mental illness. For example, an increased frequency of stressful life events and poorer coping resources may explain the higher frequency of depression in women of lower social class in inner London *(40)*. Might similar factors contribute to the general increase in physical illness that cuts across so many specific diseases?

The Black report *(23)* said that lack of personal control over one's life was likely to be an important intermediary between low social position and ill health. Further studies of civil servants in Great Britain (Table 9) found marked differences between employment grades in various measures of control and satisfaction at work, in social networks, and in personal and social activities outside work. The Alameda County study *(42)* suggests that these factors may play an important role. This is a fertile area of research and much work is now in progress.

Work or way of life

To what extent are mortality differences by social class related to work or to more general social conditions (Table 9)? Analyses in Great Britain have examined the mortality of women (classified by husband's occupation) and the variance in occupational mortality, standardizing for social class. Both occupation and general lifestyle contribute *(43)*, but they may be difficult to separate. People in jobs characterized by adverse psychosocial conditions tend to be of a lower social class and are affected by other adverse conditions off the job.

Medical care

The question posed to the Black Committee *(23)* was: after 25 years of a National Health Service in the United Kingdom, why do social inequalities in health persist? It could be that, despite the National Health Service, there are social inequalities in access to, use of, treatment by or benefit from the health services; or that health services make only a marginal difference in mortality, the main health indicator under consideration. Blaxter *(9)* concluded that

Table 9. Percentage of men reporting selected psychosocial
characteristics according to grade of employment
in the civil service in Great Britain

Characteristic	Adminis-trators	Professional and executive	Clerical	Others
Social support				
Sees confidant daily	92	86	82	80
No contact with relatives	15	17	20	22
No contact with neighbours	37	40	55	69
No social contact with people at work	55	66	72	82
No contact with other friends	20	22	20	40
Job attitudes				
Underuse of skills	50	58	68	67
Little or no control	7	14	18	33
Unfair treatment	11	16	16	33
No variety	0	4	21	37
Job of little value	2	2	6	9
Activities outside work				
Involved hobbies, solitary	46	36	26	20
Organized social, sedentary	45	39	30	29
Active, not vigorous exercise	85	86	62	40
Active sports	39	32	24	33

Source: Marmot *(41)*.

although health care systems in developed countries do not generally mitigate the health problems created by poverty, there have been some measurable effects.

Does medical care affect mortality? Does medical care reduce social differences? McKeown *(44)* found that medical care did not have much effect on mortality. Rutstein et al. *(45)* divided causes of death into those amenable and nonamenable to medical intervention. Charlton & Velez *(46)* analysed mortality trends in six countries and concluded that the fall in mortality for amenable causes was probably a result of medical care.

An analysis from Finland for 1969–1981 attributes one half of the 63% (males) and 68% (females) decline in mortality from amenable causes to health services *(47)*. Amenable causes, however, accounted for only 8.2% of all deaths in men and 13.4% in women. The reduction in total deaths from 1969 to 1981 attributable to health care was therefore 2.6% among men and 4.5% among women unless, paradoxically, health services are affecting nonamenable causes. Even if this improvement were enjoyed equally by all social classes, it would have little effect on social inequalities in mortality. In fact, in Great Britain a reduction in total mortality has been accompanied by greater social inequalities (Fig. 4 and 5).

Conclusions

1. Social class is not a variable like any other. The inverse relationship between social class and a variety of measures of ill health is important for the relationship between social structure and the determinants of health.

2. Social inequalities in mortality have probably increased in England & Wales in recent years, despite a general decline in mortality.

3. The relationship between social class and disease applies to women as well as to men, although women's occupation is not currently as powerful a predictor of mortality as other social measures.

4. There is a relationship between social class and mortality in several developed countries with a variety of mortality patterns.

5. Although the relationship between social class and mortality covers most specific causes of death, interesting discrepancies have provided etiological clues. An example is the changed distribution of heart disease by social class.

6. For the relationship between social class and mortality:

   — the observed relationships are unlikely to be a result of artefact;

   — social mobility undoubtedly exists, and health may partly determine selective social mobility, but the effect is probably not large enough to account for social differences in mortality in adult life; nevertheless, social circumstances in childhood may have a continuing effect on achieved social class and on mortality in adult life;

   — the general relationship between social class and mortality operates through such recognized pathways as health behaviour

142

and biological effects, but the truth is incompletely understood; psychosocial factors may play a role;

— the effect of medical care on reducing social inequalities is unknown, but the quantitative estimates of the effect on mortality are sufficiently small to suggest that its role is limited.

7. The current work on the relationship between different socio-economic measures and health holds promise for better understanding. Action will not necessarily follow better understanding, but it is nevertheless important to introduce effects on health into the debate on social inequalities.

References

1. **Marmot, M.G. & Morris, J.N.** The social environment. *In*: Holland, W. et al., ed. *Oxford textbook on health.* Oxford, Oxford University Press, 1984, Vol. 1.
2. **Office of Population Censuses and Surveys.** *General household survey.* London, H.M. Stationery Office, 1982.
3. **Office of Population Censuses and Surveys.** *General household survey – cigarette smoking 1972–1984* London, OPCS Monitor, 1985 (GHS 85/2).
4. **Durkheim, E.** *Suicide.* London, Routledge & Kegan Paul, 1952.
5. **Rose, G.** Sick individuals and sick populations. *International journal of epidemiology,* **14**: 32–38 (1985).
6. *Targets for health for all.* Copenhagen, WHO Regional Office for Europe, 1985 (European Health for All Series, No. 1).
7. **Jones, I.G. & Cameron, D.** Social class analysis — an embarrassment to epidemiology. *Community medicine,* **6**: 37–46 (1984).
8. **Fox, A.J. & Goldblatt, P.O.** *Longitudinal study 1971–1975: England and Wales.* London, H.M. Stationery Office, 1982 (Office of Population Censuses and Surveys, Series LS No. 1).
9. **Blaxter, M.** Health services as a defence against the consequences of poverty in industrialized societies. *Social science and medicine,* **17**: 1139–1148 (1983).
10. **Pamuk, E.R.** Social class inequality in mortality from 1921 to 1972 in England and Wales. *Population studies,* **39**: 17–31 (1985).

11. **Rose, G. & Marmot, M.G**. Social class and coronary heart disease. *British heart journal*, **45**: 13–19 (1981).

12. **Marmot, M.G. et al**. Changing social class distribution of heart disease. *British medical journal*, **2**: 1109–1112 (1978).

13. **Marmot, M.G. & McDowell, M.E.** Mortality decline and widening social inequalities. *Lancet*, **2**: 274–276 (1986).

14. **Kitagawa, E.M. & Hauser, P.M**. *Differential mortality in the United States*. Cambridge, MA, Harvard University Press, 1973.

15. **Lynge, E**. Socioeconomic and occupational mortality differentials in Europe. *Sozial- und Präventivmedizin*, **29**: 265–267 (1984).

16. **Koskenvuo, M. et al**. Differences in mortality from ischaemic heart disease by marital status and social class. *Journal of chronic diseases*, **33**: 95–106 (1978).

17. **Leclerc, A. et al**. Les inégalités sociales devant la mort en Grande-Bretagne et en France. *Social science and medicine*, **19**: 479–487 (1984).

18. **Pearce, N.E. et al**. Social class, ethnic group and male mortality in New Zealand, 1974–1978. *Journal of epidemiology and community health,* **39**: 9–14 (1985).

19. **Kagamimori, S. et al**. A comparison of socioeconomic differences in mortality between Japan and England and Wales. *World health statistics quarterly*, **36**: 119–128 (1983).

20. **Marmot, M.G. et al**. *Immigrant mortality in England and Wales, 1970–1978*. London, H.M. Stationery Office, 1984.

21. **Marmot, M.G**. Affluence, urbanisation and CHD. *In*: Clegg, E.J. et al., ed. *Disease and urbanization*. London, Taylor & Francis, 1980, pp. 127–143.

22. **Susser, M. & Stein, Z**. Civilisation and peptic ulcer. *Lancet,* **1**: 115–118 (1962).

23. *Inequalities in health*. London, Department of Health and Social Security, 1980.

24. **Blane, D**. An assessment of the Black report's explanations of health inequalities. *Sociology of health and illness*, **7**: 423–445 (1985).

25. **Office of Population Censuses and Surveys**. *Occupational mortality 1970–1972: England and Wales*. London, H.M. Stationery Office, 1978 (Office of Population Censuses and Surveys, Series DS No. 1).

26. **Marmot, M.G. et al**. Inequalities in death — specific explanations of a general pattern? *Lancet*, **1**: 1003–1006 (1984).

27. **Marmot, M.G**. Social inequalities in mortality: the social environment. *In*: Wilkinson, R.G., ed. *Class and health: research and longitudinal data*. London, Tavistock, 1986.

28. **Stern, J**. Social mobility and the interpretation of social class mortality differentials. *Journal of social policy*, **12**: 27–49 (1983).

29. **Wilkinson, R.G**. Socioeconomic differences in mortality: interpreting the data on their size and trends. *In*: Wilkinson, R.G., ed. *Class and health: research and longitudinal data*. London, Tavistock, 1986.

30. **Fox, A.J. et al**. Social class mortality differentials: artefact, selection or life circumstances? *Journal of epidemiology and community health*, **39**: 1–8 (1985).

31. **Wilkinson, R.G**. Income and mortality. *In*: Wilkinson, R.G., ed. *Class and health: research and longitudinal data*. London, Tavistock, 1986.

32. **Illsley, R**. Occupational class, selection and the production of inequalities. *Quarterly journal of social affairs*, **2**: 151–165 (1986).

33. **Illsley, R**. Social class selection and class differences in relation to stillbirths and infant deaths. *British medical journal*, **2**: 1520–1524 (1955).

34. **Forsdahl, A**. Are poor living conditions in childhood and adolescence an important risk factor for arteriosclerotic heart disease? *British journal of preventive and social medicine*, **31**: 91–95 (1977).

35. **Barker, D.J.P. & Osmond, C**. Infant mortality, childhood nutrition, and ischaemic heart disease in England and Wales. *Lancet*, **1**: 1077–1081 (1986).

36. **Marmot, M.G. et al**. Employment grade and coronary heart disease in British civil servants. *Journal of epidemiology and community health*, **32**: 244–249 (1978).

37. **Moser, K.A. et al**. Unemployment and mortality in the OPCS longitudinal study. *Lancet*, **2**: 1324–1329 (1984).

38. **Syme, S.L. & Berkman, L.F**. Social class, susceptibility, and sickness. *American journal of epidemiology*, **104**: 1–8 (1976).

39. **Cassel, J.C**. The contribution of the social environment to host resistance. *American journal of epidemiology*, **104:** 107–123 (1976).

40. **Brown, G.W. & Harris, T**. *Social origins of depression*. London, Tavistock, 1978.

41. **Marmot, M.G**. Stress, social and cultural variations in heart disease. *Psychosomatic research*, **27**: 377–384 (1983).

42. **Berkman, L.F. & Breslow, L**. *Health and ways of living*. Oxford, Oxford University Press, 1983.

43. **Fox, A.J. & Adelstein, A.M**. Occupational mortality: work or way of life? *Journal of epidemiology and community health*, **32**: 73–77 (1978).

44. **McKeown, T**. *The role of medicine: dream, mirage or nemesis?* London, Nuffield Provincial Hospitals Trust, 1976.

45. **Rutstein, D.D. et al**. Measuring the quality of medical care. A clinical method. *New England journal of medicine*, **294**: 582–588 (1976).

46. **Charlton, J.R.H. & Velez, R**. Some international comparisons of mortality amenable to medical intervention. *British medical journal*, **292**: 295–301 (1986).

47. **Poikolainen, K. & Eskola, J**. The effect of health services on mortality: decline in death rates from amenable and non-amenable causes in Finland, 1969–1981. *Lancet*, **1**: 199–202 (1986).

6

Stress, social support, control and coping: a social epidemiological view[a]

David R. Williams & James S. House

The term stress has been used in both lay and scientific literature to describe phenomena ranging from societal conditions to individual disposition. Much has been written on the subject, and much research on stress has been attempted, with varying degrees of success, to test the hypothesis that stress negatively affects health and wellbeing. Nevertheless, the research on stress and health has been neither conceptually clear nor methodologically rigorous. This chapter does not attempt to review or to resolve all of the difficult theoretical and methodological issues. Instead, it briefly assesses what is known about stress as a risk factor in morbidity and mortality, and selectively highlights important issues and problems that, if resolved, will help to advance this area.

Numerous definitions of stress have been proposed. A central notion in many of these definitions is that stress refers to demands that can challenge or tax the adaptive resources of the individual (1). Nevertheless, given that research on stress is pursued in diverse disciplines, and that some of the work is not even specifically

[a] Preparation of this chapter was supported by a John Simon Guggenheim Memorial Foundation Fellowship, a National Institute on Aging Grant, a National Institute of Mental Health Grant, and a National Institute on Alcohol Abuse and Alcoholism Grant.

147

labelled as research on stress, it is virtually impossible to find a definition that satisfies everyone. Elliot & Eisdorfer *(2)* suggest a broad approach that appears to include most major definitions. This conceptual framework divides stress into its component parts based on the response to stress. The four component parts are potential stressors, reactions, consequences and mediators.

Events and conditions that may produce physical and psychosocial reactions are potential stressors. Reactions are individual responses (biological or psychosocial) to the stressor. Many reactions are short-lived and have no long-term effects while others, such as changes in health, are sufficiently intense or numerous that they result in physical or psychosocial effects. The long-term effects of reactions are called consequences. Mediators are the filters and modifiers (genetic, psychological, social and physical) that can affect individual and group variations in stressors, reactions and consequences.

This chapter examines the effect of stressors on health, and the role of social support, control and coping as mediators or modifiers of the relationship between stress and illness. Social epidemiology studies patterns of morbidity and mortality according to social status and the social and cultural factors that cause disease. Accordingly, social context and social structure are crucial in determining the distribution and effect of stress, social support and coping. Stress does not occur in a vacuum, and paying greater attention to the environments in which stressors occur can increase understanding of the processes that link stressors to health.

Stress and Disease

Research over several decades increasingly indicates that there is a relationship between various indicators of stress and the prevalence or incidence of various diseases. Most research has focused on the impact on health of major life changes or events (such as marriage and divorce, job entry and loss, and births and deaths), but researchers have also increasingly studied more chronic role-related stresses (such as stress within marriage, on the job or in financial matters) or daily hassles and irritations *(3, 4)*. In fact, this distinction may be more apparent than real, as most life events, such as widowhood or job loss, cause periods of chronic stress, and the relationship between life events and chronic strains or hassles needs to be studied.

Acute stress or life events

There are two types of studies of life events. Researchers study the relationship between health status and such individual life events as bereavement *(5,6)*, retirement *(7,8)* or unemployment *(9,10)*. More frequently, however, studies use an inventory of life events. The social readjustment rating scale *(11)* is the most widely used indicator of this type. The key determinant of stress is purported to be the readjustment required by the individual experiencing the event. Accordingly, any event presumed to require readjustment is included, whether it is considered to be positive (marriage or a job promotion) or negative (job loss, divorce or death of a loved one). In addition, this approach weights each event by objectively rating the stress it produces.

Selye *(12)* argued that stress plays a role in the development of all diseases; the voluminous research on life events seems to support this. Stressful life events predict an increased risk of such chronic illnesses as cardiovascular disease *(13,14)* and cancer *(15,16)*. Moreover, life events have equally consistently been risk factors for mental disorders. Numerous studies confirm the role of life events in precipitating affective disorders, including clinical depression *(17–19)*, acute schizophrenia *(20,21)* and neurotic disorders *(22,23)*. The consequences of stress are relatively nonspecific for diverse diseases, and some researchers contend that physical and psychiatric illness are alternative responses to the same underlying stress *(24)*.

Despite the fact that life events are consistently linked to adverse changes in health, the association between life events and disease is clearly not as strong as might be expected. The correlations are modest, usually 0.30 or less, explaining 9% or less of the variance in health outcome *(25)*. The failure to find a stronger relationship may be caused by manifold methodological problems. There are numerous excellent reviews of these problems and some proposed solutions *(26–29)*.

Several of the basic assumptions of the approach using the life events inventory have been seriously questioned. First, in contrast to expectation, weighting schemes do not increase the predictive power of life events. Second, this approach assumes that life events are inherently stressful *(30)*, and desirable and undesirable events are thus viewed as equally stressful. Subsequent research suggests that

149

only negative life events are linked to adverse changes in health *(31)*. Further, threat or loss and not life events may be critical in precipitating illness *(17)*. Loss is interpreted broadly here to include loss of a person, a role or an idea. The key issue is that the severity of stress depends on its meaning for the individual and not on life events in general. Cross-cultural research supports the notion that the experience of loss is central in pathogenic stress *(32)*. Other features of life events that appear to be critical in determining their degree of stress include desirability, magnitude, unpredictability, time clustering and uncontrollability *(33)*.

Another major problem is that scales of life events do not discriminate between objective and subjective events. Items such as trouble with in-laws or sexual difficulties are largely subjective, and subjective events pose a serious dilemma. On the one hand, since a person's appraisal of a potential stressor is probably important in determining the stressfulness of an event *(34)*, focusing only on objective events can ignore important information. On the other hand, perceptions are not always congruent with reality and may actually be affected by pre-existing health conditions. Hudgens *(35)* noted that more than half of the stressors commonly used on scales of life events can be confounded with symptoms. Confounding has also been hotly debated in the more recent literature on daily hassles *(36, 37)*.

Several solutions to this problem have been proposed. Mechanic *(38)* suggested that researchers attempt to work at both levels, keeping the measurement of objective events distinct from the assessment of individual perceptions. Brown & Birley *(20)* developed a creative solution in their study of stress and schizophrenia, classifying events according to the probability of their independence from a person's actions. Separate analyses were then performed for potentially dependent and independent events. An association was then demonstrated between independent events and the onset of schizophrenia. Dohrenwend et al. *(39)* used and recommended a similar approach. Brown & Harris *(17)* followed another strategy. They developed objective judgements of the severity of a stressor based on careful evaluation of the detailed contextual information solicited from a person. Theorell *(14)*, House *(28)* and others advocated abandoning scales of life events in favour of studying the separate and combined effects of major negative life events (such as widowhood, divorce, job loss and bereavement).

150

Chronic stress

Studies of chronic stress can also be methodologically criticized. Most studies are cross-sectional, and often measure both chronic stress and dependent health variables by self-report. Thus, although positive associations between marital, occupational, financial, parental or other sources of stress and health are invariably found, the magnitude and causal direction of the relationships is open to question *(40)*. Nevertheless, prospective research provides sufficient evidence of relationships *(4,41)* and gives enough plausibility to the posited causal interpretation of even cross-sectional relationships to suggest the usefulness of further research on chronic stress, especially in conjunction with research on major life events.

Most reviews of the methodological problems in the literature on stress agree that there is a pressing need for prospective studies, especially on chronic stress. Although such studies are more costly than the retrospective and cross-sectional studies that are almost universally used, they could enhance detection of the direction of causation and proper estimation of the nature and strength of the association. Kasl *(29)*, for example, cited numerous examples of how supposedly well established findings from cross-sectional and retrospective studies were not substantiated in prospective investigations. The need for prospective studies is more urgent now than ever.

Prospective studies should also measure stress at more than one point in time. Stress can be fairly transient or short-lived, and stability should not be ascribed to a respondent's report of a high level of stress at one point in time. A recent study of the relationship between occupational stress and mortality demonstrated the potential usefulness of this approach. Occupational stress was measured twice, and men who had moderate to high levels of stress both times had a mortality rate three times greater than those who reported a low level of stress at one time, regardless of their stress level at the other time *(41)*.

Some Neglected Issues

Positive effects

Most studies have concentrated on how stress adversely affects health, but Selye *(12)* emphasized that stress can both damage and cure. Researchers are increasingly calling for the systematic study of both the pathogenic and the health-enhancing effects of stress *(42)*. Stress can have several positive effects. First, life events that are

151

normative over the life course may enhance individual growth and have no particular adverse effects. Second, exposure to a given stressful experience can increase self-esteem and develop skills that better equip people to deal with similar situations and to capitalize on other challenging experiences. Third, some people pursue stressful experience as a means of personal stimulation and challenge. Recent evidence indicates that physiological responses to positive and negative life events differ *(43)*, suggesting the importance of more systematic attention to these issues. At the same time, researchers must be aware of the complexity of the stress process, and design research studies that allow assessment of the effects of stress at several levels. For example, although some individuals seek out stress and find it psychologically satisfying, such stress may nevertheless adversely affect their health *(38)*.

Biological mechanisms

The study of intervening biological mechanisms is another neglected area *(2)*. Immunologists, endocrinologists and physiologists have studied the relationship between stress and biological and physiological reactions; social and behavioural scientists have studied the association between stress and changes in health. Many researchers simply assume that the physiological reactions to acute stress and to chronic stress are the same. Further, the link between physiological reactions to stress and changes in health has seldom been tested, and thus it is not known which patterns of reactions to stress lead to specific disease outcomes.

One difficulty is that many of the indicators of physiological function studied (for example, indicators of both immunological and endocrine function) do not readily predict the risk of disease. Kasl *(40)* indicated that there are even problems with the few studies that have used established risk factors such as blood pressure and serum cholesterol. While changes in these risk factors have been linked to acute stress, there are few data linking repeated exposure to stress and long-term changes in these risk factors.

Studies of the relationship between stress and disease must measure biological mechanisms and traditional risk factors, and should seek to assess the extent to which stress is independent of these factors or interacts with them. In prospective studies, for example, risk factors, indicators of physiological function and baseline morbidity must be measured. Without adequate assessment of biological risks, it is extremely difficult to evaluate the causal relationships between stress and health. Few researchers have the necessary expertise to study the complex processes linking exposure to stress and a specific disease. Multidisciplinary research is thus clearly needed to advance our understanding of stress.

The social context

Most studies of stress treat stress as an individual variable, neglecting the broader social, political and economic context in which stress is embedded. Evidence is growing that social status and roles are important determinants of the differential distribution of stress and the impact of stress on health.

Dohrenwend & Dohrenwend *(44)* found that rates of unemployment, marital difficulties, divorce, and adult and infant morbidity and mortality are all inversely associated with socioeconomic status. Achievement-oriented life events such as job promotions, community leadership responsibilities and nonroutine vacations are rare to nonexistent for people of lower socioeconomic status. Moreover, blacks of lower socioeconomic status in the United States experience higher rates of some stressors (such as health problems and unemployment) than whites of lower socioeconomic status *(44)*, indicating that exposure to both poverty and discrimination may be especially effective in producing stress *(45)*. These findings suggest that the structural arrangements in society can create life experiences that vary in terms of both type and quantity of stressors.

Nevertheless, few studies of stress have systematically examined socioeconomic and sociocultural variation in the distribution of stress. One notable exception was a longitudinal study of 2300 residents of Chicago *(46)*; stress was clearly linked to socioeconomic status, sex and age. Unemployment and divorce rates were inversely associated with socioeconomic status, but job promotion and persistent problems with parents were positively associated with socioeconomic status. More women than men reported unemployment and chronic stress within marriage, while men were more often exposed to such forms of occupational stress as work overload and depersonalization. Thoits *(47)* recently examined how life events varied according to roles (sex and marital status) using the Pearlin & Lieberman *(46)* data, and found that general life events were inconsistently related to sex and marital status. The quantity and type of life events depended on the particular roles people held. For example, network events (negative life events experienced by people important to the respondent) are more frequent among married people than among unmarried people because of the marital tie and the parental role.

House & Robbins (48) reviewed the evidence that suggests that age can also determine the levels and types of stress experienced by the individual. This age pattern in the distribution of stress is clearly illustrated by Pearlin & Lieberman (46). While marriage and divorce were inversely associated with age, other events such as illness and the death of a spouse were positively related to age. Similarly, although younger workers faced more unemployment and changing jobs, older workers experienced retirement more frequently. These results clearly illustrate that stage in life is important in determining particular life events and that the timing of a life event can determine its impact.

Non-normative and unscheduled life events are more likely to have adverse effects on health than normative ones (4). Folkman et al. (49) found that both life events and daily hassles vary by age. Older people had fewer overall life events but had more loss events than younger people. The distribution of hassles further illustrates how age variation in role-related demands affects the distribution of stress. Younger respondents reported relatively more hassles than older respondents in the areas of household, finances and work. In contrast, older respondents experienced relatively more hassles related to health, environment, social conditions and home maintenance than younger respondents.

The effects of stress may also differ between social groups. In a community study of 350 randomly selected older adults, Krause (50) found that stress had more adverse effects on mental health among women than among men. Similarly, Kessler (51) reported that comparable stressful events have stronger negative effects on people of lower socioeconomic status than on people of higher status. Nevertheless, most studies have not systematically assessed how the consequences of stress vary between different sociodemographic groups.

Psychosocial Modifiers

The literature on stress clearly indicates that illness is not an inevitable consequence of exposure to stress. In fact, the available evidence suggests that, for most people, experiencing stress does not

154

lead to adverse changes in health. Accordingly, research on stress has tried to identify factors that may compensate for or moderate the impact of stress on health. Three variables appear especially promising: social relationships and support, coping and sense of personal control. These variables can affect health by themselves, thus compensating for or counteracting the impact of stress, and they can also moderate the relationship between stress and health.

Social support
The literature on stress has catalysed intense examination of the way social relationships improve health. Whether measured as the existence or quantity of relationships (social integration), their structural properties (social networks) or the supportive content (social support), social relationships consistently display strong positive associations with physical and mental health *(52)*. In fact, social ties are associated with such a wide range of health outcomes that they presumably operate through multiple biological pathways and have a general effect of decreasing vulnerability to disease *(53,54)*.

Social relationships can improve health and reduce stress in at least three ways *(55)*. First, social ties can directly improve health by meeting basic human needs for affection, social contact, and security. Second, supportive social relationships can reduce interpersonal conflict and tensions, thereby reducing stress. Increases in social ties lead to improvements in health independent of the level of stress by these two mechanisms. The third mechanism is a buffer or interactive one. The buffering hypothesis holds that mobilizing social ties in the presence of stress protects the individual from the pathogenic consequences of stress. Social relationships thus modify the relationship between stress and health such that risks to health decline as levels of support increase.

Social support and health
Large-scale prospective studies in diverse communities have provided the most compelling evidence that social ties are linked to health *(56–61)*. These studies reported that various indicators of social relationships predicted mortality risk. In the Tecumseh Community Health Study *(58)*, for example, indices of social relationships were inversely related to mortality risk even after controlling for baseline health status, morbidity, health practices and sociodemographic variables. These findings complement earlier research on the effects of marriage on health. Marital status is a key

component of most indices that seek to measure social support and has been the most studied aspect of social relationships. Married people consistently have lower death rates than unmarried people (62, 63). Although prospective mortality studies provide impressive evidence of a positive relationship between social ties and health, they lack the data necessary to test the buffering hypothesis.

The issue of buffering has attracted considerable interest and debate in research on stress. Some have concluded that there is insufficient evidence to support the existence of buffering effects (64, 65), while most studies find either main or buffering effects (55, 66–69). We concluded a few years ago that the issue is not whether or not social support has main or buffering effects, but rather under what conditions we tend to observe main effects versus buffering effects versus combinations of main and buffering effects (69).

Buffering effects have clear patterns (70, 71). It appears that they are likely in situations of great stress in which social support is measured in terms of the perceived willingness of others to be helpful.

The dimensions of social relationships

Another prerequisite for advancing the knowledge of the association between social relationships and health is greater clarity in the conceptualization and measurement of social relationships. The term social support has been widely used to refer to any and all aspects of social relationships. Social networks and social integration are also frequently used with an equal lack of specificity. These terms, however, refer to distinct aspects of social relationships. Social ties can be described theoretically and empirically in terms of their existence, structure and functional content (68). Social integration refers to the existence, number and frequency of relationships. Social networks refers to the structural properties of a set of relationships. These characteristics include density, reciprocity and sex composition. Despite the popularity of the term network characteristics, few studies measure them.

Finally, social ties can be described in terms of their content, with social support being one aspect of the functional content of relationships. Social support involves exchanges of emotional concern, information and instrumental assistance, and is probably the central health-enhancing aspect of relationships (55). Investigators are also paying increasing attention to social conflict and social control, two other components of relationships. First, social relationships are

156

often unpleasant or conflictive, and modest evidence indicates that these negative aspects of relationships are more strongly linked to psychiatric morbidity than is social support (72, 73). Second, social ties also control people socially (74). This regulatory function of relationships can either improve or worsen health depending on the particular behaviour that is facilitated or restrained.

To assess social relationships comprehensively, a given study must include measures of social integration, social networks and social support, as well as indicators of social conflict and social control. Further, studies of this kind must assess both the relationships between these different aspects of social ties and how they change health, singly and in combination.

Structural determinants

There has been little systematic investigation of how the distribution of health-enhancing social resources is shaped by broader processes and structures. Nevertheless, the evidence available in the United States strongly suggests that the quantity and quality of social ties are linked to sex, socioeconomic status and race. Women appear to provide better social support than men (75) and seem to incur higher psychological costs for doing so (76). Further, evidence is growing that this sex difference in supportiveness is caused less by innate personal disposition and more by differential exposure to certain microstructural experiences, such as being the primary provider of child care (77).

Levels of informal contact with friends and relatives, and organizational membership and participation, increase with increasing socioeconomic status (44,78,79). Spouses of lower socioeconomic status appear to support each other less than do spouses of higher socioeconomic status, and being married is positively associated with socioeconomic status (44,80). Similarly, a recent study found that blacks were more likely than whites to be unmarried and to have low levels of both emotional and instrumental support (81). Kasl (82) has also noted that, although marriage provides more protection for blacks than for whites, the other indicators of social integration have weaker effects for blacks than for whites.

The prospective mortality studies discussed earlier illustrate well how the levels and effectiveness of social relationships are linked to macrosocial structures. Measures of social integration are more strongly linked to mortality in the urban environments of Gothenburg, Sweden and Alameda County, California than in the rural

157

environments of Tecumseh, Michigan and Evans County, Georgia *(68)*. At the same time, the level of social integration (as measured by marital status) is higher in Tecumseh than in Alameda County, which may be linked to Tecumseh's high mean socioeconomic status. Tecumseh has a low rate of unemployment and very high median levels of education and income *(83)*.

It is clearly necessary to understand the association between social relationships and the socioeconomic and sociocultural environments in which they occur and to design studies that can measure these variations. Some groups (women, poor people and minorities) are in double jeopardy, as they experience more stress and also have fewer social resources to cope with it.

Control

Along with social relationships and support, the sense of control people have in stressful situations or more generally in their lives is a second major variable, or set of variables, that may counteract or modify the deleterious impact of stress on health. As with social relationships and support, the evidence that control can enhance health comes not only from cross-sectional and retrospective studies, but also from experimental and quasi-experimental studies of animals and humans, and from a small but growing body of prospective data *(84 – 86)*. Again, this research is characterized by: varying definitions and uses of the concept of control, lack of specification of when and why control has buffering or main effects, uncertainty about the biopsychosocial mechanisms through which control affects stress and health, and a lack of attention to the social context that facilitates or inhibits the development of a sense of control *(87)*.

The literature on control has been reviewed recently by House & Cottington *(84)*, Rodin *(85)*, Rowe & Kahn *(86)*, and others. Several major lines of work can be identified. Karasek et al. *(88)* have conducted a long-term programme of research on the effects of the demands of a job (a form of stress) and decision latitude on the job (or what others might term control) on cardiovascular morbidity and mortality. Job demands were positively associated with and decision latitude negatively associated with cardiovascular disease and death in retrospective, cross-sectional, and longitudinal studies; Karasek et al. hypothesize, and sometimes find, that decision latitude can moderate or buffer the impact of job demands on health.

Langer & Rodin *(89)* and Schulz *(90)* have conducted programmes designed to increase the degree of control and predictability elderly people have in their lives, especially in nursing homes. A variety of manipulations increased people's control over and/or the predictability of: moves into nursing homes, decisions about their lives and the nursing home environment, and patterns of visits, resulting in improved physical and psychological functioning. Termination of one of the programmes resulted in increased mortality *(91)*.

Cross-sectional and longitudinal research on broader communities suggests that control is positively associated with social status *(92)*. Syme *(87)* suggests that control may be significant in explaining the greater morbidity and mortality rates of people of lower socioeconomic status *(83)*. Longitudinal research by Pearlin et al. *(4)* showed that the sense of self-esteem and mastery predicts better mental health and buffers the impact of life events on mental health.

The effects of control on stress and health, and the unresolved issues for future research in this area, are strikingly parallel to those for social relationships and support. Further, increased attention should be given to the relationship between control and social relationships and support. House & Cottington *(84)* and Rowe & Kahn *(86)*, for example, hypothesize that some of the beneficial effects of social relationships and support are realized by affecting people's sense of control over their lives and work, and Pearlin et al. *(4)* provide data that are consistent with this idea. Finally, both control and social relationships and support are presumed to affect stress and health, at least in part, by facilitating more adaptive strategies of responding to potential stressors: a process termed coping, which is the third class of potential modifiers of the relationship between stress and health.

Coping

Coping describes the strategies used in responding to a potential stressor. These strategies can be cognitive and/or behavioural responses that attempt to manage or control the psychological and physiological arousal caused by the stressor. This is accomplished by modifying the situation, modifying the meaning of the stressor, or managing the emotional response to the situation *(93)*. There is no consensus on how best to conceptualize and measure coping, and

159

definitions of coping often depend on how stress is conceptualized. Accordingly, coping is often used in a very broad and nonspecific fashion to describe any goal-directed behaviour *(94)*.

Some observers have noted that the literature on coping has shifted away from psychodynamically oriented psychology, in which coping was viewed as an unconscious defence process, to a greater current emphasis on cognitive and behavioural approaches *(94,95)*. Nevertheless, there is still considerable debate on whether coping strategies are best viewed as relatively stable personality traits or as specific responses determined by the situation *(96)*. This fundamental divergence is associated with concurrent divergences in methods of assessing coping strategies and in designs for research on the effects of coping strategies.

Measurement of coping

Studies of coping have two general approaches to measurement. The first type, originating from a concept of coping strategies as stable dispositions, asks people how they typically cope or respond in stressful situations. A theoretically generated item pool is refined through factor analysis to produce measures of a variety of coping dispositions. The Ways of Coping Checklist *(97)* is one widely used instrument that consists of several subscales, such as positive reappraisal, escape–avoidance, self-control and confrontive coping, but its major distinction is between problem-focused and emotion-focused strategies. In contrast, the concept of coping as situationally specific response strategies leads researchers to focus on a particular life event or source of stress. The cognitive and behavioural patterns of individuals who adjust well are compared with the reactions of those who are not as successful. (Singer *(96)* and Taylor *(98)* discuss the strengths and weaknesses of both approaches.)

A crucial question is whether coping strategies are conscious and can therefore be accurately reported by respondents. Frese *(99)* argues persuasively that, in coping with stress, people unconsciously use "automatic, overlearned strategies". People only consciously think about their coping efforts when these normal strategies fail. Accordingly, self-report measures of coping, while valid, capture only a small portion of coping: problematic coping *(100)*.

Coping and health

The central focus here is the relationship between coping and adaptive outcomes. Lazarus *(101)* reviewed the evidence linking coping to morbidity and mortality. Several small studies of special populations indicate that coping processes are important in determining changes in health status, but the evidence is not overwhelming. A similar assessment of the relationship between coping strategies and psychological disorder concluded that there is surprisingly little sound, empirical research that supports the assumption that the choice of coping strategies can moderate the effects of stress (95).

Moreover, several studies using the Ways of Coping Checklist or adaptations thereof have found that, regardless of the strategy used, more coping is associated with psychological distress (102). It has long been recognized that coping can sometimes have adverse health outcomes. Nevertheless, this possibility has generally been limited to inappropriate coping behaviour such as palliative strategies (for example, denial) in the face of life-threatening situations, and coping strategies associated with acknowledged pathogenic behaviour, such as type A behaviour and smoking cigarettes (101). Theorists of coping have thus been surprised that many strategies focusing on problems and emotions are positively related to morbidity (99). At the same time, a comprehensive review of intervention studies on patients coping with elective surgery came to different conclusions. This report was based only on the studies in which an experimental or quasi-experimental design was used; almost without exception, coping intervention was positively associated with emotional well-being and surgical recovery (103).

These differing results may not be as incongruous as they first appear. In nonexperimental studies, almost all types of coping probably increase with increases in the amount of stress experienced or the degree to which it is unresolved. Thus, degree of coping may be confounded with amount of stress, producing an apparent, but possibly spurious, positive association between coping and distress or ill health. In intervention studies, the type and amount of stress are generally held constant, and hence more coping reduces adverse physical or mental health outcomes. This interpretation suggests that the situationally specific approach that measures coping and its effects may ultimately prove more fruitful, and this conclusion is also consistent with the results of broader epidemiological research. In assessing the impact of coping on health, nonexperimental studies must control for the amount of stress experienced.

Specificity of coping effects
In a classic study of coping, Pearlin & Schooler (93) found that both the coping strategies employed and the relative efficacy of coping

varied by type of stress. In this study, stress was measured in the areas of marriage, parenting, household finances and occupation, and the specific strategies used in each domain were assessed. Coping strategies were found to be most important in dealing with stress within marriage. For example, the negative effect of stress within marriage was halved by the specific coping strategies used. Coping had similar but more modest effects in parenting and household finances, but it had little effect in the occupational area.

Kessler et al. *(100)* further illustrated the specificity of coping effects. First, this study of a general population sample of 1500 married people found that, although coping with chronic stress was not related to anxiety and depression, coping with recent life events did have consequences for mental health. Kessler et al. suggest that describing a chronic difficulty as a most stressful experience is an admission that previous coping attempts were maladaptive, or ineffective. Second, although such coping strategies as "avoidance, active cognitive and reappraisal" were positively associated with psychological distress, others such as "religious, active behaviour and versatile", were inversely related, while "social support and passive" were unrelated. Third, coping efficacy varied according to the type of stress. For example, although religious coping reduced psychological distress, disaggregated analyses revealed that this effect was limited to people coping with the death of a loved one.

The findings of Pearlin & Schooler and Kessler et al. are relevant to the debate in the literature on coping about the relative importance of personal and situational determinants of coping behaviour and coping efficacy. Although the results of these studies emphasize the environmental context of coping, it is also important to understand the relationship between a person and a situation. Pearlin & Schooler reported that both psychological resources (self-esteem, mastery and self-denigration) and situation-specific coping responses reduced the impact of stress on health. Nevertheless, the relative importance of personal dispositions and cognitive coping strategies varies for different kinds of stress. Since type A and type B individuals differ in their use of cognitive coping strategies *(104)*, more systematic attention to this issue is clearly warranted, including a broader assessment of coping strategies and individual dispositions.

The studies reviewed here clearly indicate the importance of a theoretically and empirically grounded concept of coping that would make it possible to identify the conditions in which particular coping strategies are likely to be effective for specific outcomes. At the same time, the study by Kessler et al. also illustrates the limitations of current knowledge and the tentativeness of the findings of any single study. First, several dimensions of coping were measured in their study, but each was assessed with only a single item. Second, and more important, although the study used a large general population sample of a major metropolitan area in the United States, it excluded blacks, single people and elderly people. The resulting respondents had a mean 13.2 years of education and mean family income of US$ 41 800 per annum in 1984. The sociodemographic profile of this community is critical because the literature on coping implies that processes of coping vary in different social groups.

The social environment
Pearlin & Schooler *(93)* emphasize the social context of both stress and the modes of dealing with it. People of similar social status display similar modes of coping. Thus, in contrast to the conventional concept of coping as an individualized response, coping is more appropriately viewed as a group response.

In one of the few studies of differences in coping between subgroups, Pearlin & Schooler found an intriguing pattern of differences according to social status. More men than women had the psychological predisposition to use the coping strategies that are effective in dealing with stress. In addition, socioeconomic position appears to lead to differential access to effective coping strategies and resources. There was a strong positive association between socioeconomic status and access to health-enhancing resources and to coping strategies. Pearlin & Schooler found no consistent pattern of age differences, but some recent studies show age differences in the use of coping strategies *(49,105)*. The issue of group differences in coping clearly deserves more careful attention than it has received.

Conclusion

Like the blind men in the fable, researchers studying stress have been busy measuring a part of the elephant and assuming that this is the entire phenomenon. Stress is clearly multifactorial in its etiology, and attempts to understand and measure it must have a similar degree of breadth and complexity. Major advances in this field can be expected when interdisciplinary research teams give coordinated attention to the complex unanswered questions in the research on stress.

Considerable progress has been made in understanding the effects on health of both acute and chronic stress, and of several key categories of variables that may counteract or buffer these deleterious effects: social relationships and support, a sense of personal control, and strategies of coping with stress. There are conceptual and measurement problems in each area, and the biopsychosocial mechanisms by which each affects stress and health need to be specified. Increasing effort must be devoted to understanding how social relationships and support, and control and coping, are related to each other and how they combine to affect levels of stress and to change health status.

Neither stress nor the resources to cope with it are randomly distributed in the population. Yet research on stress has been dominated by a clinical perspective that focuses on individual perceptions, susceptibilities and resources. The study of individual characteristics needs to be balanced by more systematic attention to stress as a socially determined phenomenon. Social processes and structures shape the lives of groups occupying different structural positions in society. Accordingly, the distribution of stress and the constraints on and options for confronting it vary according to social status. The approach of social epidemiology is thus indispensable in enhancing knowledge of the social dimensions of the stress process. Researchers should focus at least on age, sex, socioeconomic status, marital status and difference in race and ethnicity. Moreover, researchers should resist the temptation to be satisfied with descriptive epidemiology and should place greater emphasis on explanatory epidemiology. The underlying processes and mechanisms must be clearly identified and described.

One unfortunate result of the fact that research on stress focuses on individual people is that efforts to modify and alleviate stress have concentrated almost exclusively on individual change and adaptation. As larger social processes and institutions create stressful environments and conditions, however, attempts to reduce the adverse consequences of stress must also address the larger social factors that affect the development, maintenance and differential distribution of stress and the resources to cope with it.

References

1. **McGrath, J.E., ed.** *Social and psychological factors in stress.* New York, Holt, Rinehart & Winston, 1970.
2. **Elliot, G.R. & Eisdorfer, C.** *Stress and human health.* New York, Springer, 1982.
3. **Kanner, A.D. et al.** Comparison of two modes of stress measurement: daily hassles and uplifts versus major life events. *Journal of behavioral medicine,* **14**: 1–39 (1981).
4. **Pearlin, L.I. et al.** The stress process. *Journal of health and social behavior,* **22**: 337–356 (1981).
5. **Helsing, K.J. & Szklo, M.** Mortality after bereavement. *American journal of epidemiology,* **114**: 41–52 (1981).
6. **Jacobs, S. & Ostfeld, A.** An epidemiological review of the mortality of bereavement. *Psychosomatic medicine,* **39**: 344–357 (1977).
7. **Carp, F.M.** Retirement and physical health. *Advances in psychosomatic medicine,* **9**: 140–159 (1977).
8. **Kasl, S.V.** The impact of retirement. *In:* Cooper, C.L. & Payne, R., ed. *Current concerns in occupational stress.* New York, Wiley, 1980, pp. 137–186.
9. **Kasl, S.V. & Cobb, S.** Variability of stress effects among men experiencing job loss. *In:* Goldberger, L. & Breznitz, S., ed. *Handbook of stress.* New York, Free Press, 1982, pp. 445–465.
10. **Kessler, R.C. et al.** Unemployment and health in a community sample. *Journal of health and social behavior,* **28**: 51–59 (1987).
11. **Holmes, T.H. & Rahe, R.H.** The social readjustment rating scale. *Journal of psychosomatic research,* **11**: 213–218 (1967).
12. **Selye, H.** The stress concept: past, present and future. *In:* Cooper, C.L., ed. *Stress research: issues for the eighties.* New York, Wiley, 1983, pp. 1–20.
13. **Haney, C.A.** Life events as precursors of coronary heart disease. *Social science and medicine,* **14A**: 119–126 (1980).
14. **Theorell, T.G.** Review of research on life events and cardiovascular illness. *Advances in cardiology,* **29**: 140–147 (1982).
15. **Cooper, C.L.** Psychosocial stress and cancer. *Bulletin of the British Psychological Society,* **35**: 456–459 (1982).
16. **Sklar, L.S. & Anisman, H.** Stress and cancer. *Psychological bulletin,* **89**: 369–406 (1981).

17. **Brown, G.W. & Harris, T.O**. *Social origins of depression: a study of psychiatric disorder in women*. New York, Free Press, 1978.

18. **Paykel, E.S**. Contribution of life events to causation of psychiatric illness. *Psychological medicine*, **8**: 245–253 (1978).

19. **Paykel, E.S**. Causal relationships between clinical depression and life events. *In*: Barnett, J.E. et al., ed. *Stress and mental disorder*. New York, Raven Press, 1979.

20. **Brown, G.W. & Birley, J.L.T**. Crises and life changes and the onset of schizophrenia. *Journal of health and social behavior*, **9**: 203–214 (1968).

21. **Rabkin, J.G**. Stressful life events and schizophrenia: a review of the research literature. *Psychological bulletin*, **87**: 408–425 (1980).

22. **Cooper, B. & Sylph, J**. Life events and the onset of neurotic illness: an investigation in general practice. *Psychological medicine*, **3**: 421–435 (1973).

23. **Tennant, C. & Andrews, G**. The pathogenic quality of life event stress in neurotic impairment. *Archives of general psychiatry*, **35**: 859–863 (1978).

24. **Totman, R**. What makes life events stressful? A retrospective study of patients who have suffered a first myocardial infarction. *Journal of psychosomatic research*, **23**: 193–201 (1979).

25. **Rabkin, J.G. & Struening, E.L**. Life events, stress, and illness. *Science*, **194**: 1013–1020 (1976).

26. **Bloom, B**. *Stressful life event theory and research: implications for primary preventions*. Washington, DC, US Department of Health and Human Services, 1985 (No. (ADM) 85–1385).

27. **Dohrenwend, B.S. & Dohrenwend, B.P**. Some issues in research on stressful life events. *Journal of nervous and mental disease*, **166**: 7–15 (1978).

28. **House, J.S**. Chronic life situations and life change events: content discussion. *In*: Ostfeld, A.M. & Eaker, E.D., ed. *Measuring psychosocial variables in epidemiologic studies of cardiovascular disease*: proceedings of a workshop. Washington, DC, US Department of Health and Human Services, 1985 (No. (NIH) 85–2270).

29. **Kasl, S.V**. Pursuing the link between stressful life experiences and disease: a time for reappraisal. *In*: Cooper C.L., ed. *Stress research: issues for the eighties*. New York, Wiley, 1983, pp. 79–102.

30. **Holmes, T.H. & Masuda, M**. Life change and illness susceptibility. *In*: Dohrenwend, B.S. & Dohrenwend, B.P., ed. *Stressful life events: their nature and effects*. New York, Wiley, 1974, pp. 45–72.

31. **Vinokur, A. & Selzer, M.L**. Desirable versus undesirable life events: their relationship to stress and mental distress. *Journal of personality and social psychology*, **32**: 329–337 (1975).

32. **Brown, G.W. & Andrews, B**. Social support and depression. *In*: Appley, M.H. & Trumbull, R., ed. *Dynamics of stress: physiological, psychological and social perspectives*. New York, Plenum, 1986, pp. 257–282.

33. **Thoits, P.A**. Dimensions of life events that influence psychological distress: an evaluation and synthesis of the literature. *In*: Kaplan, H.B., ed. *Psychosocial stress: trends in theory and research*. New York, Academic Press, 1983, pp. 33–103.

34. **Lazarus, R.S**. *Psychological stress and the coping process*. New York, McGraw-Hill, 1966.

35. **Hudgens, R.W**. Personal catastrophe and depression: a consideration of the subject with respect to medically ill adolescents, and a requiem for retrospective life-event studies. *In*: Dohrenwend, B.S. & Dohrenwend, B.P., ed. *Stressful life events: their nature and effects*. New York, Wiley, 1974, pp. 119–134.

36. **Dohrenwend, B.S. et al**. Symptoms, hassles, social supports and life events: problem of confounded measures. *Journal of abnormal psychology*, **93**: 222–230 (1984).

37. **Lazarus, R.S. et al**. Stress and adaptational outcomes: the problem of confounded measures. *American psychologist*, **40**: 770–779 (1985).

38. **Mechanic, D**. Stress and social adaptation. *In*: Selye, H., ed. *Selye's guide to stress research*. New York, Van Nostrand Reinhold, 1983, pp. 118–133, Vol. 2.

39. **Dohrenwend, B.S. et al**. Exemplification of a method for scaling life events: the PERI life events scale. *Journal of health and social behavior*, **19**: 205–299 (1978).

40. **Kasl, S.V.** Stress and health. *Annual review of public health*, **5**: 319–341 (1984).

41. **House, J.S. et al**. Occupational stress and health among men and women in the Tecumseh Community Health Study. *Journal of health and social behavior*, **27**: 62–77 (1986).

42. **Cohen, F. et al**. Panel report on psychosocial assets and modifiers of stress. *In*: Elliot, G.R. & Eisdorfer, C., ed. *Stress and human health*. New York, Springer, 1982, pp. 147–188.

43. **Rose, R.M**. Endocrine responses to stressful psychological events. *Psychiatry clinics of North America*, **3**: 251–276 (1980).

44. **Dohrenwend, B.S. & Dohrenwend, B.P**. Class and race as status-related sources of stress. *In*: Levine, S. & Scotch, N., ed. *Social stress*. Chicago, Aldine, 1970, pp. 111–140.

45. **Kessler, R.C. & Neighbors, H.W**. A new perspective on the relationships among race, social class, and psychological distress. *Journal of health and social behavior*, **27**: 107–115 (1986).

46. **Pearlin, L.I. & Lieberman, M.A**. Social sources of emotional distress. *In*: Simmons, R., ed. *Research in community and mental health*. Greenwich, CT, JAI Press, 1979, pp. 217–248, Vol. 1.

47. **Thoits, P.A**. Gender and marital status differences in control and distress: common stress versus unique stress explanations. *Journal of health and social behavior*, **28**: 7–22 (1987).

48. **House, J.S. & Robbins, C**. Age, psychosocial stress, and health. *In*: Riley, M.W. et al., ed. *Aging in society: selected reviews of recent research*. Hillsdale, NJ, Erlbaum, 1983, pp. 287–325.

49. **Folkman, S. et al**. Age differences in stress and coping processes. *Psychology and aging*. **2**: 171–184 (1987).

50. **Krause, N**. Stress and sex differences in depressive symptoms among older adults. *Journal of gerontology*, **41**: 727–731 (1986).

51. **Kessler, R.C**. Stress, social status and psychological distress. *Journal of health and social behavior*, **20**: 259–272 (1979).

52. **House, J.S. & Kahn, R.L**. Measures and concepts of social support. *In*: Cohen, S. & Syme, S.L., ed. *Social support and health*. New York, Academic Press, 1985, pp. 83–108.

53. **Berkman, L.F. & Breslow, L**. *Health and ways of living*. Oxford, Oxford University Press, 1983.

54. **Cassel, J**. The contribution of the social environment to host resistance. *American journal of epidemiology*, **104**: 107–123 (1976).

55. **House, J.S**. *Work, stress and social support*. Reading, MA, Addison-Wesley, 1981.

56. **Berkman, L.F. & Syme, S.L**. Social networks, host resistance, and mortality: a nine-year follow-up study of Alameda County residents. *American journal of epidemiology*, **109**: 186–204 (1979).

57. **Blazer, D.G**. Social support and mortality in an elderly community population. *American journal of epidemiology*, **115**: 684–694 (1982).

58. **House, J.S. et al**. The association of social relationships and activities with mortality: prospective evidence from the Tecumseh Community Health Study. *American journal of epidemiology*, **116**: 123–140 (1982).

59. **Schoenbach, V.J. et al**. Social ties and mortality in Evans County, Georgia. *American journal of epidemiology*, **123**: 577–591 (1986).

60. **Tibblin, G. et al**. The theory of general susceptibility. *In*: Isacsson, S.O. & Janzon, L., ed. *Social support: health and disease*. Stockholm, Almqvist & Wiksell, 1986, pp. 11–19.

61. **Welin, L. et al**. Prospective study of social influences on mortality. *Lancet*, **1**: 915–918 (1985).

62. **Kitagawa, E.M. & Hauser, P.M**. *Differential mortality in the United States*. Cambridge, MA, Harvard University Press, 1973.

63. **Ortmeyer, C.F**. Variations in mortality, morbidity and health care by marital status. *In*: Erhardt, C.E. & Berlin, J.E., ed. *Mortality and morbidity in the United States*. Cambridge, MA, Harvard University Press, 1974.

64. **Kasl, S.V. & Wells, J.A**. Work and the family: social support and health in the middle years. *In*: Cohen, S. & Syme, S.L., ed. *Social support and health*. New York, Academic Press, 1985, pp. 175–198.

65. **Wallston, B.S. et al**. Social support and physical health. *Health psychology*, **2**: 367–391 (1983).

66. **Broadhead, W.E. et al**. The epidemiologic evidence for a relationship between social support and health. *American journal of epidemiology*, **117**: 521–537 (1983).

67. **Cohen, S. & Syme, S.L.** *Social support and health.* New York, Academic Press, 1985.

68. **House, J.S. et al.** Structures and processes of social support. *Annual review of sociology,* **14**: 293–318 (1988).

69. **Williams, D.R. & House, J.S.** Social support and stress reduction. *In:* Cooper, C.L. & Smith, M., ed. *Job stress and blue collar work.* London, Wiley, 1985, pp. 207–224.

70. **Cohen, S. & Wills, T.A.** Stress, social support and the buffering hypothesis. *Psychological bulletin,* **98**: 310–357 (1985).

71. **Kessler, R.C. & McLeod, J.** Social support and psychological distress in community surveys. *In:* Cohen, S. & Syme, S.L., ed. *Social support and health.* New York, Academic Press, 1985, pp. 219–240.

72. **Fiore, J. et al.** Social network interactions: a buffer or a stress. *American journal of community psychology,* **11**: 423–440 (1983).

73. **Rook, K.S.** The negative side of social interaction: impact on psychological well-being. *Journal of personality and social psychology,* **46**: 1097–1108 (1984).

74. **Umberson, D.** Family status and health behaviors: social control as a dimension of social integration. *Journal of health and social behavior,* **28**: 306–319 (1987).

75. **Belle, D.** The stress of caring: women as providers of social support. *In:* Goldberger, L. & Breznitz, S., ed. *Handbook of stress: theoretical and clinical aspects.* New York, Free Press, 1982, pp. 496–505.

76. **Kessler, R.C. et al.** The cost of caring: a perspective on sex differences in psychological distress. *In:* Sarason, I.G. & Sarason, B.R., ed. *Social support: theory, research and application.* The Hague, Martinus Nijhof, 1985, pp. 491–506.

77. **Risman, B.J.** Intimate relationships from a microstructural perspective: men who mother. *Gender and society,* **1**: 6–32 (1987).

78. **Liem, R. & Liem, J.** Social class and mental illness reconsidered: the role of economic stress and social support. *Journal of health and social behavior,* **19**: 139–156 (1978).

79. **Veroff, J. et al.** *The inner American.* New York, Basic Books, 1981.

80. **Belle, D**. The impact of poverty on social networks and supports. *Marriage and family review*, **5**: 89–103 (1982).

81. **Strogatz, D.S. & James, S.A**. Social support and hypertension among blacks and whites in a rural southern community. *American journal of epidemiology*, **124**: 949–956 (1986).

82. **Kasl, S.V**. Social and psychological factors in the etiology of coronary heart disease in black populations: an exploration of research needs. *American heart journal*, **108**: 660–669 (1984).

83. **Williams, D.R**. *Socioeconomic differentials in health: the role of psychosocial factors*. Thesis, Ann Arbor, MI, Department of Sociology, University of Michigan, 1986.

84. **House, J.S. & Cottington, E.M**. Health and the workplace. *In*: Aiken, L.H. & Mechanic, D., ed. *Applications of social science to clinical medicine and health policy*. New Brunswick, NJ, Rutgers University Press, 1986, pp. 392–416.

85. **Rodin, J**. Aging and health: effects of the sense of control. *Science*, **233**: 1271–1276 (1986).

86. **Rowe, J.W. & Kahn, R.L**. Human aging: usual and successful. *Science*, **237**: 143–149 (1987).

87. **Syme, S.L**. Control and health: a personal perspective. *In*: Steptoe, A. & Appels, A., ed. *Stress, personal control and health*. New York, Wiley, 1989.

88. **Karasek, R. et al**. Job decision latitude, job demands, and cardiovascular disease: a prospective study of Swedish men. *American journal of public health*, **71**: 694–705 (1981).

89. **Langer, E.J. & Rodin, J**. The effects of choice and enhanced personal responsibility for the aged. *Journal of personality and social psychology*, **34**: 191–198 (1976).

90. **Schulz, R**. The effects of control and predictability on the psychological and physical well-being of the institutionalized aged. *Journal of personality and social psychology*, **33**: 563–573 (1976).

91. **Schulz, R. & Hanusa, B.H**. Long-term effects of control and predictability-enhancing experiments. *Journal of personality and social psychology*, **36**: 1194–1201 (1978).

92. **Gurin, G. & Gurin, P**. Personal efficacy and the ideology of individual responsibility. *In*: Strumpel, B., ed. *Economic means for human needs*. Ann Arbor, MI, Institute for Social Research, 1976, pp. 131–157.

93. **Pearlin, L.I. & Schooler, C**. The structure of coping. *Journal of health and social behavior*, **19**: 2–21 (1978).

94. **Krohne, H.W**. Coping with stress. *In*: Appley, M.H. & Trumbull, R., ed. *Dynamics of stress: physiological, psychological and social perspectives*. New York, Plenum Press, 1986, pp. 207–232.

95. **Kessler, R.C. et al**. Social factors in psychopathology: stress, social support and coping processes. *Annual review of psychology*, **36**: 531–572 (1985).

96. **Singer, J.E**. Some issues in the study of coping. *Cancer*, **53**: 2303–2313 (1984).

97. **Folkman, S. & Lazarus, R.S**. An analysis of coping in a middle-aged community sample. *Journal of health and social behavior*, **21**: 219–239 (1980).

98. **Taylor, S.E**. Response to Singer. *Cancer*, **53**: 2313–2315 (1984).

99. **Frese, M**. Coping as a moderator and mediator between stress at work and psychosomatic complaints. *In*: Appley, M.H. & Trumbull, R., ed. *Dynamics of stress: physiological, psychological and social perspectives*. New York, Plenum Press, 1986, pp. 183–206.

100. **Kessler, R.C. et al**. *Situational determinants of coping and coping effectiveness in a general population sample*. Ann Arbor, MI, Survey Research Center, University of Michigan, 1988.

101. **Lazarus, R.S**. Stress and coping as factors in health and illness. *In*: Cohen, J. et al., ed. *Psychosocial aspects of cancer*. New York, Raven Press, 1982, pp. 163–190.

102. **Aldwin, C.M. & Revenson, T.A**. Does coping help? A re-examination of the relation between coping and mental health. *Journal of personality and social psychology*, **53**: 337–348 (1987).

103. **Johnson, J.E**. Coping with elective surgery. *Annual review of nursing research*, **2**: 107–132 (1984).

104. **Chesney, M.A. & Rosenman, R.H**. Specificity in stress models: examples drawn from type A behavior. *In*: Cooper, C.L., ed. *Stress research: issues for the eighties*. New York, Wiley, 1983, pp. 21–34.

105. **Felton, B.J. & Revenson, T.A**. Age differences in coping with chronic illness. *Psychology and aging*, **2**: 164–170 (1987).

7

Psychobiology of stress and attachment: the biobehavioural view

Holger Ursin

One of the most puzzling questions in medicine is why some people fall ill and some do not. There is no apparent consistent or linear dose–response relationship between most disease-producing agents and the resulting frequency or intensity of disease. General health status, constitution, previous life history and genetic determinants all affect resistance. Psychological factors also influence these individual differences in resistance and susceptibility: stress is one such factor and attachment (the existence of positive feelings and bonds between individuals) is another. Attachment is a resistance factor that may also have positive health-promoting effects.

This chapter reviews the contribution of these two psychological factors to individual differences in susceptibility to disease. These phenomena act through basic psychophysiological and pathophysiological mechanisms. Despite individual differences, it is still possible to formulate general principles that are common to humans and even to the rest of the animal kingdom.

Traditional medicine takes genetic variance into account, and molecular biology and molecular medicine have developed very impressive and useful methods to identify diseases caused by specific molecular mechanisms. The consequences for health of the psychological sources of individual differences are not so well understood.

One reason for slow progress is that learning and memory are the subjects of psychology and not medicine. In medicine the simple explanation is usually considered the beautiful explanation, forming a rational basis for therapy and prevention. Psychologists often develop very complex theories, but may be less effective in intervention. A stress molecule, a peptide resistance factor or a social factor that could easily be quantified would make things so much simpler. Complexity remains, however, and at least a minimum of psychology is required to understand these relationships.

There is a regrettable lack of standardization in terminology. All researchers of stress seem to prefer their own sets of definitions and I also have my own set. I will try to refer to the most widely used terminology and to emphasize the substantial consensus.

Stress

The concept of stress has too many meanings to be useful unless it is used in a specifically defined context. Stress ranges from the dramatic picture described by Selye *(1)* to the mild degree of discomfort experienced by the commuter stuck in rush-hour traffic. Stress means the stimuli that produce a certain state, the subjective feeling of discomfort in this state and the responses that occur in an organism in this state. Individuals register some of these somatic responses and may interpret and label this experience as stress. The disease-promoting effects do not seem to be related to the amplitude of the response but to its duration, and possibly to specific response types.

In this chapter, the stimuli that may produce the stress state are called load. The load may be defined in objective terms (difficulty of task, time spent, units of information per time unit) or subjectively. If the subject characterizes the load as stressful, this is called a subjective report of stress. Most people are able to quantify such experiences. Finally, the organism reacts with a general stress response affecting all systems. This response is identical to or at least indistinguishable from the general brain activation response. There is controversy about whether this response has any specificity, either for all stress responses or for types of stress.

The general activation concept is based on a brain stem system described by Moruzzi & Magoun *(2)*. Activation may be defined as a common path for all phenomena that lead to a higher level of activity in the brain. Input is received from all peripheral and central sources, producing electroencephalogram activation, muscular changes, behavioural changes and general changes to the autonomic and endocrine systems. Immunological processes are also affected. The Cannon alarm reaction (sympathetic activation), the Selye general adaptation syndrome (pituitary–adrenal activation), the cardiovascular defence reaction (mainly sympathetic activation) *(3)*, and the ergotropic response of Hess (sympathetic activation) are only parts of this general somatic response. The controversy is whether the responses in the endocrine and autonomic systems are specific responses to stress, or specific to particular emotional states or particular types of problem or personality. Only the latter seems to be reasonably well established, with a catecholamine-related (ambition, time-urgency, type A behaviour) and a control-related (defence) personality type (see Ursin *(4)* for discussion and references).

In early work, psychophysiologists postulated specific activation patterns for specific emotions, particularly for fear and anger *(5, 6)*. This has never been demonstrated consistently in individuals. The cognitive aspects of a situation seem to determine the interpretation and labelling of the changes experienced *(7, 8)*.

Pribram & McGuinness *(9)* have developed a complex model for attention processes, identifying three separate but interacting neural systems. Immediate physiological responses to sensory stimuli are called arousal, more tonic readiness to respond is called activation and the coordination between these two processes, effort. These definitions are particularly useful in work on human performance and the costs (effort) involved in solving problems (for a discussion of energetics, see Hockey et al. *(10)*). The Pribram & McGuinness postulates specify the brain mechanisms that are involved. The effort and arousal mechanisms are linked to limbic structures (amygdala and hippocampus, respectively). Henry & Meehan *(11)* have suggested that there may also be an endocrine specificity to these mechanisms. The amygdala effort mechanism may be tied to catecholamines and the hippocampus arousal mechanism to cortisol. Tucker & Williamson *(12)* have related the tonic activation system to extrapyramidal motor control, and the phasic arousal system to pyramidal motor control. Even if these hypotheses are unnecessary for now, the distinctions may be necessary for further progress in this type of research. The distinction between tonic activation and phasic arousal (also called phasic activation) is particularly important for psychosomatic pathology.

The Sustained Activation Hypothesis in Psychosomatic Pathology

If activation is a part of the normal, adaptive processes of the human organism, why should it lead to somatic disease? When is this response a healthy response, strengthening systems such as the skeletal and heart muscles (training), and when does it have a harmful effect (straining)?

The homeostatic mechanisms described in ordinary physiology are inhibited, by-passed and overridden all the time. The previous concept of invariable set values implies an overly static view of physiological processes. A psychological load activates higher brain circuits that change the gain of cardiovascular reflexes, permitting deviations from the set points observed under resting conditions. These deviations only acquire pathogenic potential when they are sustained over long time periods. The duration of such deviations is, therefore, more important than the magnitude. Slow and long-term changes in physiological processes are better indicators of stress than the traditional, short-term and phasic activation processes so often used (13).

The sustained activation hypothesis for psychosomatic disease (4) states that the tonic activation observed in all subjects confronted with a difficult task can only become pathogenic if it is sustained over time. This occurs when people realize or believe that they cannot meet and handle this threat. Sustained activation, therefore, depends on the response–outcome expectancies of each individual. Health and disease also depend on the same psychological mechanisms. An understanding of these requires an understanding of the stress-inhibiting mechanisms and the response–outcome expectancies that are developed.

Stress-inhibiting Mechanisms

The beneficial effects of attachment and social support have to be mediated via known cognitive, psychophysiological, psycho-endocrine and psychoimmunological mechanisms. Disease is assumed to be produced by sustained, tonic activation. The inhibitory mechanisms must, therefore, be understood. In humans two such mechanisms inhibit stress responses, defence and coping.

176

Defence is an old Freudian concept, but it may be regarded as a mechanism that inhibits, distorts and alters the stimulus, leading to less accurate perception of a situation. This may prove fatal in life-threatening situations *(14)* and may create additional social or inter-personal problems for the individual when the source of difficulties is projected or displaced on others *(15)*. These perceptual distortions depend on personality traits that can be measured by tachistoscopic tests *(16)* or by pencil and paper questionnaires *(17)*.

Coping is used in two different contexts. It often refers to what a person does to handle a situation, predicting nothing about the internal state of the person. Coping may also mean that the subject believes that the situation is under control, reducing activation in both humans and animals. The subject has learned not only the solution to the problem, but also that this particular solution works. This dimension, which goes beyond performance, is called coping *(18)*. Elsewhere, I have defined this as positive response–outcome expectancy *(19, 20)*. The subject learns that the response available brings the desired results. When this stage has been reached in an uncertain, threatening or difficult situation, activation is reduced, whether measured in terms of endocrine, humoral or autonomic responses *(18)*.

For both humans and animals, coping involves an individually acquired expectancy. The difficulty of the task, the reinforcing properties of the events, the predictability of the events, and the feedback that control is possible are all important for the slope of the learning curve and for the slope of the decrease in activation. Learning expectancy, however, is not identical to the learning or performance seen in the ordinary learning curve.

Coping reduces most but not all indicators of activation. The activation unaffected by coping may be called phasic activation or arousal *(9)*. Men who are coping still have an increased heart rate, increased urinary epinephrine levels and a short-term increase in testosterone levels. All these responses are anabolic. Phasic activation, therefore, may be related to physical training. The activation sensitive to the coping mechanism may be called tonic and involves increased urinary norepinephrine, decreased plasma levels of testosterone, increased blood pressure and increased plasma levels of cortisol, growth hormone, prolactin, blood glucose and free fatty acids. This tonic activation, if sustained, is assumed to be related to pathology *(4)*.

The Psychobiology of Attachment

Why is strengthening social networks and social support an essential part of health promotion? Is it really true that good friends and good family relations are essential to promote health?

Attachment refers to the bonds established between individuals, often in early life, in humans and in animals. The relationship between mother and child has been studied most. Early work concentrated on the ontogenetic aspects of attachment, which could reach across species. This was demonstrated by Lorenz *(21)* as the phenomenon of imprinting in birds and by Scott *(22)* as the socialization and taming of animals by humans. The bonds between mother, child and peers in nonhuman primates were studied in a pioneer work by Harlow & Harlow *(23)*.

Harlow & Zimmerman *(24)* showed that infantile attachment in primates was not based solely on the pleasures of feeding. The comfort from physical contact was an overriding factor. Rhesus monkey infants preferred cloth surrogate mothers to wire surrogates, even if the wire surrogate delivered milk. Pleasant physical contact somehow served to reduce emotional arousal (activation) *(25)*, and objects that have this function become the focus of emotional dependence or attachment. The mother and child are a unit that may serve to reduce emotional arousal (activation) by signifying safety for both of them. Faced with threats, mother and child seek each other out and, if they find each other, activation is significantly reduced, as measured by changes in endocrine activity in both child and mother *(26)*. The main mechanism is proximity or contact with the mother. For the infant, this is an active process: the infant achieves contact by signals or by seeking out the mother. This represents the infant's first experience of control over the environment. If it is successful, the infant copes according to the response–outcome expectancy. Loss of the mother, in fact, represents loss of control, or loss of coping, which results in marked increases in endocrine activity *(27)*. The infant's reaction to separation is modified by other environmental factors: the presence of other, familiar conspecifics will reduce its response to separation. Thus, other forms of social support also work for infants.

Human babies and their mothers follow much the same behavioural pattern. The child develops a fear of strangers, and this fear elicits attachment behaviour (28). Much effort has been spent on the question of whether humans (and animals) are inherently social or whether this behaviour is learned. Attachment behaviour was originally explained as social learning (29, 30). Primary reinforcement was offered by the mother satisfying the physiological needs of the baby. Early stages of this behaviour may be unlearned. As in all learning, reinforcement only works on responses with a certain probability of occurrence (operant level), and sets of unlearned stimuli may specify proximity. When fear and anxiety develop, they elicit attachment behaviour. This hypothesis is close to the ethological approach (31) and is also compatible with essential elements of contemporary positions in psychodynamic theory. Fear of strangers is related to separation anxiety, which is produced by the physical discomfort of being separated from the mother (28, 32).

The presence of the mother in threatening situations has a paradoxical result. A stranger is more terrifying when the mother is present and one metre away than when the mother is totally absent (31, 33). Monkey infants also cry more on separation when their mother is present, but neither close nor available, than when she is totally absent (27). These observations are strictly behavioural, however, and do not explain the internal state of the subject. Coe et al. (27) have shown that the paradox disappears when the internal state is evaluated by suprarenal cortical activity. An infant's cries and probably its emotional expressions are all instrumental responses directed towards the mother. Emitting these signals is useless if there is no mother available. Fear, as evaluated by internal state, is much greater when there is no mother present. As expected, crying is an emotional expression that may be affective or instrumental, and may be emitted both in high and low states of arousal or activation, depending on the outcome expectancy of the subject (19).

Experiences in this stage of life may influence both subsequent behaviour, and later resistance to both the psychological and biological effects of psychological or physiological loads (stress) (34). In animals, early rearing conditions are crucial for later performance as adults (35). Examples of this are the response repertoire and strategies in rats (36, 37). Early rearing conditions produce structural changes in the brain (38) and physiological changes (39, 40). The data from humans are still controversial, but suggest that enriched but safe environments are also important for the human child.

Social Networks and Health

Cassel *(41)* suggested that social support or social cohesiveness protects people against somatic disease. From a psychobiological point of view, the importance of social networks for health (see Marmot *(42)* and Chapter 5) is probably related to the attachment factor and to the psychological factors involved in attachment and establishing social bonds.

A survey of living conditions in Sweden in 1976 and 1977, which surveyed 14 000 randomly sampled men and women between 16 and 74 years of age, contained 18 measures of social network. Based on this, a social interaction index was constructed *(43)*. It was mathematically demonstrated that this index comprised two parts, one for close and intimate contacts (nuclear family: attachment) and one for more distant contacts (work colleagues, neighbours: social integration). These two parts were only moderately related. They both, however, had high internal consistency. Support from acquaintances and neighbours did not really matter, but support from work colleagues was vital for both men and women. For men, this was the strongest source of support, stronger than parents or nuclear family. Support from nuclear family members was particularly important for women in the 46–65 year age group.

In an eight-year follow-up study of cardiovascular risk factors and disease in 150 men, their social isolation and subjective rating of health predicted mortality. None of the men who had two or more social activities per week actually died during the observation period. The authors asked whether social inactivity was merely an indicator of advanced disease or perhaps an important sign of unhealthy lifestyle. Theorell *(44)* has published data on programme that promote social activity and social networks to improve the health of elderly people. He suggests that lack of social support activates long-lasting mobilization of energy and catabolism (sustained activation), which may result in a variety of psychosomatic diseases. In an disintegrated community in Newfoundland, characterized by unemployment, ineffective schools and general apathy, a social intervention programme including jobs, an improved school system and improved social relationships significantly affected health and disease *(45)*.

180

Social Stress

Before advocating that people acquire a friend a day to keep the doctor away, more should be known about the quality of the relationship. A simple head count of social contacts may not work, since it might include clear sources of stress. Conspecifics may actually induce stress. Crowding does not improve health. Increasing population density changes social relationships, increasing stress, increasing pituitary–adrenal activation and reducing gonadal function. The resulting reduction in the vitality and fertility of animals may counteract an increase in population density. An extraordinarily severe source of stress can even hinder adjustment and result in the death of the animals (46, 47).

In humans, lower social classes have always had higher death rates from all diseases. Surprisingly, this difference also seems to exist in modern welfare states, such as the Netherlands and the Scandinavian countries (48), where class now has relatively little influence on income and general standards of hygiene. The relationships seem even clearer when correlated with education rather than standard income classifications, particularly for cardiovascular death (49, 50). These variables affect nutrition, smoking and health habits. Theorell (44) and Jenkins (49) hold that social support, social instability and interpersonal conflicts are particularly prevalent among lower social classes.

The concepts of control and predictability may partially explain these relationships (51, 52). Response–outcome expectancy is assumed to be decisive for the physiological state of individuals faced with threats. This may also be true for the effects of life events on health. Again, the control and predictability of events seem really to matter (53). Undesirable life events have more pathological effect than desirable ones but the presence or absence of social support or attachment is crucial (44).

Hopelessness and Helplessness: Lack of Social Support

The decrease in sensitivity to stress produced by attachment and social support is related to establishing positive response–outcome expectancies. From the early stages of life, attachment seems to have this effect for mother and child. It seems reasonable to assume that facilitating the acquisition of positive response–outcome expectancies is an essential element in all good social relationships. Lack of social support may facilitate negative response–outcome expectancies or no expectancy at all. Helplessness exists when responses and reinforcement have no apparent relationship (54). When an animal is subjected to uncontrollable shocks, helplessness develops. The animal has great difficulty in finding proper solutions to difficult tasks, shows higher activation levels and a higher frequency of gastric ulcerations (55). Helplessness is related to external control, and coping is related to internal control (56).

Hopelessness is the expectancy that all responses will give a negative and undesired outcome: the exact opposite of coping. Individuals expect their responses to produce poor results and punishment. Therefore, this model also involves feelings of guilt and negative self-esteem. Negative response–outcome expectancies and lack of expectancy indicate a danger of risk to somatic health. They may be a sign of lack of social support and they may also produce lack of support. Noncoping people may have little to give in relationships. They lack what they need most, friends, support and hope. This not only deprives them of important life qualities, but it may also have consequences for somatic health through the sustained activation mechanism.

References

1. **Selye, H**. A syndrome produced by diverse nocuous agents. *Natura*, **138**: 32 (1936).
2. **Moruzzi, G. & Magoun, H.W**. Brain stem reticular formation and activation of the EEG. *Electroencephalography and clinical neurophysiology*, **1**: 455–473 (1949).
3. **Folkow, B**. Physiological aspects of primary hypertension. *Physiological review*, **62**: 347–504 (1982).
4. **Ursin, H**. Personality, activation and somatic health. A new psychosomatic theory. *In*: Levine, S. & Ursin, H., ed. *Coping and health*. New York, Plenum Press, 1980, pp. 259–279.
5. **Ax, A.F**. The physiological differentiation between fear and anger in humans. *Psychosomatic medicine*, **15**: 433–442 (1953).
6. **Schachter, J**. Pain, fear and anger in hypertensives and normotensives. A psychophysiological study. *Psychosomatic medicine*, **19**: 17–29 (1957).

7. **Rule, B.G. & Nesdale, A.R**. Environmental stressors, emotional arousal and aggression. *In*: Sarason, I.G. & Spielberger, C.D., ed. *Stress and anxiety*. Washington, DC, Hemisphere (Wiley), 1976, Vol. 3, pp. 87–103.

8. **Schachter, J.P. & Singer, J.E**. Cognitive, social and physiological determinants of emotional state. *Psychological review*, **69**: 379–399 (1962).

9. **Pribram, K.H. & McGuinness, D**. Arousal, activation and effort in the control of attention. *Psychological review*, **82**: 116–149 (1975).

10. **Hockey, G.R.J. et al**. *Energetics and human information processing*. Dordrecht, M. Nijhoff, 1986.

11. **Henry, J.P. & Meehan, J.P**. Psychosocial stimuli, physiological specificity, and cardiovascular disease. *In*: Weiner, H. et al., ed. *Brain, behavior, and bodily disease*. New York, Raven Press, 1981, pp. 305–333.

12. **Tucker, D.M. & Williamson, P.A**. Asymmetric neural control systems in human self-regulation. *Psychological review*, **91**: 185–215 (1984).

13. **Ursin, H. et al**. Psychological stress-factors and concentrations of immunoglobulins and complement components in humans. *Scandinavian journal of psychology*, **25**: 340–347 (1984).

14. **Vaernes, R.J**. The Defense Mechanism Test predicts inadequate performance under stress. *Scandinavian journal of psychology*, **23**: 37–43 (1982).

15. **Vickers, R.R., Jr**. Cardiovascular disease and psychological defenses: development of a working hypothesis. *In*: Ursin, H. & Murison, R., ed. *Biological and psychological basis of psychosomatic disease*. Oxford, Pergamon Press, 1983, pp. 209–221.

16. **Kragh, U**. The defense mechanism test: a new method for diagnosis and personnel selection. *Journal of applied psychology*, **44**: 303–309 (1960).

17. **Plutchik, R. et al**. A structural theory of ego defenses and emotions. *In*: Izard, C., ed. *Emotions in personality and psychopathology*. New York, Plenum Press, 1979, pp. 229–257.

18. **Ursin, H. et al., ed**. *Psychobiology of stress: a study of coping men*. New York, Academic Press, 1978.

19. **Ursin, H**. The instrumental effects of emotional behavior. *In*: Bateson, P.P.G. & Klopfer, P.H., ed. *Perspectives in ethology*. New York, Plenum Press, 1985, Vol. 6, pp. 45–62.

20. **Bolles, R.C**. Reinforcement, expectancy and learning. *Psychological review*, **79**: 394–409 (1972).

21. **Lorenz, K**. Vergleichende Verhaltensforschung. *Verhandlung der Deutschen Zoologischen Gesellschaft*, **41**: 69–102 (1939).

22. **Scott, J.P**. *Aggression*. Chicago, University of Chicago Press, 1958.

23. **Harlow, H.F. & Harlow, M.K**. The affectional systems. *In*: Schrier, A.M. et al., ed. *Behavior of non-human primates*. New York, Plenum Press, 1965.

24. **Harlow, H.F. & Zimmerman, R.R**. Affectional responses in the infant monkey. *Science*, **130**: 421–432 (1959).

25. **Mason, J.W**. A re-evaluation of the concept of "non-specificity" in stress theory. *Journal of psychiatric research*, **8**: 323–335 (1971).

26. **Levine, S**. A coping model of mother-infant relationships. *In*: Levine, S. & Ursin, H., ed. *Coping and health*. New York, Plenum Press, 1980, pp. 87–99.

27. **Coe, C.L. et al**. Endocrine and immune responses to separation and maternal loss in nonhuman primates. *In*: Reite, M. & Field, T., ed. *The psychobiology of attack and separation*. New York, Academic Press, 1985, pp. 163–199.

28. **Bower, T.G.R**. *Human development*. San Francisco, W.H. Freeman, 1979.

29. **Bandura, A**. *Principles of behaviour modification*. New York, Holt, 1969.

30. **Dollard, J. & Miller, N.E**. *Personality and psychotherapy*. New York, McGraw-Hill, 1950.

31. **Bowlby, J**. *Attachment and loss*. London, Hogarth Press, 1969, Vol. 1.

32. **Spitz, R.A**. Anxiety in infancy: a study of its manifestations in the first year of life. *International journal of psychoanalysis*, **31**: 138–143 (1950).

33. **Morgan, G.A. & Ricciuti, H.N**. Infant responses to strangers during the first year. *In*: Foss, B.M., ed. *Determinants of infant behavior*. New York, Wiley, 1969, Vol. 4.

34. **Ader, R**. The effects of early experience on the adrenocortical response to different magnitudes of stimulation. *Physiology and behaviour*, **5**: 837 (1970).

35. **Levine, S**. Infantile stimulation: a perspective. *In*: Ambrose, A., ed. *Stimulation in early infancy*. London, Academic Press, 1969.

36. **Einon, D**. Spatial memory and response strategies in rats: age, sex, and rearing difference in performance. *Quarterly journal of experimental psychology*, **32**: 473–489 (1980).

37. **Jurasha, J.M. et al**. Differential rearing experience, gender and radial maze performance. *Developmental psychobiology*, **17**: 209–215 (1983).

38. **Rozenzweig, M.R. & Bennett, E.L**. Effects of differential environments on brain weights and enzyme activities in gerbils, rats and mice. *Developmental psychobiology*, **2**: 87–95 (1970).

39. **Horn, G. et al**. Experience and plasticity in the central nervous system. *Science*, **181**: 506–514 (1973).

40. **Wilson, D.A. et al**. Early handling increases hippocampal long-term potentiation in young rats. *Behavioral brain research*, **21**: 223–227 (1986).

41. **Cassel, J**. The contribution of the social environment to host resistance. *American journal of epidemiology*, **104**: 107–123 (1976).

42. **Marmot, M.G**. Social patterns in relation to social networks in cardiovascular disease. *In*: Isacsson, S.O. & Janzon, L., ed. *Social support: health and disease*. Stockholm, Almqvist & Wiksell, 1986, pp. 59–69.

43. **Orth-Gomér, K. et al**. Social interaction and mortality in Sweden. Findings in the normal population and in cardio-vascular patients. *In*: Isacsson, S.O. & Janzon, L., ed. *Social support: health and disease*. Stockholm, Almqvist and Wiksell, 1986, pp. 21–31.

44. **Theorell, T**. On the purpose and duration of social support. *In*: Isacsson, S.O. & Janzon, L., ed. *Social support: health and disease*. Stockholm, Almqvist & Wiksell, 1986, pp. 149–160.

45. **Leighton, A**. Poverty and social change. *Scientific American*, **212**: 21–27 (1965).

46. **Christian, J.J. et al**. The role of endocrines in the self-regulation of mammalian populations. *Recent progress in hormone research*, **21**: 501–578 (1965).

47. **Henry, J.-P. & Stephens, P.M**. *Stress, health and the social environment. A sociobiologic approach to medicine*. New York, Springer, 1977.

48. **de Wolff, C.J**. Stress and strain in the work environment: does it lead to illness? *In*: Gentry, W.D. et al., ed. *Behavioral*

185

medicine: work stress and health. Boston, Dordrecht, 1985, pp. 33–43.

49. **Jenkins, C.D**. Psychosocial risk factors for coronary heart disease. *Acta medica scandinavica*, **660**(Suppl.): 123–136 (1982).

50. **Rose, G. & Marmot, M**. Social class and coronary heart disease. *British heart journal*, **45**: 13–19 (1981).

51. **Overmier, J.B. et al**. Environmental contingencies as sources of stress in animals. *In*: Levine, S. & Ursin, H., ed. *Coping and health*. New York, Plenum Press, 1980, pp. 1–38.

52. **Weinberg, J. & Levine, S**. Psychobiology of coping in animals: the effects of predictability. *In*: Levine, S. & Ursin, H., ed. *Coping and health*. New York, Plenum Press, 1980, pp. 39–60.

53. **Dohrenwend, B.P. & Dohrenwend, B.S**. *Social status and psychological disorder: a causal inquiry*. New York, Wiley, 1969.

54. **Overmier, J.B. & Seligman, M.E.P**. Effect of inescapable shock upon subsequent escape and avoidance responding. *Journal of comparative and physiological psychology*, **63**: 28–33 (1967).

55. **Murison, R. & Isaksen, E**. Biological and psychological bases of gastric ulceration. *In*: Ursin, H. & Murison, R., ed. *Biological and psychological basis of psychosomatic disease*. Oxford, Pergamon Press, 1983, pp. 239–248.

56. **Rotter, J.B. et al**. Internal versus external control of reinforcements. A major variable in behavior theory. *In*: Washburne, N.F., ed. *Decisions, values and groups*. Oxford, Pergamon Press, 1962, pp. 473–516.

8

Issues in lifestyles and health: lay meanings of health and health behaviour

Roisin Pill

A discussion document on health promotion *(1)* summarizes the case for studying the health beliefs and behaviour of lay people as viewed by advocates of health promotion:

> The predominant way of life in society is central to health promotion, since it fosters personal behaviour patterns that are either beneficial or detrimental to health. The promotion of lifestyles conducive to health involves consideration of personal coping strategies and dispositions as well as beliefs and values relevant to health, all shaped by lifelong experiences and living conditions.

These advocates perceive a need to be aware of what the people in any given community understand by health, the means by which they believe it can be achieved and maintained, and the priority they accord to behaving in a healthy manner in their daily lives. The focus is very definitely on information as the basis for more effective intervention. The obvious requirements are, therefore, for guidance on how to carry out research into these topics or guidance on what has already been done that might be relevant. What is considered relevant, of course, lies very much in the eye of the beholder; the health educator trying to mount a national or regional campaign and the health professional interested in promoting the health of individual patients are likely to want rather different information and are also likely to interpret the same information differently.

187

A cursory examination of the literature on the views of lay people about health and health behaviour in developed countries is quite likely to confuse people interested in health promotion. First, there are few available systematic studies of health, as opposed to illness beliefs and behaviour. It is only comparatively recently that large-scale surveys have been carried out that are beginning to provide an overview of both beliefs and behaviour held by national samples in Canada (2) and Great Britain (3), and behaviour only in the United States (4, 5). Second, most studies have been small-scale, often exploratory projects frequently using qualitative methods of data collection such as in-depth interviews.

The inspiration for much of this work comes from Herzlich's seminal study of the concepts of health and illness held by a sample of middle-class residents of Paris and Normandy (6). The focus on the notions held, the type of categories, language and underlying logic employed, and the host of implicit meanings communicated by the subjects provided the reference point for subsequent work in France (7–9), Scotland (10–12), Wales (13–16), and in England among both the white population (17–19) and members of ethnic minorities (20,21).

On the whole, these studies have focused on exploring the complex body of knowledge and beliefs held by the people surveyed and relating this to the social context in which the respondents live their daily lives. The samples themselves have often been selected from among those who are regarded as having an important role to play in family health and maintenance (women), and/or from groups of lower socioeconomic status, who have traditionally been viewed as posing problems for health educators and professionals. Thus, the existing published research on health beliefs is scanty and biased towards women and lower socioeconomic groups. The fact that the studies have been carried out in different countries, among different groups, by researchers with very different aims, and using a variety of techniques also makes the task of synthesis very difficult, if not impossible. Apart from Anderson's useful review (22), there have been two recent attempts to present an overview of the field; Calnan (23) examines the concepts of health of lay people under a number of different content headings, whereas Stacey (24) relates such concepts to the structure of the society in which they are found.

Research into health behaviour has been dominated by a very different approach. Apart from the straight descriptions obtained from survey data (mentioned above), a number of studies have examined the factors associated with the performance of a range of health behaviours, the aim being to determine the cluster of demographic or attitudinal variables that best explains observed differences between individuals and groups *(25 – 27)*. A number of models have been put forward *(28)*, of which the health belief model is perhaps the best known and has generated the most research *(29, 30)*. Advocates of health promotion who want a critical overview of recent research on this topic should look at the very useful report produced by Norman *(31)*.

There is probably little disagreement about the relevance to health promoters of studies focused on factors associated with health behaviour and the data obtainable from large-scale surveys. The former studies can indicate the key variables that are associated with health behaviour and enable health promoters to focus on the potentially modifiable ones. Surveys can provide quantifiable data and allow groups differing in age, sex, class and ethnic origin to be compared. Such an overview can give a snapshot of the ideas and self-reported behaviour of a community or a wider society, which might be of considerable potential interest to those trying to mobilize support for a new campaign or to target particular groups for an educational initiative.

It is perhaps less obvious exactly how the data from the small-scale qualitative studies might be used, other than in planning intervention for that particular group. There is, after all, a real danger of making unjustified generalizations on the basis of very specific data collected from a particular group at a particular time and place. What such studies can do, however, is reveal the richness and complexity of people's beliefs and the way they are shaped by characteristics such as sex, age and social position, all of which influence exposure to new ideas and the constraints operating on behaviour. Such studies can assist in understanding why some new concepts, perhaps dear to the hearts of those concerned with health promotion, are accepted and others apparently rejected. They can also help the health professional dealing with patients on a one-to-one basis to be more sensitive to their beliefs and personal circumstances, and tailor counselling for a healthier lifestyle in a more effective way.

At the beginning of this chapter, it was argued that advocates of health promotion either need help on how to carry out research into the concepts of health and health behaviour of lay people, or they need some indication of what might be relevant in the literature. The most useful approach to adopt in this chapter is to give greater attention to the former topic (issues of methodology), rather than to attempt the more traditional review of the contents of the published research. (For this, the reader is referred to the works already cited.) By examining in greater detail exactly how people have collected information on beliefs about health and health behaviour (and the implications for the type of data obtained), advocates of health promotion will get some practical guidance as to the strengths and weaknesses of the various methods. They will then be able to make more informed evaluations of the potential relevance of the research for their own needs.

If a critical look is needed at how data are collected, it is also necessary to consider critically the way they are interpreted and used. People concerned with health promotion need to examine more closely some of the assumptions underlying the literature on the subject and the research on beliefs about health and health behaviour, because it will affect the way health promotion is implemented. In particular, it is necessary to consider how people understand the relationship between the concepts of health held by lay people and *(a)* the concepts held by professionals and *(b)* actual health behaviour.

This chapter has three sections. The first examines the lay perspective on health versus the professional perspective; the second looks at the nature of the link between expressed beliefs and attitudes and actual behaviour, while the third tackles the question of methodology and its implications for the content of the data collected. In the final discussion some suggestions are put forward about the implications for those intending to embark on health promotion.

Differences in Concepts of Health

Interpretation of perceived differences
The need to describe the concepts held by members of the public arises from the perception that these concepts are often different from those held by health professionals, the people regarded as having particular skills and knowledge in the fields of health and illness. Having perceived these discrepancies, it is possible to interpret them in two ways. Different can be equated with wrong or misguided, so that these concepts of health are perceived as stemming either from

190

ignorance or wilful misunderstanding and as needing correction through the appropriate educational techniques. This approach is the basis of traditional health education, and is characterized by its uncritical adoption of the ideas currently approved by the medical establishment.

The results of the unquestioning acceptance of the medical profession's perspective can also clearly be seen in the research on health behaviour. The most notable feature of this is that the perspective of lay people has been almost totally ignored *(22,31)*, despite the fact that the definition of health behaviour most usually quoted *(32)* implies that individuals must believe that their actions will achieve the specified goals:

> Health behaviour is any activity undertaken by a person believing himself to be healthy, *for the purpose of* preventing disease or detecting it in an asymptomatic stage. [Author's italics.]

In practice, however, researchers have usually defined health behaviour according to current medical opinion and there has been no attempt, until recently, to explore self-defined health behaviour.

It was in 1979 that Harris & Guten *(33)* coined the term health-protective behaviour to describe:

> any behaviour performed by a person, regardless of his or her perceived or actual health status, in order to protect, promote or maintain his or her health, whether or not that behaviour is objectively effective toward that end.

The advantage of this approach is that it assumes that people will act with the intention of protecting their health, but it makes no assumptions about medical approval or the objective effectiveness of the behaviour cited. The question Harris & Guten asked ("What are the three most important things you do to protect your health?") was replicated by Pill & Stott *(34)* on a sample of working-class mothers in Wales. Both the recent national surveys carried out in Canada *(2)* and in Great Britain *(3)* also included questions on what respondents did, or had done in the past year, to keep themselves healthy or improve their health.

Harris & Guten *(33)* concluded that:

> people perform a wide range of activities in the belief that these activities can protect their health, that most [health-protective behaviours] do not require or involve contact with the formalized health care system and that protecting one's health is apparently a personal rather than a professional matter.

191

So far, these conclusions appear to be valid. Such findings should be welcomed by health promoters who seek to promote greater autonomy among their clients.

Knowledge of what is believed to be effective for the maintenance of health is also essential if one wishes to reinforce positive health behaviour, so it is somewhat surprising that self-defined health behaviour has received comparatively little attention. This merely emphasizes the power of the underlying assumption that the medical profession's perspective is correct and is the yardstick against which everything should be measured.

An alternative approach to the problem of perceived discrepancies between the concepts of lay people and professionals is to seek to understand how such differences have arisen and the factors that contribute to their persistence or change over time. After all, the ethos of the new health promotion philosophy strongly rejects anything that smacks of manipulation and authoritarianism, and emphasizes the need to respect people's opinions and involve them directly in decisions about their own health. Sensitive intervention must, therefore, involve some grasp of the processes involved and a clearer understanding of the nature of the relationship between the concepts of lay people and professionals in western developed countries.

Health beliefs of lay people in developed countries

An examination of developed countries can sometimes be helped by the work of anthropologists and sociologists who have researched health and illness behaviour in a variety of settings (35–37). Their findings draw attention to the intimate association of knowledge and beliefs about health with the other sets of knowledge, beliefs and values extant within a society, to the likelihood that a plurality of views may be found, and to the fact that this coexistence of apparently incompatible concepts may be associated with the presence in the society of groups that have different ideologies (38).

Parallels are found in modern western societies. Thus in her study of working-class men and women in east London, Cornwell (19) found that the people in her sample were preoccupied with the moral aspects of health and illness. Their accounts of health — the insistence that one's own health is good, the scorn for hypochondriacs — reflected the same themes apparent in their discussion of work and the nature of the individual's responsibility for work. Her subjects had little control over their working lives, and yet took upon themselves the injunction to work hard regardless of what they were doing (19):

Thus 'good' people are not only hardworking, they are also cheerful and stoical and if they feel ill, they prefer to work off their symptoms rather than give in to them. 'Bad' people, on the other hand, are people who will not work (malingerers) and who are also likely to be hypochondriacs who waste valuable medical resources.

In France, Pierret (7) has also examined how the type of work people do affects the way they interpret concepts of health and illness, by interviewing subjects differing in age, sex and socioeconomic status. She found that small farmers equated good health with good fortune, and while they saw it as an essential attribute, they felt nothing could be done to achieve it. The unskilled or semiskilled workers holding insecure jobs valued health as the way to employment and hence status within society, but thought job-related risks to health could hardly be reduced and emphasized the need for better access to health care facilities and services. Both these groups directly participate in production using their bodies as tools or implements and differed from other groups in middle-class jobs requiring knowledge and training.

For these groups the type of employer strongly affected their view of the world. Those working in the public sector were less inclined to see health as an essentially personal matter and stressed the links between environment and health facilities and health. Those working in the private sector saw health as a goal to be attained through their own endeavours. While they were well aware of their duty to be healthy, however, they also stressed that it was their right to "have fun".

A similar tension was observed in a sample of mainly middle-class people in Chicago, who often discussed health in terms of self-control and similar concepts while at the same time asserting the health-giving qualities of release — a term that suggests pleasure-seeking rather than ascetic self-denial. Crawford (39) argues that these opposing themes in the discourse on health reflect the contradictions inherent in the wider advanced capitalist society, where the dominant culture of consumption demands a modal personality that is contradictory to the personality required to produce the goods or services.

Such examples indicate the close links between beliefs relevant to health and the experiences and living conditions to which people are exposed. The work of Cornwell (19) and Pierret (7) suggests that the socioeconomic position individuals occupy in modern society will be as influential on their theories of health and behaviour as differences in ethnic or religious origin. Such concepts as social class depend crucially on categorization according to the type of job held by individuals or the head of their households. In turn, occupation is closely linked to the level of education and income received. The complex division of labour in modern societies, therefore, is one basis for anticipating a plurality of views, and the documentation of such differences between socioeconomic groups has recently begun to receive more attention in research on health beliefs *(2,3,24)*.

Anyone who lives in a modern industrial society is aware of the special role accorded to those who work with matters of health and illness. The specialist healers, the health professionals in our society, usually receive extensive training, are accorded considerable prestige and are given the authority to control and discipline the members of their own occupational group and sanction anyone else who attempts certain kinds of healing intervention *(40)*. It may therefore be rather difficult to recognize that the body of knowledge they espouse is just as much a cultural creation as the apparently more bizarre theories held by inhabitants of the "primitive" societies described by anthropologists.

Western biomedicine, defined as the system of health care that is based on the tenets of science as understood in the west and is characterized by its emphasis on a biological understanding of the human being, is the product of a particular society at a particular historical period. This is not the place to describe how the system of medical ideas that emerged in the west came to be based on the natural sciences *(38,41,42)*: it is sufficient to point out that, although biomedicine is predominant and usually provides the reference point for the theories of lay people, the concepts of professionals are by no means static, unchanging or universally agreed upon. (This is amply demonstrated by historical studies of diagnosis and treatment *(43)*.) Views can and do differ not only between various groups of health professionals but also within subgroups of a single profession. Prescriptions for the healthy life are no exception. At least part of the resistance to the theories of prevention and health maintenance currently being promulgated is attributable to the public's perception that health professionals are giving different, often conflicting messages. Moreover, they are also aware that today's messages differ from those of a decade ago, with diet and nutrition being an especially confused and contentious area.

To sum up, the way that people living in western industrialized societies, as in other societies, think and speak about their health reflects their view of themselves and their world. Sex, age, ethnic origin and religious affiliation may all exert an important influence on the kinds of experience individuals undergo, and may therefore be associated with systematic variations in health knowledge, beliefs and behaviour, although little attention has yet been paid to these issues. Socioeconomic status, that crucial feature of modern society, is receiving increased attention from people seeking to document and explain the social distribution of knowledge.

Health professionals in developed countries have generally been extremely successful in defining the terms in which health and illness are discussed, so much so that there is a danger of forgetting that other perspectives may have equal validity. It is suggested that an uncritical acceptance of the medical model by health promoters could result in victim-blaming (44) and in insensitive attempts to impose the concepts of professionals on lay people rather than attempting to understand their views. An effective counter to such a tendency is the recognition that current biomedical theories and concepts often conflict and are subject to change over time; and that many of the current debates in medicine reflect the wider social debates about the role of the state and the responsibility of the individual.

What, then, is the nature of the relationship between the beliefs held by the various groups in society and the specialist knowledge held by the professionals? Can any light be shed on the processes involved that might help the understanding of the nature of the differences between the concepts of lay people and professionals, and might be relevant to advocates of health promotion?

The relationship between lay and professional concepts

Biomedicine is predominant to the extent that its theories and concepts are seen as the only acceptable ways of understanding health and illness; its status in developed countries has even been likened to that of the established church of the medieval period (24). It is obviously a crucial influence on the system of health beliefs and practices of most of the population — the lay health system. The lay system and the professional system are not identical, however, nor is it helpful to view the lay system merely as a watered-down version of the professional system replete with all the errors arising from misunderstanding and ignorance. Chrisman (45) has suggested that one way of conceptualizing the relationship, without totally adopting

195

a biomedical standard of health beliefs, is to relate sets of beliefs and practices about health to their reference group or reference worlds. Thus many of the terms for and ideas about treatment and cause held by lay people are drawn from the biomedical professional system, but they are reinterpreted and integrated into the belief system of lay people in the context of everyday life.

Thus there is a common-sense understanding of body process and structure — the "plumbing" model or body as machine. Helman *(36)* has commented that many of these contemporary concepts of structure and function seem to be borrowed from the worlds of science and technology. For example, the constant demand for cough medicines (now clinically shown to be mostly ineffective) has been linked to the perception of the need to "flush out" the offending germ or "lubricate the tubes"; the machine metaphor includes the ideas of sources of fuel needed to provide energy for the smooth working of the body and the replacement of individual parts that may break down.

Sets of ideas about causes are also closely associated with patterns of everyday life. Chrisman *(45)* has described, for example, four categories of logic that are related to everyday behaviour and to world view:

> *Invasion*, such as the germ theory, cancer or object intrusions; *degeneration*, such as becoming run down or the accumulation of toxic substances; *mechanical*, such as blockage of digestive channels and improper placement of body structures; and *balance*, such as the maintenance of harmony in the universe or dietary requirements.

Clinicians are becoming increasingly aware that many of the communication problems they experience in managing and treating illness stem from conceptual misunderstandings between them and their patients. The same term may be interpreted very differently and hold very different associations for each party. Thus people diagnosed as hypertensive may believe that their condition is caused by acute life stress, whereas doctors usually emphasize genetic predisposition and physiological abnormalities *(46)*.

There is a growing acceptance of the value of a more systematic approach to eliciting patient beliefs in the clinical setting in order to achieve greater compliance and better outcome *(47–49)*. In contrast, most clinicians still approach preventive behaviour and health maintenance in a rather simplistic way, relying mainly on exhortation and advice, and rarely attempting to ascertain what the patient's priorities or ideas might be. Recent studies in England and Sweden show that

196

the opportunities for traditional health education or advice, linked to the problem presented in the consultation, are often not fully exploited *(50,51)*.

In keeping with the argument advanced so far, one might expect that the messages about health behaviour and health maintenance being put out by health professionals are very influential but are reinterpreted and reintegrated by the public to fit into the context of everyday life. The systematic variations in beliefs about health observed between different groups of people (particularly the variation by socioeconomic status) that was noted earlier could be the result of the very different contexts in which individuals can interpret and integrate into their daily life the biomedical messages to which they are exposed.

Applying this argument to the United States, Chrisman *(45)* points out that some ethnic groups and families of lower socioeconomic status tend to interact almost exclusively with relatives, who are also likely to be their workmates, neighbours and fellow worshippers, in a network of very close relationships. Upper- and middle-class individuals usually have a much more open and loosely knit network of relationships and hence are likely to be exposed to a greater variety of views. As they are better educated, they are also more likely to accept the premises of the biomedical system and less likely to be exposed to strong opposing views from the people with whom they come into contact. According to this approach, the observed variation in beliefs about health associated with socioeconomic status arises because of the characteristics of the networks of family, friends and acquaintances. For example, whether a network is close or loosely knit and whether it is composed mainly of better educated or less well educated people influences the degree of exposure to the scientific health system and its ideas, the types of belief about health circulating in that group, and how they are reinforced and maintained within that particular group.

Two hypotheses need further testing. The more insular or closed the individual's network is, the greater the likelihood that existing beliefs about health (whatever they are) will be maintained, because of the pressure to conform to group norms, and the greater the likelihood that the actual content of the beliefs will differ from the current biomedical view.

The above account does not do justice to the detail and sophistication of Chrisman's exposition and the wealth of illustrations he uses, and the reader is encouraged to refer to the original *(45)*. The point is that this approach begins to provide a theoretical framework in which to examine such issues as the persistence of health beliefs and the factors associated with change. It directs attention to the importance of group characteristics in the process by which beliefs and practices related to health are communicated to individuals. The potential of networks to provide social support and thus influence the health of their members has been recognized for some time; perhaps one should focus on their role in the dissemination of attitudes and knowledge.

Health Beliefs of Lay People as a Guide to Behaviour

Despite considerable empirical evidence to the contrary, researchers (and others) still tend to assume that what people say is a good indicator of their future behaviour. The implicit assumptions of those who advocate studying the health concepts of lay people are that statements are useful indicators of behaviour, and that consistency between statements and behaviour is the norm. Much of the early interest displayed by health educators in the health concepts of lay people stemmed from these assumptions, as well as from recognition of the fact that beliefs and attitudes are capable of being modified in a way that demographic characteristics associated with behaviour are not.

As noted earlier, researchers of health behaviour adopted the professionals' views about what constituted appropriate health behaviour; social psychologists were particularly active in applying the concepts of their discipline to the area of decision-making in various types of health-related behaviour. One theoretical framework, the health belief model, has been widely used. In this model, beliefs about health refer to individuals' perceptions of the severity of an illness, of their susceptibility to it, and of the costs and benefits of following a particular course of action, such as immunization.

Criticism by people working in the areas of preventive behaviour and health promotion has increasingly centred on the fact that the amount of variance explained by the health belief variables in this model is quite small and their predictive power is generally low *(52,53)*.

A more radical challenge is posed by those who claim that not only do beliefs about health not materially aid prediction, but that the

198

observed relationships between beliefs and behaviour are simply a function of the study method commonly used. In these studies, the data on beliefs and behaviour are usually collected at the same time. The respondent may simply bring attitudes into line with self-reported behaviour in a *post hoc* rationalization. It has also been suggested that, even where data were collected first on beliefs and later on behaviour, the behaviour studied has been ongoing or is sufficiently similar to other ongoing behaviour to support the proposition that past behaviour best predicts future behaviour.

Such critiques call into question the direction of the relationship between beliefs (as recorded in verbal statements) and behaviour. Instead of assuming that belief precedes, predicts or in some way causes the behaviour, it is possible that beliefs are simply *post hoc* rationalizations of behaviour or that there is a two-way interactive relationship over time. The question of the exact nature of the relationship between health-related beliefs and behaviour must await longitudinal and panel studies on the same sample of respondents. At present there is little information on the stability of concepts of health over time, nor is it understood what factors influence them.

Other models have had more success in predicting behaviour *(28)*. Fishbein's theory of reasoned action focuses on future intentions and the PRECEDE model includes a wider range of variables. In a recent review of the correlates of health behaviour, however, Norman *(31)* concluded that beliefs about health attitudes had an often inconsistent and usually weak relationship to behaviour. Such beliefs were often no more or even less important than other non-health-related beliefs in predicting action.

Current research suggests little support for any assumption that, if people are well informed about the consequences for health of particular forms of behaviour, they will develop the appropriate attitudes and act in a way calculated to promote their health. There is still less evidence that people's statements of belief, intention or attitude are strongly associated with such behaviour and can be used to predict it *(3)*.

People should not really be particularly surprised by this, since it parallels personal experience, aptly summed up by the saying, "the spirit is willing but the flesh is weak". There are a number of implications for the advocates of health promotion. First, they need to recognize that behaviour is complex, and it is unreasonable to expect any single variable or set of variables (such as beliefs about health as defined in the health belief model) to explain more than a small part of the differences observed between people. If researchers are particularly interested in understanding behaviour or the promotion of behavioural change, they must pay much more attention to situational factors that may constrain action. For example, an individual's actions often appear to be just as highly related to the behaviour of family or friends as to that individual's own attitudes *(2,54)*. The total context in which the behaviour takes place certainly needs more consideration.

Second, advocates of health promotion may need to accept that people have a right not to act in the way both they and the health promoters agree is most conducive to health. Health is not necessarily the top priority for some people *(55)*; enjoyment and gratification can be equally important goals, and some may indulge in risky behaviour, well aware of the possible consequences. Provided that health promoters are convinced that such people are fully informed when they make their choice, a decision not to act in the approved way must be accepted. Third, as noted earlier, there is a strong case for exploring what people actually do to keep themselves healthy and how to reinforce positive health behaviour. Finally, in-depth qualitative interviews can also explore the lay person's perspective much more effectively than survey techniques and, by examining attempts to reconcile conflicting goals, this approach can provide useful insights into such apparently irrational behaviour as smoking during pregnancy *(56)*.

Health beliefs of lay people as behaviour
The preceding section intended to challenge the assumptions that people's accounts of what they believe and what they should do bear a close relationship to actual behaviour, whether self-reported or observed, and also have a useful predictive function. The reader may then wonder about the value of studying what people say about health. Making statements about health is just as much an action as smoking or drinking. Like all behaviour, making verbal statements does not take place in a vacuum but in specific social contexts. Making a statement necessarily involves other people; moreover, in normal social life, people do not make statements just to inform each other of the notions they hold, but also as part of their purposive behaviour. Thus, as Holy & Stuchlik *(57)* point out, "any given verbal statement has to be considered from two different viewpoints: from the viewpoint of its contents and from the viewpoint of the reasons the speaker had for making it".

The value of this approach for those concerned with health promotion is that, instead of assuming that what people say can be taken as broadly equivalent to what people do, attention is focused on the ideas, norms and bits of knowledge that are invoked in different contexts and in connection with different actions. Those who study how knowledge is used in particular situations have usually drawn their data from direct observation of professional–patient encounters and/or patients' accounts of such encounters. Not only may knowledge be organized and presented in a particular way to achieve a particular goal during the consultation, but the patient's knowledge may be modified through interaction with health professionals (58). Concentrating on a single disease category or a particular setting, researchers have focused on the way that concepts change over time as the sufferer obtains new knowledge through interaction (59) and the way this changing model of the illness, in turn, affects behaviour and self-image (60). Although these examples are drawn from studies of beliefs about illness, it is probable that similar processes go on at health counselling sessions with professionals and in everyday situations involving friends and relatives. The practical importance of these insights for health promoters is that professionals engaging in counselling and promoting health need to be aware of the range of beliefs and ideas current in their community and the background associations of many of the concepts so that they can more effectively negotiate with their patients.

Making statements about health is a special form of behaviour and, like other kinds of behaviour, needs to be understood as the product of the total context in which it occurs. Thus, even a simple denial or declaration of knowledge may be an effort to create a specific impression of oneself. The above proposition also poses certain problems for the researcher, which shall be examined in the next section.

Studying Lay People's Beliefs about Health: Some Methodological Considerations

The context of the research interview

It is a truism that one can only learn what people know and feel about health by listening to what they say. In fact, most of the available data has been collected during interviews, rather than by direct observation during naturally occurring situations where health is the focus of conversation. One must therefore consider how the special context of the research interview might affect the nature of the data collected. After all, it is an unusual situation for most people, and it seems reasonable that the interaction with the interviewer will be governed by the same rules for social interaction with strangers that apply elsewhere in society.

Thus, in answering questions, people may reproduce what they feel is likely to be acceptable, noncontroversial and in accordance with their notions of approved medical points of view. For example, Cornwell reported that the ideas put forward by her sample varied over time as her relationship with her subjects changed. At first, they gave her what she described as "public accounts", reproducing the common social assumptions they felt were appropriate. Later on, different ideas were introduced, usually when they were asked to tell a story rather than respond to a direct question (19).

Cosminski (61) found that standardized questionnaires on illness administered in a structured interview situation produced answers focusing on immediate, single causes and empirical pragmatic treatment, whereas case studies of the same informants, using their own medical histories as a starting point, elicited more complex theories of etiology and treatment. Similarly, Blaxter (62) carried out in-depth interviews with a sample of grandmothers in Aberdeen, United Kingdom, and commented that the most notable features of the discussion were the salience of knowing about cause, the strain towards rational explanation and the importance of linking together life events.

These findings suggest that structured questions asked by a stranger are likely to produce a more stereotyped response, while if the relationship between interviewer and respondents extends over time or the respondents are encouraged to tell their own story, more complex data will emerge. The in-depth interview, in particular, often gives subjects the opportunity to reflect on issues important to them, and they may use the interview situation as an opportunity to construct a meaningful account of their experiences and seek to present themselves as morally responsible people.

The exact content of beliefs about health elicited during a research interview will vary according to the subject's interpretation of the situation, the mode of questioning employed and whether the frame of reference is general or personal. Moreover, the same individual, if observed and recorded by an anthropologist in another setting (such as a consultation with a health professional or spontaneous discussion with friends), might well produce different ideas and notions during that encounter. How are such apparent inconsistencies and contradictions to be interpreted? Are data obtained in one way or in a particular context better or more true than other data? Such questions become meaningless once one realizes that every oral statement is made for a particular purpose and has to be taken in context — the aim may be to avoid controversy with a stranger, to demonstrate to a friend that one is competent and responsible, to persuade the professional to provide a special mode of treatment, and so on.

Research interviews can provide data on respondents' general theories of health and illness — the way they think things are (which may overlap with the way they think things should be). Such data can provide an overview of the repertoire of notions, beliefs and attitudes currently in use and deemed appropriate to reproduce in a social situation. (Direct observation, of course, will show the parts of this repertoire that are invoked in particular everyday situations to achieve specific ends.)

Studies of beliefs about health and the analysis of their underlying logic, the extent to which they form a coherent system, the way they are socially distributed and this relationship with other areas of social life are often initially valuable to those concerned with health promotion because of the understanding they provide of the background knowledge and assumptions held by different groups in society. People draw on knowledge and assumptions as resources in coping with illness or seeking to maintain health, but knowledge and assumptions do not necessarily determine what is done.

Differing methodological traditions

Structured questions and in-depth interviews are two methods of obtaining data that tend to reflect a more basic dichotomy in social science between those who believe that research should take as its model the practices of the natural sciences, and those who believe that very different techniques are needed to study the social world. The former (the positivists) regard what people say about health and illness as facts to be collected in order to test a particular theory. Such an approach makes certain assumptions about the stability of attitudes and beliefs over time and ignores the possible effect of the context in which the data are being collected. The aim is to eliminate any possible bias by developing explicit, standardized sets

203

of interview procedures or scales that will aid quantification and enable comparison. For example, the questions are likely to be directed to a specific area the researcher has decided is relevant and important, and a range of responses are suggested to the respondent. (This especially applies, of course, to self-administered questionnaires.) Such an approach assumes that everyone will interpret the question in the same way and ignores the possibility that the preoccupations of the researcher may not be very salient to the respondent: on both grounds the assessment of the notions actually held risks being seriously distorted.

In sharp contrast is the work in the qualitative tradition, carried out by some social anthropologists and sociologists who stress the importance of understanding the individual's own perspective and are anxious to avoid imposing their own ideas and preconceptions. Their in-depth, ethnographic techniques allow the subjects much greater freedom to talk about what is salient for them. Open questions do not assume the type of answer that will be given; probing and cross-checking can ensure clarification of the concepts and terms used. Instead of regarding the interviewer as a possible source of bias to be controlled by standardizing the schedule, the qualitative researchers capitalize on the rapport they develop with their subjects to obtain the richest possible data. Context is important for researchers in this tradition and, typically, they are less ready to assume that beliefs are stable properties of individuals who seem free of social networks and cultural processes.

Discussion

So far I have examined some of the underlying assumptions held by those who have studied beliefs about health, and have emphasized the need for health promoters to be aware of the implications of such notions and their intimate links with the study method chosen. It has been argued that lay and professional beliefs are equally products of their own cultures and therefore reflect key preoccupations of the society at that particular time and place. Further, although the concepts of professionals are very influential and provide an important reference point for lay people, they reinterpret these concepts in the context of everyday life. Finally, systematic variation in the distribution and pattern of concepts can be understood in terms of the social position held by individuals, since the relationships they have will influence how much they are exposed to new biomedical ideas, and how great the informal pressure is to conform.

I have also challenged the proposition that individual beliefs are stable properties that do not change with time and context and that, once described, they are good indicators of subsequent action. Instead I put forward the view that oral statements of knowledge, belief and attitudes are in themselves actions that occur in a given context. The research interview is a special case of such interaction. The relationship of statements to self-reports and direct observations of other behaviour is problematic. The type of questioning used might materially influence the content of the statements and produce apparent inconsistencies.

This is not intended to dissuade people from undertaking research into beliefs about health or to imply that there is one correct way to investigate this area; rather, the intention is to warn them about possible traps for the unwary.

Finally, after the data have been obtained on the perspectives of lay people in a particular community, how this information is used remains an open question. I distinguished at the beginning between advocates of health promotion working at the level of countries, regions or communities, and health professionals concerned more with the health of individual clients, their families and the immediate community. For the former, large-scale surveys might seem to offer most because they can potentially provide an overview of the variety, combination and demographic distribution of the concepts held in a particular community or society. There are three main ways in which such data might be used.

It has been argued that, without understanding the dimensions and boundaries of popular conceptions, advocates of health promotion cannot gauge the potential support for policies; nor can they judge from where that support is likely to emanate, the likely participation in health promotion activities or the potential of various kinds of social interaction.[a] The emphasis is, therefore, on intervention and change: using the data to pinpoint the groups that might be most receptive to the views of the advocates and thus prepared to collaborate in formulating policy and bringing pressure to bear on other government and environmental agencies.

---

[a] *Vienna dialogue on health policy and health promotion towards a new conception of public health*: report on a WHO meeting, Copenhagen, WHO Regional Office for Europe, 1987 (unpublished document ICP/HSR 623).

Health promoters may also wish to raise the consciousness of the groups that are least in tune with current WHO policy, and target these groups for educational initiatives to make them more aware of the way that powerful social and economic forces encourage health-denying lifestyles. It could be argued that such consciousness-raising is necessary before any effective collaboration, involving all sectors of the community, can take place.

A third possibility is that advocates of health promotion may wish to use evidence of changes in health-related beliefs and behaviour over time to indicate the success of specific interventions in the community or society, whether these have been implemented as the result of collaboration or imposed from above.

Whatever approach is taken, the problem of how to implement the aims of collaboration with all sections of the community to co-produce health remains a very real one. Sensitivity to the perspective of lay people is a necessary but not a sufficient condition for success.

Awareness of the theories held by various groups in the community is also necessary for health professionals interacting with clients on a daily basis. Such data (derived from surveys) give the professionals background information on the knowledge and beliefs that may be invoked during interaction and will certainly influence the whole encounter. Studies using qualitative methods hold out greater promise for understanding the processes by which people come to accept or reject ideas emanating from the medical establishment, and hence for understanding the factors underlying change. This may encourage more sensitive intervention. Moreover, qualitative in-depth studies have revealed considerable individual variation within groups homogeneous in age, social class, and occupational and educational background. Such apparently contradictory findings carry considerable implications for people working in clinical settings.

The danger is that health professionals will use survey research findings to create oversimplified stereotypes and then use those stereotypes as a basis for interaction (63). In other words, they could apply generalizations about groups inappropriately in a one-to-one clinical situation. Survey methods and in-depth studies can provide insights into the range of beliefs and attitudes current in a community, but to achieve effective health promotion in primary care, professionals need to be able to elicit the beliefs and attitudes of each particular client (64) in order to negotiate properly. Negotiation, a

206

concept that implies a more equal relationship between professional and client, is the key to patient-centred care, where the clients or patients are more involved in decisions affecting their health care. Primary health care professionals need to be simultaneously aware of the broad trends and the considerable complexity and apparent inconsistency of individuals, and use both types of research findings to promote health during interaction with their clients.

References

1. A discussion document on the concepts and principles of health promotion. *Health promotion*, **1** (1): 73–76 (1986).
2. *The active health report — perspectives on Canada's health promotion survey 1975*. Ottawa, Department of National Health and Welfare, 1987.
3. *The health and lifestyle survey*: preliminary report of a nationwide survey of the physical and mental health, attitudes, and lifestyle of a random sample of 9003 British adults. Cambridge, Health Promotion Research Trust, 1987.
4. **Schoenborn, C.A. & Danchik, K.M**. *Health practices among adults: United States 1977*. Washington, DC, US Department of Health and Human Services, 1980 (Advance Data, No. 64).
5. **Gohlieb, N.H. & Green, L.W**. Life events, social network, lifestyle and health: an analysis of the 1979 national survey of personal health practices and consequences. *Health education quarterly*, **11**(1): 91–105 (1984).
6. **Herzlich, C**. *Health and illness*. London, Academic Press, 1973.
7. **Pierret, J**. Les significations sociales de la santé: Paris, l'Essone, l'Herault. *In*: Auge, M. & Herzlich, C., ed. *Le sens du mal: anthropologie, histoire, sociologie de la maladie*. Paris, Editions des Archives contemporaines, 1984, pp. 217–246.
8. **d'Houtaud, A. & Field, M**. The image of health: variations in perception by social class in a French population. *Sociology of health and illness*, **6**(1): 30–60 (1984).
9. **d'Houtaud, A. & Field, M**. New research on the image of health. *In*: Currer, C. & Stacey, M., ed. *Concepts of health, illness and disease*. Leamington Spa, Berg, 1986, pp. 223–256.
10. **Blaxter, M. & Paterson, L**. *Mothers and daughters: a three-generation study of health attitudes and behaviour*. London, Heinemann, 1982.

11. **Williams, R.G.A**. Logic analysis as qualitative method. *Sociology of health and illness*, **3**(2): 141–187 (1981).

12. **Williams, R.G.A**. Concepts of health: an analysis of lay logic. *Sociology*, **17**(2): 185–205 (1983).

13. **Pill, R. & Stott, N.C.H**. Concepts of illness causation and responsibility: some preliminary data from a sample of working class mothers. *Social science and medicine*, **16**: 43–52 (1982).

14. **Pill, R. & Stott, N.C.H**. Choice or chance: further evidence on ideas of illness and responsibility for health. *Social science and medicine*, **20**(10): 981–991 (1985).

15. **Pill, R. & Stott, N.C.H**. Preventive procedures and practices among working class women: new data and fresh insights. *Social science and medicine*, **21**(9): 975–983 (1985).

16. **Pill, R. & Stott, N.C.H**. Development of a measure of potential health behaviour: a salience of lifestyle index. *Social science and medicine*, **24**(2): 125–134 (1987).

17. **Calnan, M. & Johnson, B**. Health, health risks and inequalities: an exploratory study of women's perceptions. *Sociology of health and illness*, **7**(1): 55–5 (1985).

18. **Calnan, M**. Maintaining health and preventing illness: a comparison of the perceptions of women from different social classes. *Health promotion*, **1**(2): 167–177 (1986).

19. **Cornwell, J**. *Hard-earned lives: accounts of health and illness from East London*. London, Tavistock, 1984.

20. **Currer, C**. Concepts of mental well- and ill-being: the case of Pathan mothers in Britain. *In*: Currer, C. & Stacey, M., ed. *Concepts of health, illness and disease*. Leamington Spa, Berg, 1986, pp. 181–198.

21. **Donovan, J**. We don't buy sickness, it just comes. *In*: *Health, illness and health care in the lives of black people in London*. Aldershot, Gower, 1986.

22. **Anderson, R**. *Health promotion: an overview*. Edinburgh, Scottish Health Education Group, 1984, pp. 1–126 (European Monographs in Health Education Research, No. 6),

23. **Calnan, M., ed**. *Health and illness: the lay perspective*. London, Tavistock, 1987.

24. **Stacey, M**. Concepts of health and illness and the division of labour in health care. *In*: Currer, C. & Stacey, M., ed. *Concepts*

of health, illness and disease. Leamington Spa, Berg, 1986, pp. 7–26.

25. **Steel, J.L. & McBroom, W.H.** Conceptual and empirical dimensions of health behaviour. *Journal of health and social behavior*, **13**: 382–392 (1972).

26. **Coburn, D. & Pope, C.R.** Sociodemographic status and preventive health behaviour. *Journal of health and social behavior*, **15**: 67–78 (1974).

27. **Langlie, J.K.** Social networks, health beliefs and preventive health behaviour. *Journal of health and social behavior*, **18**: 244–260 (1977).

28. **Mullen, P.D. et al.** Health behaviour models compared. *Social science and medicine*, **24**(11): 973–981 (1987).

29. **Becker, M.H. et al.** The health belief model and preventive health behaviour. *Health education monographs,* **2**: 324–473 (1974).

30. **Janz, M.K. & Becker, M.H.** The health belief model: a decade later. *Health education quarterly*, **11**: 1–47 (1984).

31. **Norman, R.M.G.** *The nature and correlates of health behaviour.* Ottawa, Health Promotion Directorate, Department of National Health and Welfare, 1986 (Health Promotion Studies Series, No. 2).

32. **Kasl, S.V. & Cobb, S.** Health behaviour, illness behaviour and sick-role behaviour. *Archives of environmental health*, **2**: 245–266 (1966).

33. **Harris, D.M. & Guten, S.** Health-protective behaviour: an exploratory study. *Journal of health and social behavior*, **20**(1): 17–29 (1979).

34. **Pill, R. & Stott, N.C.H.** Looking after themselves: health protective behaviour among British working class women. *Health education research*, **1**(2): 111–119 (1986).

35. **Loudon, J.B., ed.** *Social anthropology and medicine.* London, Academic Press, 1976.

36. **Helman, C.** *Culture, health and illness.* Bristol, Wright, 1984.

37. **Foster, G.M. & Anderson, B.G., ed.** *Medical anthropology.* New York, Wiley, 1978.

38. **Unschild, P.** The conceptual determination of individual and collective experiences of illness. *In*: Currer, C. &

Stacey, M., ed. *Concepts of health, illness and disease*. Leamington Spa, Berg, 1986, pp. 51–70.

39. **Crawford, R**. A cultural account of "health": control, release and the social body. *In*: McKinlay, J.B., ed. *Issues in the political economy of health care*. London, Tavistock, 1984.

40. **Freidson, E**. *Profession of medicine*. New York, Harper & Row, 1970.

41. **Armstrong, D**. *Political anatomy of the body: medical knowledge in Britain in the twentieth century*. Cambridge, Cambridge University Press, 1983.

42. **Foucault, M**. *The birth of the clinic: an archaeology of medical perception*. London, Tavistock, 1973.

43. **Gabbay, J**. Asthma attacked? Tactics for the reconstruction of a disease concept. *In*: Wright, P. & Treacher, A., ed. *The problem of medical knowledge: examining the social construction of medicine*. Edinburgh, Edinburgh University Press, 1982.

44. **Crawford, R**. You are dangerous to your health: the ideology and politics of victim blaming. *International journal of health services*, **7**: 663–680 (1977).

45. **Chrisman, N.J**. The health seeking process: an approach to the natural history of illness. *Culture, medicine and psychiatry*, **1**(4): 351–378 (1977).

46. **Blumhagen, D.W**. Hypertension: a folk illness with a medical name. *Culture, medicine and psychiatry*, **4**(3): 192–227 (1980).

47. **Katon, W. & Kleinman, A**. Doctor–patient negotiation and other social science strategies in patient care. *In*: Eisenberg, E. & Kleinman, A., ed. *The relevance of social science for medicine*. London, D. Reidel, 1981.

48. **Pendleton, D. & Hasler, J**. *Doctor–patient communication*. London, Academic Press, 1983.

49. **Pendleton, D. et al**. *The consultation: an approach to learning and teaching*. Oxford, Oxford University Press, 1984.

50. **Tuckett, D. et al**. *Meetings between experts: an approach to sharing ideas in medical consultations*. London, Tavistock, 1985.

51. **Larsson, U.S. et al**. Patient–doctor communication on smoking and drinking: lifestyle in medical consultations. *Social science and medicine*, **25**(10): 1129–1137 (1987).

52. **Calnan, M**. The health belief model and participation in programmes for the early detection of breast cancer: a

comparative analysis. *Social science and medicine*, **19**(9): 823–831 (1984).

53. **Dean, K**. *Influence of health beliefs on lifestyles: what do we know? In*: Edinburgh, Scottish Health Education Group, 1984, pp. 127–149 (European Monographs in Health Education Research, No. 6).

54. **Gatherer, A. et al**. *Is health education effective?* London, Health Education Council, 1979.

55. **Calnan, M**. Lay conceptions of health. *In*: Calnan, M., ed. *Health and illness: the lay perspective*. London, Tavistock, 1987, pp. 117–140.

56. **Graham, H**. Smoking in pregnancy: the attitudes of expectant mothers. *Social science and medicine*, **10**: 399–405 (1976).

57. **Holy, L. & Stuchlik**, M. *Actions, norms and representations*. Cambridge, Cambridge University Press, 1983.

58. **Young, A**. When rational men fall sick: an inquiry into assumptions made by medical anthropologists. *Culture, medicine and psychiatry*, **5**(4): 317–335 (1981).

59. **Posner, T. & Vessey, M**. *The consequences of an abnormal cervical smear: women's experiences*: report for the Cancer Research Campaign. Oxford, Department of Community Medicine, 1985.

60. **Williams, G**. The genesis of chronic illness: narrative reconstruction. *Sociology of health and illness*, **6**(2): 175–200 (1984).

61. **Cosminski, S**. The impact of methods on the analysis of illness concepts in a Guatemalan community. *Social science and medicine*, **11**: 325–332 (1977).

62. **Blaxter, M**. The causes of disease: women talking. *Social science and medicine*, **17**(2): 56–69 (1983).

63. **Pill, R. & Stott, N.C.H**. The stereotype of "working-class fatalism" and the challenge for primary care health promotion. *Health education research*, **2**(2): 105–114, (1987).

64. **Stott, N.C.H. & Pill, R**. Health promotion and the human response to loss — the clinical implications of a decade of primary health care research. *Family practice*, **4**(2): 278–286 (1987).

Part III

Families, workplaces and hospitals as settings for health promotion

9

The role of the family in creating and maintaining healthy lifestyles

Geneviève Cresson & Agnès Pitrou

Although all societies, since time immemorial, have used specialists such as healers and witch doctors to avert sickness and disease, the responsibility for health and for the practices that safeguard it has always been assigned to the family and, more specifically, to women.

Even today, despite the virtually automatic recourse to specialists whose ever-increasing diversity and technical skill often elicit unquestioning faith, the family continues to act as a link with these specialists and to promote or impair the physical and mental development and wellbeing of family members. Habits of cleanliness, hygiene and nutrition are forged in the home. Individuals learn to relate to their bodies and the daily and annual rhythms of life are inculcated; knowledge of the many forms of self-medication is acquired in the home, and relationships with specialists are developed that involve both trust and tolerance of a certain degree of control.

This process of inculcation within the family, which is stronger than is often suggested, nevertheless conflicts with other often contradictory influences in other areas of life.

The Autonomy of the Family in Developing its Own Lifestyle

The first issue is the ability of the family to choose its own lifestyle and to resist pressure to adopt patterns of behaviour likely to injure health. This ability is linked with the structure of the family unit and with the constraints and normative influences to which it is subject within its environment.

Family structure and family practices

The current evolution of family units modifies the strength and continuity of their normative capacity in health matters. Relationships between couples are becoming increasingly unstable,[a] which threatens to undermine the continuity of the practices agreed between them, particularly for children whose family environment changes when the parents divorce or separate. Although both parents continue to play an important role in ensuring continuity, the changes experienced by the family increase the need for support from other members of the family; however, this sometimes involves practices and norms developed by previous generations, which have not always kept pace with modern knowledge about health, hygiene and child care. Moreover, the authoritarian power of one spouse over the other and of parents over children has been severely weakened in favour of more open discussion and more autonomy for individual family members; each individual leads a more independent life, even at the level of meals, recreation and leisure activities. This may result in behavioural pluralism, respected or at least tolerated by each family member; the individual is considered, rightly or wrongly, to be the only person affected by personal matters. This may, in turn, expose the family to external influences transmitted by each family member from the daily environment.

Further, in health and other areas of life, adults are often uncertain about the principles, values and patterns of behaviour that should be transmitted. They find it difficult to see why they should make their children (or spouse) give up a particular habit or adopt a different one, when they themselves are unsure of their own responsibilities and torn between conflicting lifestyles and advice.

Nevertheless, these structural and relational changes within the family unit have not reduced the mutual concern shared by individual family members. Public opinion polls show that health is still the most cherished asset, and the prerequisite for all others. It is therefore

---

[a] This instability should not be exaggerated, however, compared with that of certain sections of society in the past: working-class families that developed out of the migration from the countryside or that experienced the hardships of the early stages of industrialization, or families broken up by premature deaths and widowhood *(1)*.

214

the primary concern of partners for each other[a] and particularly of parents for their children. The fall in the number of children per family to between one and two in developed countries enables parents to supervise closely and overprotect their children; every effort is made, even before birth, to detect all deficiencies and abnormalities and to eliminate them. Moreover, some parents are very reluctant to entrust their children to other educators (for example, in nurseries or summer camps) for fear that the children will not be properly looked after — which often means being less pampered than in the family cocoon.

Constraints on the family

The freedom of each family to choose its own lifestyle is more illusion than reality. Although we do not wish to be narrowly deterministic, free choice is often exercised through a series of conditioning processes that restrict choice, especially for people with few financial and cultural resources and little power within society.

The major structuring elements that shape families' lives are very often conceived and organized so that they conflict with the requirements of maintaining each person's mental and physical health and with the practices that are likely to develop this biological capital. Work is necessary not only to live but also to become integrated into society and contribute to it (this applies to both men and women). What, then is the effect of work schedules that are designed to keep machines rolling and services being delivered, with no consideration for the rhythm of family life or for biological requirements (2)? What stress is caused by poor working conditions (including noise, the handling of contaminating materials, indoor air pollution and excessively rapid and repetitive work rates) or a poor environment? What of the required geographic mobility that is so disruptive to the family? Even worse, a lifestyle cannot encourage individual development when one partner is deprived of a job by unemployment, or reduced to taking an insecure, intermittent job that pays badly because it is only part-time.

Second, the family environment influences the acquisition of healthy habits, the opportunities for peace, quiet and rest, and the facilities for living healthily and preparing food in good conditions.

---

[a] This concern does not, of course, exclude aberrant patterns of behaviour harmful to health or to life itself, such as alcohol abuse, smoking, overexertion during leisure activities, or careless driving.

The housing accessible to families does not always meet these requirements. Except for a very destitute minority (which has increased in size recently) and for certain immigrants, slums (in the traditional sense of the term) have been virtually eliminated in cities in developed countries. But the size, location, layout and facilities of the housing built recently in large towns and suburbs do not promote a healthy and well balanced daily lifestyle.

The same could be said of the environment; the natural environment as well as the goods and services available have been polluted and damaged. Consumer choice is often limited to the packaging of products rather than including any health criteria, and even people who try to consume only natural products have difficulty finding unadulterated products, even among "health foods".

It is very important for the family to be able to choose how to organize its own time, as the family can then establish a calm atmosphere in which individual rhythms can be respected. Yet this is unattainable because of the restrictions imposed by school and working hours and the organization of leisure and entertainment activities, which tend to impose constant pressure and to lead to hyperactivity. Children's schedules outside school hours, are divided into lessons, group participation in sporting and cultural activities, and the watching of addictive television programmes. This clearly illustrates the contradictions inherent in attempting to develop a balanced pace of life while confronted with attractions that are totally incompatible with this need.

The facilities offered by the system of medical and paramedical care are fundamental to maintaining and restoring health within families. Regardless of the type of health system, informed choice of medical practitioners and the place at which medical care is provided is an illusion, particularly for less well informed parents. Families depend on medical authority for cure or advice (particularly for children). This dependence is virtually absolute — even if the widespread availability of health care resulting from the social progress achieved in various countries is a major step forward. Families still have few opportunities to participate in changing the way this care is organized and dispensed, or even in choosing the type of medicine they use.

Contradictory influences?
The health of individuals is influenced by practices and patterns of behaviour that are largely outside their control. The state makes

demands to ensure that the national "health capital" develops satisfactorily. Expectant mothers are required to undergo repeated examinations; there are compulsory vaccination programmes; alcohol is forbidden for young people, and the public is advised to use less tobacco (which is completely inconsistent with cigarette advertising). Different social milieus transmit norms that are not always consistent with those desired by families: the food served in schools or workplaces, advice given on hygiene, and the physical activities offered or imposed (and often badly managed). At certain stages in the life cycle, individuals find themselves in collective accommodation (in holiday camps, hospitals, maternity units or barracks) where the hygiene and living conditions are not necessarily inspiring and do not allow for any debate or exchange of views for everyone's benefit. The advertising industry constantly bombards people with images that encourage some clearly harmful or dangerous consumption and practices. The impact of advertising on children in particular has been well established. Moreover, this influence is exerted in the home, where family life unfolds. Television programmes that depict heroes and lifestyles that contradict some of the principles maintained elsewhere by the family and by society also have an insidious influence.

It is Utopian to think that the family exerts its influence outside this social context, which also includes the social relationships that exert peer group pressure. In some families that are more susceptible to new developments, successive contradictory fads are adopted: diets, physical and sporting activities, naturism and patterns of baby care.[a]

All these outside influences, particularly the instructions issued by institutions, are based on a dual assumption that families are not able to define what is good for their health and must therefore be guided and checked and, further, that families are not capable of assuming real autonomy in health care or of judiciously using the appropriate techniques. At most, they may be delegated certain tasks, such as checking and carrying out instructions (3).

Of course, this suspicion may only strengthen the conviction of families that it is too difficult to take responsibility for one's own

---

[a] These successive fads are not entirely unconnected with the whims of certain paediatricians and doctors, who are also subject to succeeding and sometimes contradictory doctrines that are always characterized by a certain degree of dogmatism based on arguments presented as scientific.

physical and mental wellbeing. This conviction may be further strengthened by the fact that experts of all kinds do not seem able to agree and send contradictory messages.

Coping with contradiction

These inconsistencies may actually define the margin of freedom within which individuals and families can exercise a certain degree of autonomy. It should be positive that a variety of behaviour patterns is presented and proposed, on the condition, of course, that the recipients of these messages are able to make rational choices and put forward their own viewpoint. Families that depend on the social security system are extremely vulnerable, clearly showing the limits of the capacity for making real choices.

Families have access to very different resources to deal with the various models that are put forward or with norms that are virtually imposed. It is therefore a misuse of language to speak of a family lifestyle common to all families. People who are highly educated, speak the same language as medical specialists and have a social status that eases their relationship with medical technicians or people in charge of hospital departments have the tools and the resources to filter the information that bombards them from all directions. People who have the money to choose what is best from the goods and services that contribute to maintaining health can obviously recover a certain degree of autonomy in managing the family's health, even though these factors retain significant influence and the medical profession continues to try to impose its judgement. But people who have no money and, in particular, people whose cultural traditions conflict with the demands of hygiene and health, obviously become heavily dependent not only on the institutions that exert social and medical control but also on influences and statements expressed in specialized language.

Some families know how to operate within these constraints and influences to achieve the objectives that correspond to their ideological aims or priorities, while others are only capable of living from hand to mouth.

Moreover, even the best informed families may disagree, particularly the parents, about the best lifestyles to adopt, the principles to be observed and the daily practices to be implemented. It is then no longer possible to cope consistently with these internal contradiction.

Nevertheless, because of the influence that the family exerts on a continuous, daily basis, it is impossible to deny that the family plays a synthesizing role or to ignore the fact that, because the most basic health and hygiene practices are usually implemented in the family, it represents an irreplaceable link in health education, which may be positive or negative for any particular family.

The family provides more emotional support than anyone else, except for the support provided at certain well defined stages, such as adolescence, when the family's role is taken over by friends and partners. Nevertheless, people initially turn to the family when they experience a temporary or permanent problem that affects their physical (and, to some extent, mental) wellbeing.

Women are at the centre of the family structure, whose role it is to ensure this continuity and consideration for the development of each family member. Women are still largely responsible (although this varies according to social class and age) for teaching and supervising daily health and hygiene practices: sustenance, treatment and care of children and sick people. Women also suffer more than men from the contradictory instructions received from outside institutions and the conflicts between contradictory constraints or aspirations. It is absurd to continue to single women out as solely or mainly responsible for the family's wellbeing, and thus to blame them in the event of trouble in the family (illness, accident, children's physical or psychological problems), since women do not usually have the power to choose the patterns of behaviour of those around them (husband, children, grandparents). This is obvious for smoking, drug use, road accidents and alcohol abuse.

If people's awareness of behaviour patterns in daily life that are likely to affect health has to be increased, such information should be addressed to each person who is considered autonomous, regardless of age or sex. It will then be more clearly understood that not only should the family be encouraged to develop a healthy lifestyle, but the entire mechanism of social relationships with its contradictions and effects on the health of individuals should be examined. Individuals should also be encouraged to confront their behaviour patterns and the assumptions on which they are based, particularly within the family in which most of the practical arrangements for daily life are implemented. The more open, less authoritarian exchanges currently developing between parents and children should have a positive influence; nevertheless, the family still requires the basic principles and resources to conduct this exercise.

Creating a Healthy Lifestyle: What Does it Mean?

This section centres on three main questions. Is there, and can there be, any consensus on what a healthy lifestyle is, and how to evaluate this? Is health the only (or the main) objective pursued by families, and if it is not, how can it be reconciled with other family objectives? One dimension is often ignored in discussion about lifestyle: health education carried out at home by family members. Can the relationships between lifestyle and health be clarified by referring to the health education carried out in the family?

The difficulties of evaluating a healthy lifestyle
The very concepts of what is healthy and what is good for health, vary according to historical period, social class and the particular specialties of professionals.

The age is now past when dirt was thought to protect the health of children (and adults) and people were very suspicious of using water for personal hygiene. Recently, the virtues of breastfeeding, feeding on demand or at fixed times, and supposed "wonder" drugs have fluctuated with changing fashions. Childcare is subject to the rapid expansion of knowledge and constantly changing attitudes (3–5). As children are the principal focus of medical attention to the family, this attention will tend to be provisional and characterized by fads and change. There is no reason to condemn this, except when those responsible for the health services, as is too often the case, attempt to conceal the provisional nature of the medical process by supposedly authoritative assertions that merely reflect the cult of progress.

Differences in concept and practice
There is no commonly accepted concept of what is healthy, of what constitutes illness or of the action that should be taken in the event of pain or illness (6). One of the keys to explaining these divergences lies in the differing relationships between individuals and their bodies depending on social situation, occupation, age and sex. The entire socialization process influences these different relationships to the body and different concepts of health and sickness. It would not,

therefore, be realistic to attempt to influence these concepts without at the same time accepting the need for change in the social and occupational situation of these individuals.

In any case, nonspecialists are being increasingly deprived of the fundamental power of defining what sickness is, and what is and is not the proper concern of the health care system and the medical profession.

As Freidson (7) points out, the medical profession defines both sickness and treatment and also what is conducive to good health, just as legislative or religious authorities define crime or sin, punishment or penitence. This is an abuse of power. This does not mean, however, that there are no differences of opinion within the medical profession, depending on the institute, country, specialty or generation of the specialists. Parents are aware of this when deciding whether to have their youngest child's tonsils taken out or when choosing an effective treatment for their oldest child's warts. Sometimes, specialists do reach consensus, and the diversity of opinions need not be a problem in itself. After all, it is reassuring to know that it is possible to choose between several different procedures, treatments or even diagnoses. It is not difficult to conceive of a doctor–patient relationship in which doctors would fairly regularly suggest a range of treatments from which the patient could then choose, but this requires breaking the power relationship between the medical profession and society and between doctor and patient (8). From the doctor's point of view, the responsible patient follows medical advice to the letter and voluntarily submits to treatment.

Assessing effectiveness

Any attempt to assess whether a lifestyle encourages good health faces the difficulty of evaluating the techniques and practices implemented. Thus Freidson (7) has analysed the paradoxes of controls within the medical profession. It is very difficult to verify the effectiveness of particular practices and techniques, even if responsibility for such verification remains with the medical profession, because of: the inherent uncertainty of medical practice, the differences of opinion between different schools of thought, developments in knowledge and techniques (and the difficulties encountered by doctors in keeping their training up to date), the complexity and uniqueness of each patient, and the great emphasis on personal judgement and responsibility.

221

Nevertheless, the most remarkable thing is that, despite the reluctance of the medical profession to have its own practices supervised, it is willing to exercise control or to assess the activities of paramedical workers or lay people. Several historians have stressed the role of doctors in socially controlling mothers and families in the disadvantaged social classes. Through children, the family itself is scrutinized, not only by medical or social institutions, but also by the schools, the legal system and social workers *(9)*.

At present, the preventive institutions tend to impose a socially biased model that does not take into account that some people do not share the characteristics that form the basis of the proposed model *(10,11)*. The initial factors at work in prevention, and subsequently in medical care, are not solely related to health but are also socio-political in nature. Mortality rates still vary according to social class (Desplanques *(12)* for France; Townsend & Davidson *(13)* for the United Kingdom) and children's health is likely to be more threatened if their parents are in a lower social class. What conclusions can be drawn from this about families' lifestyles? How can lifestyles help to cause these illnesses and premature deaths? Differences related to class are fundamental and are not a product of areas in which the family is autonomous.

Assessing lifestyles based on results also poses problems at the individual level. Is it sufficient simply to propose that families that produce healthy adults and children are healthy? There is a risk of blaming the family for the development of illnesses it cannot control. A multitude of factors are at work, including genetic diseases, inadequate schools, poor urban or material environments, and the possibility of diagnostic or treatment errors by professionals. Responsibility for the consequences of these factors cannot be attributed to families alone, even if they provide the framework within which these consequences evolve. This allocation of blame is even more tempting when little is known of the causes of a particular illness. It has been particularly easy, for instance, to attach stigma and blame to the mothers of asthmatic or schizophrenic children and, interestingly, they make little effort to reject the blame attributed to them.

Nevertheless, some of the contradictions inherent in imposing norms cannot easily be removed. To do so, everybody would have to benefit as much as possible from the undeniable progress made in science and from medical and biological discoveries and each individual would have to have several alternatives. In particular, two divergent situations would have to be taken into account: medical and social emergencies, ranging from road accidents to battered and abused children, which should receive an appropriate and rapid response from society as a whole, and in particular from the social services, and all other situations, for which the aims of democratization and free choice are largely contradictory.

But when does a situation become an emergency and at what point do unheeded daily practices create that emergency? Any answer must necessarily be a socially dated and located compromise, particularly in defining a healthy lifestyle and the choice of authorities qualified to make such a definition.

Is health in family life a single cogent objective for all?

Maintaining the physical and mental health of family members is not a self-contained goal to be pursued in isolation from other objectives. This can be demonstrated by examining the occasions and means devoted to maintaining family health. Meal times and food have a role that goes far beyond maintaining (or threatening) the health of family members to include education, the transmission of cultural, religious or regional heritages and family knowledge, and the establishment of a forum for intense emotional exchange; economic resources and work schedules significantly influence the preparation and consumption of meals. Similarly, sporting activity is much more than just a means of keeping fit.

Is it reasonable, in the name of a particular concept of child health, to ask parents to stop travelling long distances to visit relatives living in far-flung places? Is it reasonable to advise young North Africans not to observe Ramadan for health reasons, when this practice and its religious, cultural and family connotations are an important factor in determining their personal and relational equilibrium?

Calculated risks

When two objectives conflict, what level of risk to health is acceptable to the family, particularly for the most vulnerable members? The gradual and continuous transmission from adult to child of responsibility for the risks that face the child is part of educating the child. Family life is a surprising mixture of overprotection and inordinate risks (road accidents, for example, and thoughtless behaviour). It is not a question of justifying risk, but education cannot possibly eliminate all dangers.

223

Moreover, family members cannot really control the biggest risks, comprising occupational hazards, traffic accidents, epidemics and accidents at school or at play. Families are once again asked to cope with risks arising outside the family structure (and which, should the opportunity arise, will be blamed on them).

The medical or epidemiological definition of risk fails fully to account for the reality of risk. Medical approaches have only identified as risks the factors for which it seemed immediate medical action was possible *(14)*, or they have emphasized the individual aspects of risk and ignored the collective and social aspects. Using the term risk factors may foster a limited view of the real risks.

Differing needs within the same family
The family is not simply one unit. It comprises a variety of people of different ages and sexes and (sometimes) social conditions whose needs cannot possibly coincide at all times. The same lifestyle or behaviour may not be good for all members of the family. Family life protects men's health, for example, while it tends severely to strain women's health. What is decreed to be good for children's health is not necessarily always good for the health of their mothers. It is good for a baby to have an adult wake up at night to tend to it, feed it and comfort it; is it also good for the mother or father to be dragged from sleep? Professionals and mothers usually implicitly agree that children's health should be given priority over parents'. But the women most involved in caring for their families (or for others, such as nurses) risk compromising their own health *(15)*. Little research has been done in this area, as if there is only room for one patient at a time in the family and as if what is good for one member of the family must necessarily be good for the others. Similar questions could be raised with respect to diet, the consumption of certain foods, educational practices and entertainment, which may be necessary for some people and harmful for others in the same family.

A favourable environment but a heavy work burden
Taking responsibility for the physical and mental health of a family is too often equated with simply providing emotional support, particularly when it involves caring for elderly, infirm or sick people. Nevertheless, obtaining a working knowledge of the principles, knowledge and skills involved in maintaining or restoring health is also correctly emphasized. A further issue that receives less

224

prominence is the recommendation that people should avoid a prolonged stay in hospital by convalescing at home. This recommendation ignores all the work involved in caring for convalescents and in general in establishing and maintaining a healthy lifestyle.

A healthy lifestyle can only be maintained through a multitude of tasks that are relegated to the level of household chores, although they are essential to health and survival. The health of children depends on changing nappies, washing clothes, properly maintaining housing and preparing meals. In addition to these unavoidable material tasks are tasks related to relationships and education. The care given by a good nurse is assumed to include being concerned about the psychological wellbeing of patients and making sure they understand instructions. Equal recognition must be given to such tasks when they are performed by lay people in the home.

A parent who telephones a professional (or decides not to) has already carried out some sort of diagnosis and often has some idea, however incomplete and provisional, of the treatment that is required. Doing these tasks in the home requires time, knowledge and skills that are not really socially recognized for several reasons. First, the expertise applied within the family to ensure or promote the health of family members is not presented as a range of acquired skills but as a set of innate qualities that develop and flourish in a primarily emotional context. As Collière (16) makes clear, however, this is a significant misunderstanding, since the caring functions carried out by family members require the most time and energy.

Second, women have mainly been responsible for caring and health-related tasks. Male family members, whether children, husbands, fathers or others, play a marginal role in these tasks. These functions and all other household and educational tasks are left mainly to women. The availability of women for domestic tasks, however limited their autonomy in health, is increasingly limited by paid employment outside the home, which will probably lead to a more equal distribution of domestic responsibilities.

Finally, tasks carried out in hospitals for pay are performed in the home without financial compensation. This is not a matter of regret, nor a demand that mothers and fathers be paid. Nevertheless, work carried out without remuneration thereby becomes invisible, without value or recognition. Indeed, even mothers state that they are doing nothing in particular for the health of their children and often share the blindness of society towards their health-related tasks. Asking

which lifestyle encourages health in terms of the work required —
including training, information, time, availability, materials,
relationships and finances — makes possible the genuine recognition
of what families do, rather than merely passing judgement on what
they are, or on what they do not do.

In the division of health-related labour, recognizing and increasing the status (even if not in monetary terms) of what women and, let
us hope, men do could be the first stage in families' recapturing
initiative and power over their own health.

Conclusion

The role of the family in establishing and maintaining healthy
lifestyles is both fundamental and limited. Social policies and health
care professionals oscillate between two contradictory attitudes that
either overburden families with tasks and responsibilities or
emphasize their inadequacies, which the professionals then attempt
to improve. These two attitudes have dangers and limits. The family
has only limited autonomy in matters of health and lifestyle and the
health of family members is largely determined outside the family
structure. This suggests that it is necessary to examine and improve
the family environment and living conditions rather than the family
itself. Establishing healthy lifestyles requires time, work, knowledge
and skill and this re-establishes the value of the health care work
carried out in the home, while highlighting the disparities in the
resources available to different families. The notion of family health
is ambivalent and contradictory, and varies in meaning depending on
time, the people involved, the functions being considered, and sex
and social categories. This shows the social and political issues at
stake in matters related to health.

One should not throw the baby out with the bath water by
entrusting each family with its own norms and values, as if they were
inviolable, but the autonomy of families must be acknowledged, even
in defining the objectives and priorities they establish for themselves.
The efforts and the quality of the feelings families devote to
establishing a healthy life for family members should also be recognized. Finally, the real needs of families in establishing a healthy
lifestyle should be recognized and expressed not in medical terms,
but primarily in terms of living conditions. The wellbeing of
individuals and of families and the behaviour patterns they follow

ensure that wellbeing cannot be isolated from the whole range of socioeconomic and political measures that also determine it.

References

1. **Flandrin, J.L.** *Familles, parenté, sexualité dans l'ancienne société*. Paris, du Seuil, 1984.
2. **Reinberg, A. et al.** *L'homme malade du temps*. Paris, Pernoud/ Stock, 1979.
3. **Boltanski, L.** *Prime éducation et morale de classe*. Paris, Mouton, 1969 (Cahiers du Centre de Sociologie Européenne).
4. **Boltanski, L.** Les usages sociaux du corps. *Annales E.S.C.*, **16**(1): 205–233 (1971).
5. **Delaisi de Perseval, G. & Lallemand, S.** *L'art d'accommoder les bébés*. Paris, du Seuil, 1980.
6. **Herzlich, C. & Pierret, J.** *Malades d'hier, malades d'aujourd'hui : de la mort collective au devoir de guérison*. Paris, Payot, 1984.
7. **Freidson, E.** *Profession of medicine*. New York, Harper & Row, 1970.
8. **Guyot, J.C.** *Quelle médecine pour quelle société ?* Toulouse, Privat, 1982.
9. **Meyer, P.** *L'enfant et la raison d'Etat*. Paris, du Seuil, 1978 (Collection Points).
10. **Crawford, R.** You are dangerous to your health: the ideology and politics of victim blaming. *International journal of health services*, **7**: 663–680 (1977).
11. **Gottraux, M.** La logique sociale de la prévention. *In*: Fragnier, J.P. & Gilliand, P., ed. *Santé et politique sociale*. Vevey, Delta, 1980.
12. **Desplanques, G.** *La mortalité des adultes. Résultats de deux études longitudinales (1955–80)*. Paris, INSEE, 1985.
13. **Townsend, P. & Davidson, N.** *Inequalities in health*. Harmondsworth, Penguin, 1982.
14. **Morton, G. & Ebel, R.** *Epidémiologie et biostatique*. Paris, Doin, 1983.
15. **Finch, J. & Groves, D.** *A labour of love. Women, working and caring*. London, Routledge & Kegan Paul, 1983.
16. **Collière, M.F.** *Promouvoir la vie. De la pratique des femmes soignantes aux soins infirmiers*. Paris, Interéditions, 1982.

10

The social support functions of the family

Lois Pratt

Efforts to promote health and prevent disease have been directed increasingly towards enlisting the family to foster sound health practices. The family is a powerful agency for promoting physical and emotional wellbeing, and much social science research has been based on this assumption. This research has generally focused on how family support influences the outcomes of health and wellbeing *(1 – 3)*. Less conceptual and empirical attention has been paid to how social support may influence personal health practices.

This chapter attempts to assess and explain how families support or promote eating, exercise, smoking and sexual practices, especially among children and adolescents. These practices are known or strongly suspected to affect health; individuals can carry them out themselves, and they fall at least partly within the family's sphere of responsibility.

No single principle or underlying mechanism explains how the family influences various types of health behaviour. The actions involved in one type of health-promoting or health-damaging behaviour (eating, for example) bear little resemblance to the actions involved in another (such as smoking), and people practising one healthful form of behaviour do not necessarily practise other forms. More important, the family's involvement varies for different health behaviours: norms prescribe quite different parental responsibilities for a child's eating than for the child's sexual conduct. This chapter examines several family functions, capabilities and structural features that may be used in developing and maintaining these varied health practices. Most of the evidence cited is based on United States samples.

The Structure and Functions of Family Support

The structure and functions of family support may be distinguished. The structure is the organizational properties and capabilities that enable families to support sound health practices, while functions are the dynamics or mechanisms by which families provide support for members' health practices.

Structure

The structural characteristics of the family include: durable relationships, frequent and regular contacts between members, intense relations (both deep and manifold), openness and accessibility of members to each other, normative prescriptions of responsibilities to each other, and common location in a household in which basic activities of sustenance and health maintenance are carried out. These characteristics provide the family with a unique capacity to promote health protective behaviour.

Interest in how the structure of relationships affects wellbeing developed from Durkheim's (4) research on the association between suicide and the degree to which people are integrated into a social group. The major indicator of this was marital status. Much subsequent work has been based on the hypothesis that married people have health advantages over single, divorced or widowed people, because marriage provides opportunities for regular interaction in a close and stable relationship. Other structural features that may be related to health and health behaviour include the two-parent versus the single-parent household, the division of household tasks according to sex, the employment status of the wife and/or mother, and child-rearing methods.

More complex models of family structure have been used to predict the level of health and health behaviour. The key ingredients in some of these models are the family's resources and capabilities to cope and adapt. In the circumplex model (5), families with balanced cohesion tend to function more adequately on behalf of family members than families at either extreme — disengaged or enmeshed. In the energized family model, the rationale is that improved health

230

behaviour is achieved in families in which the members interact frequently in a variety of contexts, maintain contacts with other groups, actively attempt to cope with and master their lives, and have flexible role relationships and high autonomy *(6)*.

Functions

The central hypothesis on social support is that it affects health and wellbeing by mediating stress. Underlying the impressive research in this field is the view that support may be provided by any social relationship or network, so the family has not been treated as a distinctive agency of support. While neither the family nor health behaviour has been the focus, this work has implications for the functions of family support in health practices.

A source of confusion is that social support refers to both the aid given to another person and the effect of that aid on the recipient. X gives affection and approval (support), and Y derives self-esteem and confidence (support). As it is important to distinguish between cause and effect — what families do that results in certain health behaviours — the aid provided is called forms of support, and the effect, functions of support.

Social support includes socioemotional, instrumental, informational and appraisal support *(7,8)*. Socioemotional support comprises expressions of love, caring, esteem, reassurance, trust, empathy and concern. This type of support reinforces self-esteem, a sense of worth and a feeling that one matters to others, and may thereby convey a sense that one's person and body are worth caring for and protecting. It may also enable the recipient to control stress and thereby focus constructively on maintaining health rather than engaging in aimless or harmful activity *(9)*. Communication of trust and approval reinforces a sense of mastery and builds confidence and pride in one's coping efforts. It may encourage people to take control of their health and wellbeing by developing health-promoting regimens.

Instrumental support consists of supplying goods, equipment, money, time or effort to assist with tasks or activities. Such aid, which is a foundation of family life, may directly facilitate health practices by supplying the means to translate intentions into action. Instrumental support may also contribute indirectly to healthy behaviour by demonstrating that the helping person is dependable and will assist when asked *(8)*.

Informational support is communication of facts or opinions relevant to a person's needs, finding information sources, informing

231

about available services and techniques, and giving advice, suggestions and directives. Health education may facilitate health practices by providing a blueprint or guidelines for health behaviour, and by developing a coping style of seeking information and applying it in decisions on health care. Appraisals of health problems and how to handle them, feedback on how the person is performing, criticism, and comparisons with performances of the others may also provide behavioural guidance and enhance the person's motivation to protect health. While information processing has not been regarded as a family specialty, members of a family quite regularly offer advice and evaluate each other's health behaviour.

Focusing on the family as a particular agency of social support means recognizing additional forms or modes of support that may be relevant to health behaviour (10). The family has an essential role in linking the members to groups and resources outside the family that can support the member's activities and needs. This family function is related to, but should be distinguished from, instrumental support. This role ranges from the use of libraries and museums to camping excursions, coaching a children's sports team, visiting a restaurant and using the health care system.

Another basic family function is providing companionship or partners for activities. By doing things together and for each other, people learn to carry out behavioural routines and develop expectations about how each person will perform. Moreover, companionship is a stimulus to act and to persist in activities, because it is a reward in itself. Companionship may be a vehicle for generating and mobilizing health behaviour, particularly the types of behaviour that involve interaction.

Parents also shape children's behaviour by modelling or exhibiting appropriate health practices for children to imitate. The child's behaviour is presumably shaped by internalizing the image of how a role is performed.

The family is also responsible for the lifelong process of inculcating ocial norms and values that enable people to adapt. Much body care behaviour is regulated by social norms that define what is correct, decent, tasteful, chic and attractive, what is proper regard for one's health, and what are appropriate forms of behaviour to protect health. The family's role in inculcating body care norms may not unequivocally promote health because certain norms prescribe behaviour that may have harmful effects on health.

Families manipulate powerful cultural symbols in their activities, and thereby lend deep cultural meanings to their actions. Serving a child a hamburger, apple pie and Coca Cola, for example, infuses the eating experience with "American" meanings, while serving milk lends additional connotations of wholesomeness and purity, and steak conveys manly vigour. Families shape and reinforce children's health behaviour by exposing them to basic symbolic images and meanings from the broader culture.

Family Support of Health Practices

Eating behaviour
The influence of families on eating practices is profound and pervasive. The dynamics are so complex, however, that it is difficult to sort out which mechanisms are most significant. In fact, the mode of family influence may differ for various aspects of eating, such as eating a balanced diet, avoiding high-risk foods, observing regular mealtimes, and avoiding excessive consumption. The family influences eating habits in many ways: informational support and health education; participating in the food-processing cycle and interacting during meals; parental modelling of behaviour and manipulating cultural food symbols.

Health educators operate on the principle that imparting information about good nutrition practices and the importance of nutrition for health is an effective means of establishing sound eating practices, especially if this begins in childhood. A frequently asserted extension of this principle is that families can contribute substantially to developing good eating practices by learning and teaching the facts about an appropriate diet and its effects on health. Several conditions must be met for this to occur, and there appear to be weak links in the sequence.

First, if parents are to be effective health socializers, they must have appropriate knowledge themselves. Most parents know some of the basic facts about nutrition. For example, three quarters of adults cited eating fewer calories as one of the two best ways to lose weight (11). Three quarters of adults are aware of the principal dietary factors that are strongly suspected to be related to heart disease and high blood pressure (12), and 71% of adults believe that the most important thing that they do to protect their health involves eating (13).

233

Second, parents must actively try to teach children about nutrition. Over 90% of parents in one study explained to their children aged 9–13 years the kinds of food that are proper to eat (6).

Third, communication must be effective and children must absorb the information accurately. Indeed, children at all ages are aware that personal behaviour affects health. Whether it is the parents that have accomplished this teaching is indicated by whether children's knowledge and beliefs reflect those of their parents. In fact, however, they are not closely related. Parents' beliefs about susceptibility to illness, for example, are not related to their children's beliefs (14).

There are other indications that the communication process may be faulty. Thompson et al. (15) found that parents had little accurate knowledge of what their child thought about various matters, and the level of open communication parents reported that they had with the child had no relation to the parent's ability to assess the child's opinions on issues accurately. Mothers' beliefs about what foods their child liked best were found to be inaccurate (16).

Fourth, the knowledge about nutrition must be converted into action. If the communication of health information between parents and children is flawed, parents' efforts to educate for health will not be very successful in developing sound eating behaviour in children. Even if nutrition information is imparted effectively so that children achieve an understanding of nutrition facts and principles, this knowledge still may not be translated into behaviour. Mechanic (17) concluded that there is little evidence that the family influences children's health behaviour by influencing children's health beliefs. Parents' efforts to instruct children about the proper foods to eat are not related to children's eating practices (6). There are isolated findings that support the notion that beliefs about nutrition are related to health behaviour. A study of children aged 11–16 in Northern Ireland (18) reported that knowledge of good nutrition was related to good eating practices. For example, for children with the highest knowledge scores, 31% had the highest ratings on eating behaviour, while for children with the lowest knowledge scores, only 12% scored in the highest category of eating behaviour. In addition, opinions of obese children about the benefits of dieting are related to their current weight loss efforts (19). Most of the evidence, however, suggests that nutrition education is not parents' most important influence on children's eating behaviour.

234

Eating practices are shaped in the food-processing cycle — selecting, shopping, storing, preparing, serving, consuming and cleaning up. Food and eating are a significant part of family life and a primary way members act out their responsibilities to each other. The family division of labour is grounded in the roles members play in feeding activities. The nurture of infants centres on feeding. Manners are schooled at the table. Courtship and romance are played out in candlelight dinners. Food and eating routines provide abundant and regular opportunities for family members to influence each other by providing information and advice, modelling behaviour, companionship and instrumental assistance with tasks, instilling normative standards, and expressing the cultural meanings of food.

Significant relationships are found between body weight in spouses, parents and children, siblings, and even over generations from grandparents to grandchildren. Neither homogamy nor genetic patterns are the principal causes. Longitudinal studies show a consistent marital synchrony in body weight over nine years of marriage, with weight gain or loss by one family member related in time to gain or loss by another member. Genetically related pairs who no longer live together do not exhibit these similarities in weight, while unrelated adult pairs and child pairs who live together do resemble each other in weight (20). Social aspects of family life, such as modelling, are predominant (21).

Family members influence each other's body weight by exhibiting a pattern of calorie consumption and also an image of desirable body shape and weight. Both the parents and children in a weight loss programme who were trained to praise each other for desired dietary changes and to act as models for each other lost more weight than other groups (22). Preparing a proper diet is a major influence; 83% of the total calories consumed by children and teenagers come from foods eaten at home (23), and parents' and children's consumption of carbohydrates, saturated fats and calories (but not cholesterol) were found to be related (24). Spouses show close similarity in caloric intake (25).

The availability of family companionship is a significant factor in shaping meal patterns. Older people who live with a spouse or other family members are more likely to eat three meals a day than people who live alone, and having a meal partner is largely responsible (26). While mealtime companionship is not provided uniquely by families, it is provided most frequently by them.

235

Instrumental support in feeding tasks is another way families influence eating behaviour. About 45% of mothers breastfeed their babies at hospital discharge, but many stop and only 21% still breastfeed after six months *(12)*. After the first month, maintaining breastfeeding depends in part on the assistance the mother receives, which enables her to balance her responsibilities to the infant and to other family members *(27)*.

Families influence eating habits by manipulating potent food symbols. The fundamental meanings of food — what is considered good or unfit to eat, what constitutes a meal, what are proper foods for different ages and sexes, what are the appropriate menus for particular eating occasions, what foods go together, the meanings of hot and cold foods — are embedded in national cultures and ethnic subcultures. Families do not create these basic meanings: they use and transmit them. Thus, families express unity by serving birthday and anniversary cakes, and integration into the national culture by preparing the traditional foods of the national holidays. Family influence is sustained by tapping the deep meanings of food in family life and enhancing the family's role in transmitting the basic eating patterns of the culture — both harmful and healthful practices.

This may explain why weight-control programmes for adolescents that involve parents are often unsuccessful. Not only does parental involvement exacerbate strains between the parent and the adolescent, but the issue is food and eating, the reason for much of the family strain. Nevertheless, involving a spouse in a weight-reduction programme is important not only because of the support provided in changing behaviour, but because values about food and eating shared by husband and wife have become an important element in their marital relationship *(22)*.

Exercise habits
The family influences children's exercise behaviour by providing parental modelling, companionship, instrumental support, and support and encouragement, and by linking family members to resources outside the family. Exercise habits appear to depend more on physical exercise carried out within the family than on supportive attitudes.

A national survey suggests that behaviour modelling is extremely important in promoting physical exercise. Subjects who said that their mother was involved in sports and athletics when they were growing up were significantly more likely to be currently active in

236

sports (80%) than subjects whose mothers were not interested in sports when they were growing up (55%). The findings were similar for fathers' interest in sports participation *(28)*. This effect may begin in early childhood, because mothers' participation in and satisfaction with physical leisure activities is associated with their preschool child's playfulness *(29)*.

Despite the significance of parental modelling in shaping children's exercise habits, the United States national children and youth fitness study *(30)* found that less than 30% of parents of children in grades 1–4 (aged 6–9 years) engaged in appropriate physical exercise (moderate to vigorous physical activity for 20 continuous minutes at least three times a week) and 50% never exercised.

Providing willing and reliable companionship is a prominent family contribution. Interaction between family members is one of the most significant influences on children's exercise habits *(6)*. Yet the national children and youth fitness study found that a majority of parents of children in grades 1–4 (58% of mothers and 62% of fathers) did not exercise at all with their child in a typical week, and less than one quarter exercised at least two days a week with their child for 20 minutes or more. A report on attitudes toward sports in the United States *(31)* found somewhat higher rates of participation by parents and children. Only 25% of parents of children aged 3–18 said that they did not participate in sports with their child, while 40% frequently did. In addition, two thirds of the parents said that they were the ones most likely to accompany their children to sports events.

Parents cannot be expected to participate directly in many of children's physical activities, particularly those requiring a team, but they can provide other forms of direct support. Parents can provide instrumental assistance, such as obtaining sports and exercise equipment and teaching athletic skills. Parents' greatest contribution may be in using resources and organizations outside the family. Parents can coach a junior athletic team, transport children and equipment to games, and attend children's athletic events. In the report on attitudes to sports, 61% of parents surveyed said that one or both parents always watched their children's sports activities and only 6% never did *(31)*. Parents send children to camps, locate outdoor recreation areas, and organize outdoor excursions. This mobilization of activities by parents has lifelong effects on children's physical exercise. In another survey, individuals' activities were traced through three time periods; individuals who frequently participated in outdoor activity from ages 6 to 11 years and ages 12 to 17 years continued to be active as adults, and individuals who were inactive during childhood were inactive as adults. The activities that involved family participation were the ones most likely to persist in adulthood *(32)*. The aspects of family life that contributed most to children's exercise habits were family members' active participation in activities and groups outside the home and a high level of interaction between family members *(6)*.

Parents may also contribute to their children's exercise habits by encouraging and supporting physical activity. Three quarters of parents surveyed said that they often encouraged their children to participate in sports, and nearly as many encouraged their children to practise their skills away from the games *(31)*. Recent cohorts of parents tend to be more supportive of exercise than earlier cohorts. In a Harris survey *(28)*, 46% of young people aged 18–24 reported that their fathers had encouraged them to participate in sports, compared with only 13% of the oldest group surveyed. Nevertheless, parents' encouragement does not have as much effect on whether children actually engage in sports as parental actions: being active themselves, participating in physical activity with children, and using community resources to enable the child to engage in physical activity.

Smoking

Considerable research has gone into trying to trace the influence of the family on children's smoking behaviour. Mechanisms that have been examined are health education, expressing normative standards and applying sanctions, parental modelling of appropriate (nonsmoking) behaviour, and the quality of family relationships. Mechanisms that succeed in childhood are different from those that are effective in adolescence.

Parents have played an active role in education about smoking. Over three quarters of fathers and mothers explained to their children aged 9–13 years about the effects of smoking, and three quarters of the children also acknowledged that their parents had instructed them *(6)*. Young people increasingly believe that smoking has dire consequences. Between 1975 and 1985 the proportion of high school seniors (in the last year of school) who accepted this rose from 51% to 66% *(33)*, although 90% of adults believe that smoking poses grave

238

health risks *(11)*. Nevertheless, there is little evidence to link the belief among youth that smoking is hazardous to health with lower rates of smoking among youth, although a moderate relationship has been found among adults *(34)*.

Directly expressing disapproval of smoking is more influential than inculcating beliefs. If neither parent is upset about the child smoking, the child is about five times more likely to smoke than if both parents are upset *(35)*. The rate of smoking by teenagers is higher when parents give normative support to smoking by offering cigarettes to their children *(34)*. Parental disapproval is also associated with the child giving up smoking.

Evidence supports the modelling hypothesis of parental influence on children's smoking behaviour. In 1965, 43% of adults in the United States smoked. The rate dropped to 30% by 1985. The percentage of high school seniors smoking dropped from a peak 27% in 1976 to 19% in 1985, and the rise among teenage girls that occurred in the 1970s was curbed *(11)*. This suggests that youth were responding to the behavioural change exhibited by adults. The modelling hypothesis is supported more directly by evidence that children of smokers are more likely to smoke than children of nonsmokers *(36)*. A study in the United States reported that children are twice as likely to smoke if both parents smoke and twice as likely not to smoke if neither parent smokes *(35)*.

Parents' influence on smoking behaviour diminishes significantly when children reach adolescence. Parental influence is foremost among children in grades 4 and 6 (aged about 9 and 11 years); by grades 11 and 12 (children aged 16 and 17 years) this is no longer the case *(37)*. The continuing influence parents have on adolescent smoking is through expressing normative standards rather than as models of behaviour. The influence of peers on smoking behaviour increases; peers exert their influence more by their behaviour than by expressing normative standards. Parents have a longer time than peers in which to instil general cultural standards, whereas peers are omnipresent behavioural models during adolescence *(38, 39)*.

While generally proscribed by adults, smoking has positive cultural meanings that especially attract young people. Ironically, adolescents call upon the image of the cigarette smoker that was portrayed in the movies of an earlier era: the Humphrey Bogart and Lauren Bacall image of being tough, cool, sophisticated, attractive, dangerous and romantic. Adolescents tend to admire spontaneity and risk-taking and are not easily reined in by fears of long-term consequences for health, tending to view good health as an intrinsic quality of young people. Hence, peer influence is more likely than parental influence to promote smoking.

While parents generally influence the smoking behaviour of adolescents less than do peers, some aspects of parent–child relationships especially influence the incidence of smoking in adolescence. Involvement of the teenager in family decision-making *(40)*, attachment to the father and mother *(41)*, family adjustment *(42)*, and a low level of family stress and strain *(43)* are associated with a low incidence of smoking among teenagers. McCubbin et al. *(43)* propose that family tensions may cause adolescents to search for alternative means of managing their discomfort. Instead of working out the problems within the family, they smoke as a coping strategy. Smoking numbs the distress adolescents feel and also wins the approval of friends to whom they turn for comfort. Close and amicable parent–adolescent relationships thus protect the adolescent from developing a need for such a coping device.

Adolescent sexual behaviour

The sexual behaviour of children and adolescents is generally viewed as something to be prevented. Phase one is restraining the first sexual intercourse until an acceptable age, and phase two is preventing pregnancy, promiscuity and sexually transmitted diseases when young people become sexually active. The task has thus been defined as a paramount responsibility of the family, and the strategies prescribed for families in preventing unsafe sexual behaviour by young people are providing a stable and caring family environment, regulating conduct and transmitting information and values on sex and reproduction.

There is modest evidence that a stable and caring family environment contributes to restrained and responsible sexual behaviour among adolescents. Both black and white adolescent girls whose parents were very concerned about their lives were significantly less likely than others to give birth out of wedlock *(44)*. Additionally, for white adolescents, having parents who often talked with them also reduced the likelihood of a birth out of wedlock.

Household structure (two parents versus one parent) has been used as a rough indicator of a family's resources for providing care and supporting children. White teenage girls who lived in two-parent households were less likely than those in single-parent or no-parent households to begin sexual intercourse at an early age, but this did not apply to black girls or to males *(45)*. Girls who were living with two parents at age 14 were more likely to use birth control at their first premarital intercourse (50%) than girls living with one or no parents (39%) *(46)*.

The findings on the role of parental regulation and control of children's conduct are limited and inconsistent. White teenage girls whose parents monitored their homework were less likely than others to give birth out of wedlock *(44)*, but mothers' efforts to control their daughters' conduct (by restricting going out at night and the people the child sees) and whether the child is allowed to make decisions were not related to the daughter's early initiation of coitus *(45)*.

Another mode of influence on teenagers' sexual activity is parental modelling of appropriate sexual behaviour. Mothers who were less sexually active as adolescents had a higher percentage of daughters who delayed initiation of intercourse *(45)*. Early childbearing by mothers who kept the child increased the likelihood of early childbearing by the daughter.[a] In addition, girls whose sisters had teenage pregnancies and girls who lived in households with over nine members had an elevated risk of teenage pregnancy *(47)*. Studies have found anywhere from a doubled risk to a four-fold risk among sisters. The original model for early childbearing is the mother, and when a daughter has an early pregnancy, she serves as an additional model for that behaviour among her sisters.

The mode of parental influence that has been examined most extensively is sex education. Parents usually acknowledge the norm that they are responsible for teaching children about sex at home *(48)*. High percentages of fathers and mothers expect to discuss various sexual topics with their male and female children, although the proportions range widely by topic and by the sex of parent and child *(49)*. For example, about 90% of mothers surveyed expected to talk to their daughters about birth, reproduction, body differences, sexual morals and menstruation, but fewer planned to discuss intercourse, abortion, homosexuality or masturbation. Significantly fewer fathers planned to talk to their daughters or sons about any of these topics.

Actual communication about sex between parents and children falls far short of these intentions. There is little direct communication

---

[a] **Presser, H.B.** *Social consequences of teenage childbearing.* Paper presented at the Conference on Consequences of Adolescent Pregnancy and Childbearing, Bethesda, Maryland, 1975.

from parents to children, and what little does occur is between mothers and daughters (50). Fewer than half of the mothers and one quarter of the fathers reported that they had explained to their child aged 9–13 years how reproduction takes place. Fewer parents had discussed reproduction than had discussed any of seven other health care topics (6). Much of the discussion that takes place is not successful. Parents have reported discussing reproduction with their child, but the child reported that such discussions had not taken place (6), and some mothers and teenage daughters do not agree on whether birth control has been discussed (51).

Parents may be reluctant to discuss sex with children when they are young, because the principal objective of the parents is to prevent sexual activity. Parents may fear that if they advise the child about sex, the child may interpret this as encouragement and begin sexual activity. The parents do not, at this stage, want to tip their hand and disclose prematurely that they will later accept a revised agenda and promote safe and responsible sex. The children perceive that their parents' objective is to prevent sexual activity, and when the children become sexually active, they are reluctant to discuss sex with their parents, fearing that disclosure of this sexual activity will bring parental disapproval (48). Girls often find such discussions stressful (52) and are less likely to talk about sex with their mothers than with a girlfriend. A majority of daughters who went to a family planning clinic had not told their mothers about the visit or that they had had sex. Very few of the daughters who visited a clinic had been encouraged by their mothers to initiate birth control and only 9% came with their mothers (48, 53).

When parents learn that their child has become sexually active, they usually acknowledge the pragmatic agenda — safe and responsible sex. Four out of five daughters surveyed said that their mothers ultimately supported their visit to the clinic (48). At this stage, however, there are other factors that restrain communication about sex between parents and sexually active adolescents. The norms of sexual privacy restrain parents from intruding into their child's sexual thoughts, deeds and relationships. Parents are also proscribed from becoming too closely involved in their child's sex life (especially mothers with sons and fathers with daughters) to eliminate implications of an incestuous relationship. Another major limitation on parental efforts to guide their children towards responsible sexual behaviour is the nature of adolescent life and the adolescent subculture. Teenagers tend to perceive themselves as being invulnerable to such health problems as pregnancy and sexually transmitted diseases *(14)* and they value spontaneity, excitement and romance. From the frame of reference of adolescents, contraceptives may be viewed as distasteful and inhibitive. Most teenagers know about contraception, but may not find the information to be a compelling basis for action *(54, 55)*.

Given this flawed communication about sex and reproduction, sex education by parents would probably form a shaky foundation for shaping children's sexual conduct. When mothers and daughters discussed menstruation (before the girl was 18), the daughter was more likely to use contraception at her first premarital intercourse (50% as against 37%) *(46)*, and when there were frequent conversations about sexual matters, the daughter was more receptive to using birth control *(50)*. A longitudinal study found, however, that the causal sequence was the reverse. Communication was more likely to follow than precede contraceptive use, as daughters who had become effective contraceptive users were better able to discuss sex with their mothers *(56)*. The failure of sex education by parents to influence teenagers' sexual behaviour decisively may not entirely be the result of faulty parent–child communication, but may be a problem with sex education as a mode of influence on sexual behaviour. Some studies have found no relationship between prior sex education or knowledge of contraception and the likelihood of a birth out of wedlock *(44)*.

Families do influence children's sexual behaviour, including the time at which they begin intercourse, their use of contraceptives, and the likelihood of a birth out of wedlock. The most effective modes of influence appear to be parental modelling of appropriate sexual behaviour and providing a stable and caring family environment.

It is important to recognize how limited this family influence is. Even among teenagers who lived in more favourable family situations (in two-parent households in which parents discussed sexual development with the child), 50% of the daughters did not use contraception at their first premarital intercourse *(46)*.

Conclusions

The family provides significant support for various health practices, including eating, exercise, nonsmoking and responsible sexual practices, but it is impossible to conclude whether the family is more successful in shaping one health practice than others.

The literature on social support has stressed the socioemotional function of family support. Love, esteem and trust may not even be the most influential mode of family support for health practices. The conception of the social support functions of the family should be extended to include other support mechanisms, such as parental modelling of appropriate health behaviour; providing companionship, informational support, health education and instrumental support; instilling normative standards; linking members to community resources; establishing stable and equable family relationships; and manipulating cultural symbols.

Certain modes of family influence are less effective and others are more effective, regardless of what kind of health practice is involved. Compared with other mechanisms, informational support and health education do not appear to have much effect on children's health practices. Parental modelling of appropriate health behaviour, however, is an important mechanism for promoting various health practices.

There are important differences in the effectiveness of different family support mechanisms in shaping various health practices. Instrumental support, linking members to resources outside the family, and companionship are essential ways that families assist in developing proper eating habits and engaging in sports and physical exercise. Families also manipulate cultural food symbols to support eating habits. Inculcating normative standards and providing a stable and caring family environment are especially important in developing safe and responsible sex practices and for maintaining nonsmoking by teenagers.

The family's influence on children's health behaviour diminishes in adolescence, and the effectiveness of various mechanisms of family support changes. Direct influences such as parental modelling of appropriate behaviour are less effective. A stable, caring and non-stressful family environment becomes an important support, which helps adolescents to cope constructively and to resist seeking immediate gratification in smoking, junk food and spontaneous sex.

What are the prospects for and limitations on family support for health-promoting behaviour in children and adolescents? Families have enormous opportunities to foster sound health practices, but parental influence needs to be exerted early and strongly by setting a

244

positive example, actively discouraging harmful practices, mobilizing the resources that facilitate sound health behaviour, and (in adolescence) by providing secure and accepting relationships.

Accomplishing this depends on several factors. If parents are to be positive role models for their children, future parents must establish estimable health practices that they can then project to their children. Stronger negative cultural images of such harmful practices as smoking, risky sex, overeating and physical indolence will have to evolve to counterbalance the positive images that are attractive to adolescents. Even the most resourceful families are left confused by professional guidelines for health behaviour that are often inconsistent, in dispute among professionals, and constantly changing. While this is how scientific knowledge is developed, perhaps families would become less discouraged and less likely to stop trying to cope if new health warnings were presented less dogmatically to the public.

Needed research
Many questions remain about family support and personal health practices. It is essential to study the family as a unit rather than as an aggregate of separate individuals to understand the dynamics of family support. Support is interactional and involves costs and gains to both giver and recipient. Family support has negative consequences along with its beneficial effects, but mainly the positive effects have been examined. Researchers also need to examine family support at various stages of the life cycle, including old age. Additional work is needed on other health practices including sleep, alcohol and drug use, home safety and accidents, dental and body hygiene, and care of illness at home.

References

1. **Cohen, S. & Syme, S.L., ed**. *Social support and health*. New York, Academic Press, 1985.
2. **Lin, N**. *Social support, life events, and depression*. New York, Academic Press, 1986.
3. **Sarason, I.G. & Sarason, B.R., ed**. *Social support: theory, research and applications*. Dordrecht, Martinus Nijhoff, 1985.
4. **Durkheim, E. Suicide**. Glencoe, IL, Free Press, 1951.
5. **Olson, D.H. & McCubbin, H.I**. Circumplex model of marital and family systems V: application to family stress and crisis

intervention. *In*: McCubbin, H.I. et al., ed. *Family stress, coping, and social support*. Springfield, IL, Charles C. Thomas, 1982, pp. 48–68.

6. **Pratt, L**. *Family structure and effective health behavior: the energized family*. Boston, Houghton Mifflin, 1976.

7. **Thoits, P.A**. Social support and psychological well-being: theoretical possibilities. *In*: Sarason, I.G. & Sarason, B.R., ed. *Social support: theory, research and applications*. Dordrecht, Martinus Nijhoff, 1985.

8. **Wills, T.A**. Supportive functions of interpersonal relationship. *In*: Cohen, S. & Syme, S.L. ed. *Social support and health*. New York, Academic Press, 1985, pp. 61–82.

9. **Wilcox B.L. & Vernberg, E.M**. Conceptual and theoretical dilemmas facing social support research. *In*: Sarason, I.G. & Sarason, B.R., ed. *Social support: theory, research and applications*. Dordrecht, Martinus Nijhoff, 1985.

10. **Caplan, G**. The family as a support system. *In*: McCubbin, H.I. et al., ed. *Family stress, coping, and social support*. Springfield, IL, Charles C. Thomas, 1982, pp. 200–220.

11. **US Department of Health and Human Services, Public Health Service**. *Health United States 1986 and prevention profile*. Washington, DC, US Government Printing Office, 1986.

12. **US Department of Health and Human Services, Public Health Service**. *The 1990 health objectives for the nation: a midcourse review*. Washington, DC, US Government Printing Office, 1986.

13. **Harris, D.M. & Guten, S**. Health-protective behaviour: an exploratory study. *Journal of health and social behaviour*, **20**: 17–29 (1979).

14. **Gochman, D.S**. Family determinants of children's concepts of health and illness. *In*: Turk, D.C. & Kerns, R.D., ed. *Health, illness and families: a life-span perspective*. New York, Wiley, 1985, pp. 23–50.

15. **Thompson, L. et al**. Do parents know their children? The ability of mothers and fathers to gauge the attitudes of their young adult children. *Family relations*, **34**: 315–320 (1985).

16. **Weidner, G. et al**. Family consumption of low fat foods: stated preference versus actual consumption. *Journal of applied social psychology*, **15**: 773–779 (1985).

246

17. **Mechanic, D**. The influence of mothers on their children's health attitudes and behaviour. *Pediatrics*, **39**: 444–453 (1964).

18. **McGuffin, S.J**. The nutritional knowledge and behaviour of 11 to 16-year-old school pupils in Northern Ireland. *Health education journal*, **45**: 155–159 (1986).

19. **O'Connell, J.K. et al**. Utilizing the health belief model to predict dieting and exercising behaviour of obese and non obese adolescents. *Health education quarterly*, **12**: 343–351 (1985).

20. **Garn, S.M. et al**. Obesity and living together. *Marriage and family review*, **7**: 33–47 (1984).

21. **Baranowski, T. & Nader, R**. Family health behaviour. *In*: Turk, D.C. & Kerns, R.D., ed. *Health, illness and families: a life-span perspective*. New York, Wiley, 1985, pp. 51–80.

22. **Baranowski, T. & Nader, R**. Family involvement in health behaviour change programs. *In*: Turk, D.C. & Kerns, R.D., ed. *Health, illness and families: a life-span perspective*. New York, Wiley, 1985, pp. 81–107.

23. **Evans, M.D. & Cronin, F.J**. Diets of school-aged children and teenagers. *Family economics review*, **3**: 14–21 (1986).

24. **Laskarzewski, P. et al**. Parent–child nutrient intake inter-relationships in schoolchildren ages 6 to 19: the Princeton School District study. *American journal of clinical nutrition*, **33**: 2350–2355 (1980).

25. **Sobal, J**. Marriage, obesity and dieting. *Marriage and family review*, **7**: 115–139 (1984).

26. **Pratt, L**. The family and health promotion among the elderly. *In*: Ramsey, C.N., Jr., ed. *Family systems in medicine*. New York, Guildford Press, 1988.

27. **Graham, H**. Family influences in early years on the eating habits of children. *In*: Turner, M., ed. *Nutrition and lifestyles: proceedings of the British Nutrition Foundation*. London, Applied Sciences Publishers, 1980, pp. 169–178.

28. **Harris, L. and Associates, Inc**. *The Perrier study: fitness in America*. New York, Great Waters of France, Inc., 1979.

29. **Barnett, L.A. & Chick, G.E**. Chips off the ol' block: parents' leisure and their children's play. *Journal of leisure research*, **18**: 266–283 (1986).

30. *Summary of findings from National Children and Youth Fitness Study II*. Washington, DC, Office of Disease Prevention and-

Health Promotion, US Department of Health and Human Services, 1987.

31. *The Miller Lite report on American attitudes towards sports.* Milwaukee, WI, Miller Brewing Company, 1983.

32. **Cheek, N.H., Jr. et al.** *Leisure and recreation places.* Ann Arbor, MI, Ann Arbor Science, 1976.

33. **Johnston, L.D. et al.** *Drug use among American high school students, college students, and other young adults. National trends through 1985.* Washington, DC, US Government Printing Office, 1986 (National Institute on Drug Abuse, DHHS Publication No. (ADM) 85–1394).

34. **Reid, D.** Prevention of smoking among schoolchildren: recommendations for policy development. *Health education journal*, **44**: 3–14 (1985).

35. **Nolte, A.E. et al.** The relative importance of parental attitudes and behaviour upon youth smoking behaviour. *Journal of school health*, **53**: 264–271 (1983).

36. **Boddewyn, J.J.** *Why do juveniles start smoking? An international study of the role of advertising and other contributory factors in Australia, Hong Kong, Norway, Spain and the United Kingdom.* New York, International Advertising Association, Inc., Children's Research Unit, 1986.

37. **Pederson, L.L.** Changes in variables related to smoking from childhood to late adolescence: an eight year longitudinal study of a cohort of elementary school students. *Canadian journal of public health*, **77**: 33–39 (1986).

38. **Biddle, B.J. et al.** Parental and peer influence on adolescents. *Social forces*, **58**: 1057–1079 (1980).

39. **Kandel, D.B. & Adler, I.** Socialization into marijuana use among French adolescents: a cross-cultural comparison with the United States. *Journal of health and social behaviour*, **23**: 295–309 (1982).

40. **Mittelmark, M.B. et al.** Predicting experimentation with cigarettes: the childhood antecedents of smoking study. *American journal of public health*, **77**: 206–208 (1987).

41. **Skinner, W.F. et al.** Social influences and constraints on the initiation and cessation of adolescent tobacco use. *Journal of behavioural medicine*, **8**: 353–376 (1985).

42. **Dielman, T.E. et al.** Susceptibility to peer pressure, self-esteem, and health locus of control as correlates of adolescent

248

substance abuse. *Health education quarterly*, **14**: 207–221 (1987).

43. **McCubbin, H.I. et al**. Adolescent health risk behaviours: family stress and adolescent coping as critical factors. *Family relations*, **34**: 51–62 (1985).

44. **Hanson, S.L. et al**. The role of responsibility and knowledge in reducing teenage out-of-wedlock childbearing. *Journal of marriage and the family*, **49**: 241 (1987).

45. **Udry, J.R. & Billy, J.O.G**. Initiation of coitus in early adolescence. *American sociological review*, **52**: 841–855 (1987).

46. **Mosher, W.D. & Bachrach, C.A**. First premarital contraceptive use: United States, 1960–82. *Studies in family planning*, **18**: 83–95 (1987).

47. **Friede, A. et al**. Do the sisters of childbearing teenagers have increased rates of childbearing? *American journal of public health*, **76**: 1221–1224 (1986).

48. **Furstenberg, F.F., Jr. et al**. Family communication and teenagers' contraceptive use. *Family planning perspectives*, **16**: 163–170 (1984).

49. **Koblinsky, S. & Atkinson, J**. Parental plans for children's sex education. *Family relations*, **31**: 29–35 (1982).

50. **Fox, G.L**. The family's role in adolescent sexual behaviour. *In*: Ooms, T., ed. *Adolescent pregnancy in a family context*. Philadelphia, PA, Temple University Press, 1981.

51. **Furstenberg, F.F., Jr**. Birth control experience among pregnant adolescents: the process of unplanned parenthood. *Social problems*, **19**: 192 (1971).

52. **Philliber, S**. Socialization for childbearing. *Journal of social issues*, **36**: 30 (1980).

53. **Nathanson, C.A. & Becker, M.H**. Family and peer influence on obtaining a method of contraception. *Journal of marriage and the family*, **48**: 513 (1986).

54. **Silverman, J. et al**. Barriers to contraceptive services. *Family planning perspectives*, **19**: 94–102 (1987).

55. **Trussell, J. & Kost, K**. Contraceptive failure in the United States: a critical review of the literature. *Studies in family planning*, **18**: 237–283 (1987).

56. **Herceg-Baron, R. & Furstenberg, F.F., Jr**. Adolescent contraceptive use: the impact of family support systems. *In*: Fox, G.L., ed. *The childbearing decision: fertility attitudes and behaviour*. Beverly Hills, CA, Sage Publications, 1982.

11

Health promotion in the workplace

Töres Theorell

Occupational health care teams focused on improving the health habits of employees are increasingly active in most countries in the western hemisphere. This is considered to be financially important because absenteeism from work is an increasing financial burden for many employers. An occupational health care team has an extraordinary opportunity to improve health habits because people are more easily accessible at the workplace than at home. Thus, a large number of antismoking, physical exercise and relaxation programmes have started, and the effects of such programmes have been documented *(1–3)*. The workplace is a practical site to distribute health propaganda. One of the largest health promotion programmes carried out by the WHO European Collaborative Group *(4)* took place in factories in several countries. The study showed that it is possible not only to influence health habits favourably, but also to lower the incidence of coronary heart disease during the follow-up period. A screening procedure identified individuals at risk. Groups of high-risk individuals were then formed for regular meetings at the workplace involving antismoking propaganda and diet counselling. The results clearly showed, however, that the participants' degree of enthusiasm and willingness to pursue the programme was of central importance to its success. In Belgium, where enthusiasm was great, risk factors improved markedly *(4)*.

The programmes that teach employees relaxation techniques, and various stress management programmes are also very important. The controlled studies at the New York Telephone Company showed that it was possible and useful to teach employees the Benson relaxation technique (2). Another example is the controlled study of the effects of teaching employees a combination of yoga and biofeedback (5). A follow-up after four years showed that the programme had lasting effects in lowering blood pressure. In both studies all the health education in groups took place at the workplace.

The Work Environment

Many of the programmes aimed at individual teaching in the workplace have been based on insufficient analysis of the possible effects that the work environment itself has on health habits. The work environment could influence the risk of disease either by effects on the mechanisms that produce physiological stress or by effects on health habits. A person who has a boring life may not be interested in acting now to prolong life by five years at some time in the remote future. Studies (6) have shown that people in occupations in which a large proportion of workers find their jobs monotonous and boring are more likely to smoke cigarettes. Other mechanisms besides boredom may also influence health habits in the workplace. For instance, the personnel in a cancer ward are fully aware of the dangers of smoking cigarettes and yet many of them still smoke. One reason for this "disobedient" attitude towards antismoking propaganda may simply be that the psychosocial work environment in the cancer ward is very demanding because of all the suffering among the patients and their relatives. Employees may be able to relieve the tension by going to the smoking room with some of their workmates who smoke and discussing the current situation. This example clearly shows that, in some cases, health habits can only be improved if the process starts in the work environment itself. A greater knowledge of psychology as well as organized opportunities for personnel to discuss psychological problems could remove some of the reason for smoking cigarettes. Supervisors could also allow employees to take a tension-releasing pause for reasons other than smoking.

Psychosocial and Physiological Correlates of Hypertension

A study recently performed on a sample of 28-year-old men (7, 8) explored the psychosocial and physiological correlates of early stage (mainly asymptomatic) elevated blood pressure (Fig. 1). The results indicated that high resting blood pressure could mostly be explained by two physiological factors, overweight and plasma adrenaline. The psychosocial factors that explained high plasma adrenaline level were a poor social network (few friends) and a boring type of job (jobs had been classified using national surveys *(9)*). Overweight was associated with lack of employment security (a combined dimension constructed by factor analysis of four self-reported items concerning risk of redundancy). Elevated blood concentration of liver enzyme (a possible indicator of longstanding excessive alcohol consumption) was also correlated with both elevated blood pressure and poor social network. The relationship between excessive eating and drinking and elevated blood pressure in young men, who may then become early victims of coronary heart disease in the future, indicates that the psychosocial environment should be a prime target in the efforts to prevent coronary heart disease, and that propaganda to improve health habits should never be an isolated educational effort *(7, 8)*.

Improving the Psychosocial Work Environment

The psychosocial work environment can be improved as part of a health-promoting programme in the workplace. Increased awareness of the interaction between the environment and risk factors may even be necessary to attain lasting effects in a health-promoting programme. Our research programme *(7, 8)* and others *(10 – 12)* have shown that combinations of excessive demands, lack of intellectual discretion and authority over decisions, and lack of social support may be decisive in many adverse health outcomes. For instance, in a large epidemiological study *(13)*, scores for demands, decision latitude and social support in the workplace were standardized and then multiplied together. A cross-sectional analysis showed that men in the upper third of this combined score prematurely developed symptoms of heart disease at least five years earlier than men in the lower third of the combined score. The effect was strongest in male blue-collar workers.

It is not surprising that lack of support and decision latitude and excessive demands at work can have adverse effects on health and health habits. Methods to record these dimensions and strategies to improve them are being developed. Several large-scale occupational health care teams in Sweden have used this knowledge. Questionnaires constructed to measure these dimensions have been used

Fig. 1. Psychosocial and physiological factors in elevated resting systolic blood pressure in 28-year-old men

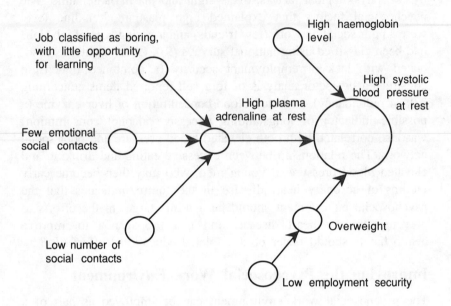

Source: Adapted from Knox et al. (7).

anonymously in many workplaces. The responses have been compared with large reference groups, and this comparison has been fed back to each workplace in a joint meeting. This strategy has beneficial effects only if key people at the workplace have been properly prepared, and if the proposals for changes that may result can be handled constructively by all parties involved. Examples of occupational health care teams operating on this principle are Volvo (14), Statshälsan (the Swedish Foundation for Occupational Health and Safety for State Employees) (15) and Bygghälsan (the Construction Industry Organization for Working Environment, Safety and Health) (16).

Involving People at the Workplace: A Study

One key element in prevention is activating people at the workplace. It may not be sufficient to conduct a questionnaire survey, make some proposals for improvement and then ignore the issue. Recent studies

254

have assumed that cardiovascular risk factors are perceived as vital, and that a programme to increase awareness and knowledge of the interaction between the work environment and these risk factors may have stronger effects on both of these than an either/or strategy. We *(17)* used the following method to fulfil this goal.

The method
The study involved seven groups of employees, each in a different occupation. Its purpose was to explore psychosocial and cardiovascular risk factors in the workplace. The employees were invited four times in one year to participate in the study. The fact that the study takes time is important in itself. The team returned several times to facilitate discussion about the work environment and risk factors.

The employees were trained to measure their own blood pressure using self-operated equipment approximately hourly (as close as possible) during an ordinary working day, at leisure and at work. For each measurement they also recorded what they had been doing during the previous hour and their mood during measurement.

The employees filled out questionnaires for each measurement. From the replies we calculated indices of psychological demands and decision latitude, according to Schwartz et al. *(18)*. We also calculated other psychosocial indices, such as positive factors, roughly corresponding to social support in the workplace.

Blood samples were drawn in the morning before work started and before breakfast. The blood was analysed for lipid (total cholesterol and triglycerides) and liver enzyme concentration. Smoking habits and the ratio of body weight to height were recorded.

Individual feedback
After each examination the subject received information about possible pathological results and other important medical comments. After all four examinations were finished, the subject received a summary including all the conventional risk factors: serum lipids, smoking habits, blood pressure (average at work and at leisure), overweight and liver enzyme, and self-reported alcohol consumption. This information was tabulated with the data on demands and decision latitude and also with percentage calculations for each occurrence of the emotional states sadness, anger, worry and rush, and calmness.

The subjects received considerable feedback. First, they were able to see all the self-recorded information in the protocol. For example, each person who tended to have elevated blood pressure in stressful situations was able to see the type of emotion and activity that was associated with elevated blood pressure. Second, the summary showed whether alcohol consumption, smoking habits or blood pressure was affected by the workplace situation. Important life events outside the workplace were recorded in the summary. Tables 1–3 show individual examples of parts of such a summary.

Table 1. Summary statement of risk and lifestyle factors for a 40-year-old airport baggage handler supervisor

Risk and lifestyle factors	Oct. 1984	Feb. 1985	May 1985	Sept. 1985
Reported frequency of a particular emotion during the recording day (%) (somewhat or very much):				
— joy	57	23	0	10
— sadness	0	0	0	0
— anxiety	35	53	0	0
— irritation	0	0	0	0
Serum cholesterol (mmol/litre)	6.9	7.7	7.2	7.2
Self-recorded average blood pressure at work (systolic/diastolic, mmHg)	126/93	142/96	129/90	133/90
Number of cigarettes smoked per day	0	0	0	0
Demands score (0–15)	7	13	7	6
Decision latitude score (0–18)	11	10	10	13
Sleeping disturbance score (0–30)	8	12	11	11

Table 1 shows a 40-year-old airport baggage handler who was a supervisor in his team. There were four recordings during the year. In February 1985 his work demands dramatically increased and his decision latitude was relatively low. At that time his average blood pressure at work was higher, he reported more anxiety and less joy, and in the questionnaire he reported more sleeping disturbances than at other times. The person in Table 2 was a 45-year-old nonsupervisor baggage handler whose decision latitude was very low and blood pressure at work relatively high. This person had continual difficulties in sleeping caused by family problems. The person in Table 3 was a 50-year-old chief surgeon. His blood pressure was low in the morning, but it was markedly elevated at some measurements. His highest blood pressure was recorded immediately after a telephone call from the administration that threatened the resources provided to

Table 2. Summary statement of risk and lifestyle factors
for a 45-year-old airport baggage handler

Risk and lifestyle factors	Oct. 1984	Feb. 1985	May 1985	Sept. 1985
Reported frequency of a particular emotion during the recording day (%) (somewhat or very much):				
— joy	35	20	0	0
— sadness	0	0	6	92
— anxiety	12	0	6	50
— irritation	0	0	6	0
Serum cholesterol (mmol/litre)	6.90	6.10	5.60	5.66
Self-recorded average blood pressure at work (systolic/diastolic, mmHg)	145/95	149/106	144/96	150/108
Number of cigarettes smoked per day	0	0	0	0
Demands score (0–15)	6	7	7	6
Decision latitude score (0–18)	5	4	3	3
Sleeping disturbance score (0–30)	17	17	17	17

Table 3. Summary statement of risk and lifestyle factors
for a 50-year-old chief surgeon

Risk and lifestyle factors	Sept. 1984	Feb. 1985	May 1985	Sept. 1985
Reported frequency of a particular emotion during the recording day (%) (somewhat or very much):				
— joy	0	0	0	38
— sadness	0	0	0	0
— anxiety	0	0	0	0
— irritation	0	0	0	0
Serum cholesterol (mmol/litre)	6.2	6.2	5.3	5.5
Self-recorded average blood pressure at work (systolic/diastolic, mmHg)	151/96	152/91	144/85	139/79
Number of cigarettes smoked per day	11–20	11–20	11–20	11–20
Demands score (0–15)	6	7	7	6
Decision latitude score (0–18)	5	4	3	3
Sleeping disturbance score (0–30)	17	17	17	17

the clinic. In the group of physicians, the protocols clearly indicated that acute problems with patients were not the only factors that induced peaks in blood pressure. The problems that arose because of personnel conflicts frequently caused elevated blood pressure.

257

Group feedback

After the individual feedback there was also group feedback. Some of our data could be compared with a very large reference group, while for other variables the seven groups we studied were compared. For instance, the baggage handlers had a lower level of intellectual discretion than the other groups. They also had more cardiovascular risk factors than others: high blood pressure levels both at work and at leisure, a relatively high rate of cigarette smoking and high body mass index. The physicians studied had few cardiovascular risk factors and a high level of intellectual discretion, but they reported a high frequency of rush and worry and anger, mostly transient states in the daily protocols. Interestingly, male physicians also had higher morning levels of plasma cortisol than other men. Physicians frequently had problems at work: too much variation and too many difficult decisions in ambiguous situations. This is consistent with previous studies that show that physicians in Sweden have a relatively low incidence of cardiac deaths but a high incidence of suicide *(19)*. In addition to the baggage handlers, waiters and orchestral musicians reported very unfavourable combinations of high demands and low decision latitude. The waiters' situation was further complicated by the fact that there was little psychosocial support at work. These psychosocial problems were reflected in excessive smoking and high alcohol consumption (but not high liver enzyme levels). This group also reported frequent gastrointestinal symptoms.

In the feedback sessions, we found statistical evidence that the ratio between scores for demands and for decision latitude was significantly associated with increased blood pressure at work, particularly among people with a positive family history of hypertension *(20)*.

During the study, several group interviews were organized at all the workplaces. The goal was to discuss strategies for collective coping or how the group handles a crisis situation. This exploration showed that physicians very often used denial to cope with the emotional problems they encountered, and also that some of their collective coping strategies may be regarded as destructive. Air-traffic controllers, who have a very demanding and difficult job, had been forced to develop effective collective coping ("otherwise we kill people"), and this was reflected in low levels of negative emotions in the daily protocols and low levels of cardiovascular risk factors.

Participation

What are the effects of a combined psychosocial and medical cardio-vascular exploration in the workplace? The participation rate varied somewhat in the groups studied. Table 4 shows the percentage of men and women from seven different occupational groups that partici-pated at least once.

Table 4. Participation rate for different groups[a] in
the combined exploration of psychosocial environment
and cardiovascular risk factors

Occupational group	Participation rate (%)	
	Men	Women
Orchestral musicians	78	100
District nurses	—	98
Air-traffic controllers	66	81
Aeroplane mechanics	59	—
Baggage handlers	58	—
Physicians	53	74
Waiters	50	69

[a] The total number of participants was 208.

Women participated more often than men. The participation rate for men varied from 50% and 53% (waiters and physicians, respec-tively) to 78% (orchestral musicians). For women the corresponding numbers were 69%, 74% and 100% in the same groups. An important factor that explains some of the differences between the groups is the availability of a person who can take responsibility for all the follow-up contact work and blood samples. All groups that had a reliable contact person had very high participation rates. In our experience blue-collar workers are less interested in psychosocial factors than white-collar workers.

About half of the participants endured all four measurements. The participation rate varied slightly for different kinds of measurement: blood tests were more popular than questionnaires, and the least popular was self-measurement of blood pressure. The more activity required, the less people participated. Some interesting improve-ments in health parameters were observed among people who partici-pated four times (Table 5).

Table 5. Significant changes in risk factors in subjects who participated in four measurements during one year

| | Self-measured blood pressure at work (mmHg) | | Blood pressure measured by medical personnel after 10 minutes' rest (mmHg) | | Liver enzyme[a] | Smoking index[b] |
	Systolic (N = 79)	Diastolic (N = 77)	Systolic (N = 68)	Diastolic (N = 68)	(N = 110)	(N = 91)
Measurement 1	128.2	84.5	121.9	80.5	0.57	0.67
2	125.9	83.3	119.7	77.3	0.53	0.71
3	126.5	82.4	119.7	77.7	0.49	0.66
4	123.7	81.4	117.0	76.5	0.49	0.69
Analysis of variance, effect of measurement occasion	$P < 0.001$	$P < 0.01$	$P < 0.01$	$P < 0.01$	$P < 0.01$	NS
Interaction between measurement occasion and group (two-way analysis of variance)	NS[c]	NS	NS	NS	NS	$P < 0.03$

[a] Log blood concentration of glutamyl transferase.
[b] 0 = 0 cigarettes smoked per day; 1 = 1–3 cigarettes per day; 2 = 4–10 cigarettes per day; 3 = 11–20 cigarettes per day; 4 = > 20 cigarettes per day.
[c] NS = not significant.

The self-measured blood pressure levels at work and those measured conventionally (by trained personnel after 10 minutes' rest in the supine position) significantly decreased during the study. Subjects who had blood samples taken four times showed significant decreases in liver enzyme concentration. The smoking habits of the groups did not change in any consistent direction, but there were significant differences in the direction of change between the groups. The members of the group with the highest rate of smoking, waiters, decreased their smoking dramatically.

Subjects who participated four times in the measurement of blood pressure formed only 38% of the total study population. For liver enzymes the figure was 53%, and 44% for smoking. Still, we believe that the programme may be effective in promoting health. Of course, we cannot prove which components of the programme may be effective, but Glasgow et al. *(21)* have shown that self-monitoring of blood pressure may cause reductions by itself.

We do not yet know whether the programme induced any changes in the work environment itself. According to a follow-up survey in the group of subjects that participated in the fourth measurement (Table 6), the amount of discussion that arose at the different workplaces varied considerably. This group comprised 31% of the men and 25% of the women (or 94 men and 103 women).

Only 14% of the physicians participating claimed that the project induced discussions about the work environment, the lowest percentage of any group. The baggage handlers reported the highest percentage of discussion (35%). Perhaps this was because this group of low-status blue-collar workers was not used to such attention. One

Table 6. Participants in the fourth measurement who claimed that the combined exploration of psychosocial environment and cardiovascular risk factors triggered discussions about the work environment

Occupational group	Participants	
	Percentage	Number
Orchestral musicians	32	25
Air-traffic controllers	33	21
Physicians	14	29
Baggage handlers	35	17
Waiters	27	22
Aeroplane mechanics	21	19
District nurses	31	64

year after all the data had been collected and thus after all the groups had participated in group feedback, the participants were asked again whether discussions about conditions at work were taking place. Interestingly, discussions had increased; 28–61% of the participants in the different workplaces reported such discussions, and they also reported a significantly elevated level of skill discretion. Thus the whole procedure may have acted as a stimulus to some beneficial psychosocial changes, but we still do not know how durable these changes will be or what caused them (17).

This kind of study must be prepared well in advance and all parties involved, including employers, unions, and occupational safety and health committees, should not only be informed before the study starts but should also be prepared to implement changes if necessary. It is also important that recommendations be based on continual discussion with workers and not on sudden statements by experts. It is important to avoid making consultations that are entirely negatively focused. There are always positive aspects in the environment that can be explored and further developed.

Increasing Awareness

The occupational health care team deals both with the environment and the individuals in it. The interaction between them could be described as in Fig. 2.

It is important to differentiate the individual programme (the coping strategy) from the environment and from the reactions to an adverse situation. Reactions to the environment can be physiological, behavioural or psychological, or a combination of the three, and all of these can be either conscious or unconscious. The primary goal of the occupational health care team should be to increase the level of consciousness in all three categories and to strengthen the knowledge of the interaction between the environment and reactions to it. The principles of the study on cardiovascular risk factors could be used in several other situations, such as electromyographically recording muscular tension along with recordings of activities and feelings in daily life in the workplace, and generating protocols on eating habits, including detailed accounts of food intake and reasons for intake. These procedures can always be combined with observing the work environment.

An important aspect of Fig. 2 is that it emphasizes the dynamic character of the individual programme. New strategies will always

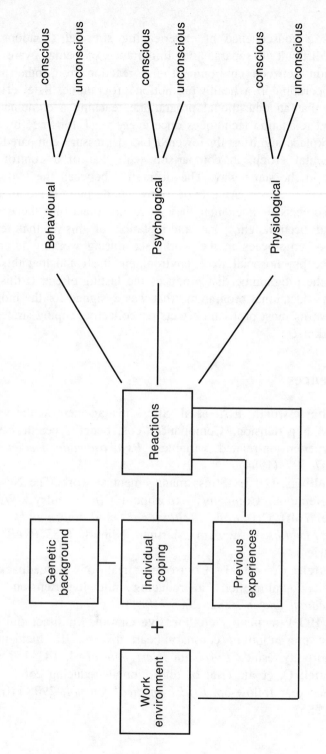

Fig. 2. Theoretical model of the interaction between the environment, the individual and his or her reactions

Source: Adapted from Kagan & Levi (22).

263

arise as a consequence of experiencing stressful situations. It is always difficult to separate the importance of being aware of the interaction between environment and reaction from other mechanisms operating in a health promotion programme. Patel et al. *(3)* showed that an educational programme teaching a combination of yoga and relaxation techniques once every week for three months in the workplace significantly lowered blood pressure compared in the experimental group, in comparison with that of a control group selected in the same way. The difference between the two groups persisted even after four years of follow-up, despite the fact that many of the subjects claimed that they were not practising the exercises they had been taught. One interpretation of this is that teaching groups of employees in the workplace during working hours may affect the psychosocial work environment itself and that this is the part of the programme that produces the lasting effect. If this is the case, an educational programme that was designed for the individual may have its most profound effects on collective coping strategies in the workplace.

References

1. **Charlesworth, E.A. et al**. Stress management at the worksite for hypertension. Compliance, cost–benefit, health care and hypertension-related variables. *Psychosomatic medicine*, **46**: 387–397 (1984).
2. **Collings, G., Jr.** Stress management at work. The New York Telephone Company experiment. *In*: Gentry, W.D. & de Wolff, C.J., ed. *Behavioral medicine: work, stress and health*. Amsterdam, Martinus Nijhoff, 1985 (NATO, ASI series).
3. **Patel, C. et al**. Controlled trial of biofeedback-aided behavioural methods in reducing mild hypertension. *British medical journal*, **282**: 2005 (1981).
4. **WHO European Collaborative Group**. Multifactorial trial in the prevention of coronary heart disease. III. Incidence and mortality results. *European heart journal*, **4**: 141–159 (1984).
5. **Patel, C. et al**. Trial of relaxation in reducing coronary risk: four year follow-up. *British medical journal*, **290**: 1103–1106 (1985).

6. **Alfredsson, L.** *Myocardial infarction and environment: use of registers in epidemiology.* Thesis, Stockholm, Karolinska Institute, 1983.

7. **Knox, S. et al.** The relation of social support and working environment to medical variables associated with elevated blood pressure in young males: a structural model. *Social science and medicine,* **21**: 525–531 (1985).

8. **Theorell, T. et al.** On the interplay between socioeconomic factors, personality and work environment in the pathogenesis of cardiovascular disease. *Scandinavian journal of work, environment and health,* **10**: 373–380 (1984).

9. **Alfredsson, L. et al.** Type of occupation and near future hospitalization for myocardial infarction and some other diagnoses. *International journal of epidemiology,* **14**: 378–384 (1985).

10. **Orth-Gomér, K. et al.** *Psychosocial factors and cardiovascular disease — a review of the current state of our knowledge.* Stockholm, National Institute for Psychosocial Factors and Health, 1983 (Stress Research Report No. 165).

11. **Johnson, J.** *The impact of workplace social support, job demands and work control upon cardiovascular disease in Sweden.* Stockholm, Department of Psychology, Division of Environmental and Organizational Psychology, University of Stockholm, 1986 (Report No. 1).

12. **Orth-Gomér, K. & Johnson, J.** Social network interaction and mortality. A six-year follow-up study of a random sample of the Swedish population. *Journal of chronic diseases,* **40**: 949–957 (1987).

13. **Johnson, J. et al.** Combined effects of job strain and social isolation on cardiovascular disease morbidity and mortality in a random sample of the Swedish male working population. *Scandinavian journal of work, environment and health,* **15**: 271–279 (1989).

14. **Wallin, L. & Wright, I.** Psychosocial aspects of the work environment: a group approach. *Journal of occupational medicine,* **28**: 384–393 (1986).

15. **Moser, V.** *A programme for teaching psychosocial aspects of the working environment.* Eskilstuna, Statshälsan, 1985.

16. *Efficiency, working environment and health.* Stockholm, Bygghälsan, 1984.

17. **Theorell, T. et al**. *Arbetstagarens egen kartläggning av arbetsmiljö och hjärt-kärlrisk — ett sätt att stimulera diskussion kring förbättring av den psykosociala arbetsmiljön* [The worker's own exploration of the work environment and risk of heart disease — one way of stimulating discussion about improving the psychosocial work environment]? Stockholm, Swedish Work Environment Fund, 1988.

18. **Schwartz, J. et al**. A procedure for linking psychosocial job characteristics data to health surveys. *American journal of public health*, **78**: 904–909 (1988).

19. **Arnetz, B. et al**. Suicide patterns among physicians related to other academics as well as to the general population. Results from a national long-term prospective study and a retrospective study. *Acta psychiatrica scandinavica*, **75**: 139–143 (1987).

20. **Theorell, T. et al**. Changes in job strain in relation to changes in physiological state — a longitudinal study. *Scandinavian journal of work, environment and health*, **14**: 189–196 (1988).

21. **Glasgow, M.S. et al**. Behavioral treatment of high blood pressure, II. Acute and sustained effects of relaxation and systolic blood pressure biofeedback. *Psychosomatic medicine*, **44**: 155–165 (1982).

22. **Kagan, A.R. & Levi, L**. Adaptation of the psychosocial environment to man's abilities and needs. *In*: Levi, L., ed. *Society, stress and disease. The psychosocial environment and psychosomatic diseases*. London, Oxford University Press, 1971, pp. 388–404.

12

Health promotion in hospitals

Carolyn I. Speros & Neil Sol

Hospitals in the United States are increasingly positioning themselves as the leading provider of health promotion services within the community. As consumer demand for health information and preventive services intensifies, hospitals are re-evaluating their traditional focus on sick care, and considering optional ventures that will mobilize and satisfy an expanding market of health-conscious, apparently well people.

Traditionalists argue that hospitals should maintain their long-established role as centres for acute care, relegating the responsibility for health promotion to the public health sector and other community agencies. Progressive hospital leaders, however, are establishing integrated health care systems as a strategy for long-term survival *(1)*. By diversifying and expanding their traditional revenue base, hospitals can increase their revenue from diversified services to offset the losses incurred by declining inpatient population, while assuring sufficient capital to provide high-technology, labour-intensive and costly acute care.

Hospitals are targeting health promotion and wellness services as a viable diversification strategy. In addition to the potential for generating revenue, health promotion activities contribute positively to patient satisfaction, the hospital's image within a community and relations with medical staff *(2, 3)*. Hospitals can benefit by taking an active and leading role in ensuring the good health of the community they serve.

In a statement on health promotion in 1979, the American Hospital Association *(4)* recommended the following:

> In addition to their primary mission of providing health care and related education to the sick and injured, hospitals have a responsibility to work with others in the community to assess the health status of the community, identify target health areas and population groups for hospital-based and cooperative health promotion programs, develop programs to help upgrade the health in those target areas, ensure that persons who are apparently healthy have access to information about how to stay well and prevent disease, provide appropriate health education programs to aid those persons who choose to alter their personal health behavior or develop a more healthful lifestyle, and establish the hospital within the community as an institution which is concerned about good health as well as one concerned with treating illness.

In today's health-conscious environment, physicians continue to be perceived as the primary source of useful and reliable health information, but few people are satisfied with the information they receive from their physicians *(5)*. Most people associate hospitals with physicians and transfer this perceived reliability and credibility to hospital-based activities. In many communities the hospital is identified as a centre for health. It seems likely, therefore, that people would want hospitals to take a leading role in health promotion.

In order to provide quality health information and guidance, hospital-based health promotion services are multidisciplinary, relying on the expertise of a variety of health professionals, typically physicians, nurses, physiotherapists, physiologists and nutritionists. Each member of the health care team works with individuals as inpatients, outpatients or in the community to assist them in achieving their health-related goals.

The professional practice standards established by many professional organizations specifically refer to the role and responsibilities of hospital-based practitioners in promoting health as an integral component of quality care. Many institutions include health education and health promotion responsibilities in performance standards, and evaluations, promotions and salary increases are then based on compliance with these standards. Because hospitals have not emphasized prevention and health promotion in the past, these standards serve as important reminders and incentives to the staff to look beyond treatment protocols.

Hospital-based health promotion programmes typically include patient education and counselling services, clinical rehabilitation

268

programmes, and community and corporate wellness services. All the activities in each programme area are consistent with the goals of health promotion and are designed to (4):

foster awareness, influence attitudes, and identify alternatives so that individuals can make informed choices and change their behavior in order to achieve an optimum level of physical and mental health and improve their physical and social environment.

Hospital-based health promotion programmes support individual efforts to achieve a state of optimal health and physical, mental and emotional wellbeing.

Patient Education

One of the earliest health promotion initiatives within a hospital was the establishment of formal programmes for patient education. The Joint Committee on Health Education Terminology (6) defined patient education as:

the health experiences designed to influence learning which occurs as a person receives preventive, diagnostic, therapeutic and/or rehabilitative services, including experiences which arise from coping with symptoms, referral to source of information, prevention, diagnosis and care, and contacts with health institutions, health personnel, family and other patients.

Patient education services include a variety of activities designed to inform patients about their illnesses and the effect of those illnesses on their daily lives, to prepare patients for diagnostic and treatment procedures and the experience of being in hospital, to assist patients in managing their diseases after discharge, and to modify their bahaviour to promote optimal health and prevent further illness.

The goal of patient education is to foster an active partnership between patients, their families and their health care providers so that collaborative decisions can be made about care, treatment plan, and lifestyle after discharge.

Many social factors led to the increased interest in patient education observed in the late 1960s and 1970s, including: the increased prevalence of chronic diseases requiring long-term and continuous management, often self-administered; a growing social concern about containing costs, the utilization of health services, and quality care; the consumer movement, public demand for influence in medical care decisions, and frustration with the complexities of the health care

269

delivery system; documented evidence that patient education helps attain treatment goals; legislation related to informed consent; and malpractice issues *(7)*. In response to these factors and others, supportive documents, mandates and guidelines have evolved to further entrench patient and family education as an integral component of quality care and professional practice in hospitals.

Patient education programmes are typically planned and coordinated at three levels within hospitals: the institutional level, involving the entire facility or hospital; the programmatic level, targeting specific patient populations or groups having a similar disease, in-hospital experience, or demographic characteristic; and the patient level, involving direct contact and interaction with the patient *(7)*.

The activities at each level directly affect people at the other levels. For example, an institution-wide policy that specifies the role of nursing service personnel in patient and family education can greatly support the bedside teaching activity conducted by nurses. Lesson plans developed for specific patient groups enhance the consistency of the patient teaching provided by a variety of care givers working with any one patient. Programme planning at all three levels enhances the quality and quantity of patient education and decreases the likelihood of duplication of effort and inefficient use of resources *(8)*.

Developing and designing a comprehensive inpatient education programme encompasses four sequential and interrelated steps: assessment of need, planning and objective setting, implementation and evaluation. Each step of this process has a different focus for each level of programming being considered.

In assessing the needs of institutions, existing policies, roles and responsibilities, resource allocation and the strategic goals of the organization must be assessed. At the programmatic level, disease profiles, staff capacities and medical staff idiosyncrasies must be analysed. At the patient level, the learning needs of patients and their families should be assessed, focusing on their current knowledge, skills and attitudes. A comprehensive needs assessment at any level of programming becomes the foundation and justification for the activities being planned.

After the needs of the institution, patient population or individual are assessed, a plan of action with specific and measurable objectives should be established. The objectives may be short- or long-term and should guide subsequent programme evaluation.

Throughout implementation, teaching must be documented in the medical record and evidence of learning must be monitored. Effective communication, both written and verbal, is critical. For institutions, communication between work groups and between providers such as physicians, nurses and pharmacists enhances receptivity to innovative programming strategies and new or revised policies and procedures. Skill in leading groups and communicating concepts and information is an essential part of teaching patients effectively.

Evaluation at the institutional level measures the success of the overall plan. The parameters often monitored are the satisfaction of patients, medical staff and providers, and quality audits related to documentation and compliance with predetermined standards of practice. For patients, behavioural outcome prior to discharge is the measure of successful intervention. At all levels of programming, the objectives of the plan form the basis for an effective evaluation system.

Many studies have demonstrated the benefits that patients realize from a planned and coordinated approach to patient education. Reductions in length in stay *(9–11)*, reductions in complications *(12, 13)*, and reductions in admissions and readmissions to hospital *(14, 15)* are the benefits to patients most widely documented in research on patient education.

Clinical Rehabilitation

Clinical rehabilitation programmes that incorporate exercise therapy and health education enhance the continuity of care and treatment of people moving from the inpatient unit to the outpatient unit or home treatment. Following the treatment and stabilization of an illness, a rehabilitation programme is designed to return the person to a level of health equal to or greater than the level before the illness. The goal of clinical rehabilitation programmes is to improve stamina and strength, return people to their homes and activities of daily living, and at the same time prevent recurrence of the illness or injury.

Clinical rehabilitation programmes typically provided by hospitals include: cardiac rehabilitation and pulmonary rehabilitation; exercise therapy to rehabilitate mental health patients and those suffering from substance abuse and eating disorders; and sports medicine.

Clinical rehabilitation programmes are discussed collectively in this chapter, but cardiac and pulmonary rehabilitation programmes are the best-established rehabilitation conducted at hospitals. They reduce risk factors, increase functional capacity, return individuals to work sooner, and reduce the incidence of heart disease (16). Exercise therapy for mental health and related problems has been initiated more recently. Early indications are that exercise is a prudent augmentation of traditional forms of treatment (17). Sports medicine programmes use aggressive forms of physical therapy, progressive resistance training, and education in prevention, to return the athlete to competition and other activities.

Clinical rehabilitation programmes begin with inpatients and continue when they become outpatients. These programmes provide a continuum of supervised care and treatment until the patient is trained in self-care skills and ready for discharge from the programme.

All patients must be referred to the clinical rehabilitation programme by their attending physician. Typically, the referring physician prescribes exercise and education. The success of clinical rehabilitation programmes depends on the patient's relationship with the referring physician. Physicians frequently resist referring their patients to rehabilitation programmes for fear of losing control of the treatment plan. The personnel of the rehabilitation programme are responsible for involving referring physicians in the rehabilitation process. Encouraging the physician to prescribe graded levels of exercise and education for the period of rehabilitation, and assuring periodic feedback and consultation with the physician encourage medical staff to support the programme.

Patient entry into rehabilitation usually begins with a physiological and medical evaluation. For example, in cardiac rehabilitation programmes, the patient undergoes a battery of tests that can include a graded exercise test, blood chemistry analysis, determination of body composition, and nutritional analysis (18). This information offers a baseline for developing an individualized prescription for exercise and education. Similar assessments are made for patients entering other types of rehabilitation programme. An exit evaluation is compared with initial test results, documenting the progress made.

Outpatient rehabilitation programmes vary in length. The period of time depends on: the physician order, the type of rehabilitation, the patient's response to the rehabilitation, the patient's motivation and interest, and the patient's ability to pay for the service (19).

To participate in a medically supervised programme, people must live within a reasonable distance of the rehabilitation site. Accessibility is a critical factor in adherence to the rehabilitation regimen. Often people live an unreasonable commuting distance from the hospital or rehabilitation centre. It is best to refer these people to a home rehabilitation programme.

Self-directed, home rehabilitation programmes are prudent alternatives to structured hospital-based programmes. Typically, the guide for the home programme is provided on discharge from the hospital. Rehabilitation professionals carefully educate people in exercise and lifestyle modification. Home programmes require frequent follow-up to evaluate progress, encourage adherence, and provide support.

Since professionals are not in direct contact with the patient, home programmes are less effective than supervised programmes in achieving rehabilitation. The disadvantages of home programmes are the risk of nonadherence, reliance on self-motivation, and the patient's fear of unsupervised activity. Peer camaraderie and the sense of security provided by trained personnel are strong advantages of participating in hospital-based rehabilitation programmes. Discharge criteria are established collaboratively by the patient, the physician and the rehabilitation team. These criteria depend on the type and severity of the patient's initial illness. Continuous documentation of patient progress is essential to determine appropriate discharge points. Clinical rehabilitation is a systematic and progressive process that assists individuals in making the transition from acute illness through recovery to an optimal state of health and fitness.

Community and Corporate Wellness

Motivated by changes in the market and potential new revenue, hospital decision-makers are targeting community and corporate wellness services as a form of diversification (20). As hospitals capitalize on growing consumer interest in health practices and fitness, they target the apparently well population for a variety of hospital-based health promotion services.

Wellness programmes are designed to educate and motivate individuals to reduce their risk of preventable diseases. By adopting healthy lifestyle practices, the individual decreases the risk of premature death and disability, and the costs associated with medical care. The enhanced community relations and direct revenue resulting from providing health promotion services can justify entry into the wellness arena for many hospitals.

Hospital-based programmes are typically directed at three audiences: apparently well groups or individuals within the community, employees of local businesses and industries (and their dependants), and the health professionals and other staff employed by the hospital. The programmes encompass a broad spectrum of activities and services, and are planned to address the health-related needs and interests of the target population.

Many hospitals with well established inpatient education and clinical rehabilitation programmes have moved quickly into the market for apparently well people. Inpatient education programmes focusing on disease management, self-care skills, and prevention have great appeal to nonpatient groups. By 1984, 67% of all hospitals in the United States offered some type of wellness programme for the community (21). This number is expected to increase as more hospitals recognize the potential benefits of a community-wide campaign.

The motives for hospitals to initiate a community wellness programme are varied and are based on the institution's outreach objectives. The objectives that can be attained include: improving the hospital's image, promoting specific services, recruiting physicians and marketing their services, and establishing a presence within a target service area (22).

Most community wellness services are marketed to individuals within the primary service area of the hospital. Many hospitals are segmenting their market, as they focus health promotion activities on specific groups such as women, old people and young people. Once the target population is identified, its health needs can be more precisely assessed. Segmenting the community in this manner facilitates advertising and promotional efforts, and enhances the meaning and value of the activity for the target audience.

A study by Miaoulis (23) profiled the health-seeker segment of the disease prevention and health promotion market. Health-seeking individuals actively participate in fitness programmes and frequently use preventive medical services. They tend to be opinion leaders for health-related issues, and thus stimulate positive health behaviour among other people. They are usually well educated and have high incomes. Designing hospital-based health promotion services for health-seekers helps to nurture a socially and medically desirable attitude among large numbers of people and leads to improved public health via word of mouth. In addition, it increases the satisfaction of health-seekers and prevents them from abandoning the traditional health care delivery system for alternative services that may be of questionable benefit.

Participation in these programmes also appears to be related to individual health status and how recently care was received at a hospital. People in fair or poor health and those who have been in hospital within the last three years are most likely to participate in hospital-based health promotion programmes (24).

The needs and interests of the target audience determine the components of the programme. Nutrition education, stress management, smoking cessation, cardiopulmonary resuscitation, aerobic exercise and prenatal education are a few of the typical popular offerings in the wellness market.

Activities and services should be designed to achieve three objectives: assessing the risks to the health of the individual or group, intervening appropriately, and providing continuing support to maintain healthy behaviour. Assessment is most often accomplished through appraisals of health risk. These are screening tools or programmes that identify individual health risks before illness or symptoms of disease become apparent. Assessment is based on a quantitative measurement of a variety of physiological, spiritual, psychological and sociological parameters related to health habits and lifestyle. These are combined to present a composite of the individual's risk of illness. Aggregate data for groups compiled from the assessment of health risks can be used to set priorities among intervention strategies.

A myriad of intervention strategies are used to modify unhealthy behaviour and practices. Health education classes and fitness activities, typically led by health care professionals, are designed to inform, motivate, and substitute healthy forms of behaviour for unhealthy ones. Health professionals from the hospitals, such as physiotherapists, nutritionists, exercise physiologists, nurses and counsellors, contribute their expertise in planning and developing wellness curricula. All intervention strategies are based on the results of the assessment, focusing on reducing risk factors and modifying behaviour.

Continuing support is crucial. In the past decade, 500 000 self-help groups have been formed in the United States, reaching more than 15 million people (25). More than half of all American hospitals currently sponsor or co-sponsor support or self-help programmes for individuals and their loved ones. Self-help groups provide education, counselling and peer support over an extended period of time, services that hospital departments typically cannot offer to patients whose stays are limited.

Hospitals can obtain several benefits by associating closely with such groups as Alcoholics Anonymous and Overeaters Anonymous (for people with substance abuse and eating disorders), Mended Hearts (for people recovering from open-heart surgery), and Resolve (for people afflicted with life-threatening illnesses). Some of the cost-effective ways that a hospital can support the work of a self-help organization are by offering space at the hospital for meetings, assigning health professionals on the staff to be guest speakers, and initiating referrals for episodic care. In return, the hospital realizes many benefits in its relations with patients and the public, inpatient referrals, and visibility in the community. Hospitals can thus redirect their resources to narrow the gap between patient needs and available medical services.

Many hospitals are able to reach their target group through existing networks in the community. Local YMCAs, churches, community agencies, and racket and health clubs offer promising opportunities for joint nventures with hospitals. The medical expertise and resources within a hospital are an attractive incentive for existing fitness programmes conducted through local agencies. Facilities that are suitable for recreational activities are often an investment too expensive for hospitals. Hospitals can join community agencies in offering health promotion programmes at locations that are convenient and accessible to the target population, decreasing duplication of service and reducing needless competition between other provider groups.

More and more employers are demonstrating a commitment to promoting the health of their employees, in the hope of reducing the spiralling costs associated with acute inpatient care. Many employers lack the number of employees needed to justify an in-house department of occupational medicine and health promotion, and are therefore contracting with local hospitals to provide the necessary medical expertise and resources to create a safe and healthy workplace environment (26).

Corporate health promotion programmes are designed to protect the health and safety of employees at the workplace, prevent

276

work-related illness and injury, and create an environment that promotes healthy living. Services hospitals often provide to employers include: environmental assessment of health hazards, screening for health problems related to specific work tasks, and education focused on preventing accident and injury. Other typical services include diagnosis and emergency care for work-related accidents, disability evaluation, and processing workers' compensation claims *(27)*.

A combination of occupational health and wellness services provided by hospitals at the workplace is a highly attractive alternative for employers considering offering a health promotion benefit to their employees. Companies view health promotion initiatives as a strategy to reduce costs. Combining occupational health and wellness services addresses the employees' perception that the company is interested in their wellbeing, and the employer's needs to cut the cost of episodic care. The goal of all health promotion programmes marketed to employers is to improve the relations between the hospital and employers, a critical need in today's health care marketplace. The private sector is demanding that health care costs be more effectively controlled. By promoting prevention, self-care and outpatient treatment, hospitals can actively help in containing health care costs, which is highly appealing to insurance companies and employers.

The hospital work environment presents unique challenges to health promotion programmes that target hospital workers. Burnout, inferior working conditions, rotating shifts, and frequent exposure to communicable diseases increase the hospital employee's risk of stress, disease and on-the-job injury.

Successful workplace health promotion programmes within hospitals are often linked directly to employee benefits, as the employee benefit plan provides incentives for participation. Top management must assure release time for participation and implement institution-wide policies that create a healthier working environment for the programme to be successful. The typical workplace health promotion activities provided to non-hospital employees can be supplemented by: banning smoking in designated areas of the hospital, educating staff about preventing back injury and controlling infection, and providing counselling services to employees so that they can better cope with grief, stress and burnout. A model initiative schedules activities around the clock, reaching all staff with risk-reducing activities that target the unique needs of hospital employees.

Benefits to Providers

Hospitals can realize numerous benefits by providing comprehensive health promotion services. It is essential, however, that the goals of the health promotion programme are linked to the goals of the hospital.

Health promotion programmes can improve the profitability of a hospital by generating new revenue *(28)*. Revenue from health promotion services can help replace revenues lost because of declining inpatient admissions.

Health promotion programmes also improve the community's image of the hospital *(29)*. Historically, this was the primary reason for hospitals to enter the health promotion arena. Hospitals provided free education and preventive services in an effort to fulfil their leadership role as providers of health promotion services. The outreach programmes continue to enhance awareness of the hospital and its medical staff.

Health promotion services help hospitals to obtain patients. Highly popular community screening programmes (health fairs) identify varying percentages (2.6–47.9%) of participants with abnormal test results *(30)*. These participants are typically referred to their physicians or to a physician on the staff at the sponsoring hospital. One hospital found that 1.5% of the participants screened at a health fair used hospital services or were admitted to the hospital within five months of the fair *(31)*.

Relations with medical staff are often improved through health promotion programmes. In areas with a surplus of physicians, hospitals have used community education and other health promotion services to market staff physicians' practices. Collaborative ventures between physicians with a preventive orientation and hospital-based health promotion programmes are becoming more common.

Conclusion

Many hospitals in the United States appear to be re-evaluating their mission as they begin to provide disease prevention and health promotion services. Prompted by people frustrated with the cost and complexities of the traditional system of health care delivery, hospitals are instituting nontraditional services oriented towards consumer education, self-care, rehabilitation and wellness.

278

Because hospitals have been slow to enter the health promotion arena, there has been little research to support the benefits of diversification. Early indications, however, are that hospital-based health promotion initiatives can save money and improve the quality of health care.

The long-term effect of the commitment of hospitals to health promotion will only be realized if health care professionals begin to enter hospitals oriented towards prevention. The success of a programme directly depends on the values and skills of the physicians, nurses and other health professionals who provide the services. Hospitals that actively recruit this new breed of practitioner, and that manage the programmes in a customer-oriented way will be leaders in the health care system of the future.

References

1. **Coddington, D. et al**. Strategies for survival in the hospital industry. *Harvard business review*, **63**(3): 129–138 (1985).
2. **Ardell, D.B**. And what's in it for the hospital. *Promoting health*, **1**(1):1–2 (1980).
3. **Kernaghan, S. & Giloth, B**. *Working with physicians in health promotion*. Chicago, American Hospital Publishing, 1983.
4. *Policy and statement on the hospital's responsibility for health promotion*. Chicago, American Hospital Association, 1979.
5. **Seuntjens, A**. The role of hospitals in health promotion: an administrative diagnosis. *Hospital and health services administration*, **28**(4): 73–84, (1983).
6. **Joint Committee on Health Education Terminology**. New definitions: report of the 1972–1973 Joint Committee on Health Education Terminology. *Health education monographs*, **33**: 63–69 (1973).
7. **Deeds, S. et al**. *A model for patient education programming*. Washington, DC, APHA Public Health Education Section, 1979.
8. *Policy and statement — the hospital's responsibility for patient education services*. Chicago, American Hospital Association, 1982.
9. **Devine, E.C. & Cook, T.D**. A meta-analytical analysis of effects of psychoeducational interventions with surgical patients. *Nursing research*, **32**: 267–274 (1983).

10. **Evans, R. & Robinson, G**. An economic study of cost savings on a care-by-parent ward. *Medical care*, **21**: 768–782 (1983).

11. **Fuqua, L**. Diabetes care and education: a creative approach. *In*: Bartlett, E.E. & Peples, D. ed. *Patient education: a solution to the challenge of prospective payment*. Birmingham, AL, University of Alabama, 1983.

12. **Karam, J. et al**. A cost/benefit analysis of patient education. *Hospital and health services administration*, **31**(4): 82–90 (1986).

13. **Lane, D. & Liss-Levenson, W**. Education and counselling for cancer patients. *Patient counselling and health education*, **2**(4): 154–160 (1980).

14. **Alogna, M**. CDC diabetes control programs — overview of diabetes patient education. *Diabetes educator*, **10**: 32–36 (1985).

15. **Assal, J.P. et al**. Patient education as the basis for diabetes care in clinical practice and research. *Diabetologia*, **28**: 602–613 (1985).

16. **Fox, S.M. III, ed**. *Coronary heart disease — prevention, detection, rehabilitation with emphasis on exercise testing*. Denver, International Medical Corporation, 1974.

17. **Dishman, R.K**. Medical psychology in exercise and sport. *Medical clinics of North America*, **69**: 123–143 (1985).

18. **American College of Sports Medicine**. *Guidelines for exercise testing and prescription*. Philadelphia, Lea & Febiger, 1985.

19. **Wilson, P.K., ed**. *Adult fitness and cardiac rehabilitation*. Baltimore, MD, University Park Press, 1975.

20. **Moore, B**. CEO's plan to expand home health, outpatient services. *Hospitals*, **59**(1): 74–77 (1985).

21. **Ross, C. et al**. Health promotion programs flourishing: survey. *Hospitals*, **59**(16): 128–135 (1985).

22. *Community health promotion resource kit*. Chicago, American Hospital Association, 1984.

23. **Miaoulis, G**. Benefit segmentation for health promotion. *In*: *Proceedings of the Conference of the Association for Consumer Research in Health Care*. Ann Arbor, MI, Association for Consumer Research, 1982.

280

24. **Jensen, J. & Heitbrink, R**. Consumer interest in health programs often related to individuals' health. *Modern healthcare*, **17**(2): 56–57 (1987).
25. *Sharing/caring*. Chicago, American Hospital Association, 1987.
26. **Gardner, S. et al**. Big business embraces alternate delivery. *Hospitals*, **59**(6): 81–84 (1985).
27. **Bader, B. et al**. *Planning hospital health promotion services for business and industry*. Chicago, American Hospital Publishing, 1982.
28. **Sol, N**. Defining the measure of success. *Optimal health*, **3**(3): 8–9 (1987).
29. **Sweeny-Bills, S**. In crowded market, hospitals look to wellness for competitive edge. *Promoting health*, **5**(1): 1–3 (1984).
30. **Berwick, D**. Screening in health fairs. *Journal of the American Medical Association*, **254**(11): 1492–1498 (1985).
31. **Sol, N. & Speros, C**. Health fairs: a lucrative product. *Optimal health*, **1**(1): 24–26 (1984).

Part IV

Population-oriented health promotion

13

Promoting
women's health

Lesley Doyal

The move towards health-promoting policies that has been documented elsewhere in this book is potentially of great value to women. Indeed, empowering people through creating a healthier environment, more effective support networks and better educational programmes has been a priority of feminist health activists since the early 1970s *(1,2)*. The particular needs of women, however, have received very little attention so far in the establishment of health promotion policies. Most medical decisions are still made by the male doctors controlling the medical establishment, and health promotion policies are being created mainly by men, many of whom have little awareness of the lives of the women for whom decisions are being made.

If this situation is to change, the effect of gender on health needs to be more carefully explored and the findings will have to be incorporated into policy-making. This will necessitate creating a more accurate information base about women's health and developing a better understanding of the relationship between women's health and the social and economic roles of women. Women also need to be more directly involved in both formulating and implementing health promotion strategies to reap the greatest possible benefit from these new developments.

Methodological Problems in Explaining Women's Health and Illness

Traditional approaches to women's health have been based on the biomedical model. Doctors are defined as the experts and medical knowledge is the only acceptable form of expertise. As a result, very little attention has been paid to the social or environmental aspects of women's ill health. Where sex differences have been explored, the focus has been on the physical differences between male and female reproductive systems, or on assumed differences between male and female psychology. If health promotion policies are to be effective for women or for men, they must be based on more accurate information about the relationship between health and gender roles.

In developing an information base, existing epidemiological knowledge must be critically assessed to find any systematic bias in the way research is done. Alcoholism is a recent example of such work. Several studies *(3,4)* have pointed out that: men and women do not experience alcoholism similarly, their reasons for drinking are often different, the physiological consequences vary, and society reacts to drinking by males and females in different ways. Yet these issues are largely overlooked in planning prevention and treatment strategies and in evaluating their outcomes.

A very different example is the debate about the causes of cervical cancer. In the 1860s it was discovered that nuns almost never contracted cervical cancer while prostitutes relatively often did. This apparently misled generations of epidemiologists into thinking that women's sexual habits — their promiscuity — were entirely to blame for the disease *(5)*. The sexual activity of the male partners of cervical cancer victims has only recently received any attention at all, despite clear evidence about the etiology of other sexually transmitted diseases. As a result, thousands of women have been made to feel guilty and responsible for contracting a distressing and sometimes fatal disease. Committed delving on the part of Jean Robinson *(6)* — a feminist without formal epidemiological training — has also uncovered evidence that had been around for at least 50 years that links some cervical cancers with certain female occupations but also, very importantly, with the jobs of the victims' male partners. These two examples indicate the need to look carefully at existing epidemiological findings to identify the assumptions doctors tend to make about women when investigating their health and illness. Research that ignores real differences between the sexes or makes erroneous judgements about women's lives is unlikely to succeed in producing knowledge beneficial to women's health.

In creating the information base necessary for health promotion, women's experiences, both of their own health and of the health problems of others, should be given much greater status in what is effectively a hierarchy of knowledge. Almost every time people visit a doctor they are reminded that there are two kinds of knowledge — clinical expertise and their own common-sense experience — and the former is given much more prestige than the latter. This is especially true for women, who are often allowed even less credibility than men in similar circumstances. The height of absurdity this can reach is illustrated by a true story from a book by Ann Oakley *(7)*. A doctor commented to a pregnant woman that she already had a boy and a girl. When the woman replied that she had two girls the doctor said, "Really, are you sure?", and checked his notes. Of course the doctor immediately recognized his mistake, but that is not the point. His training led him to believe that his clinical knowledge was superior and only the absurdity of the example forced him to admit his error. If health promotion policies are to maximize women's wellbeing, they will need to take women's knowledge and experience seriously. This is not to suggest that there is no place for expertise, but rather that privileged status should not automatically be given to formal medical knowledge in all circumstances.

It is obvious but frequently forgotten that people who have experienced a health problem often understand it better than people who have not. They may not fully grasp the physiology or bio-chemistry of the condition (though some people develop as great a clinical understanding as their doctors), but they often have greater knowledge of the day-to-day experience of their particular health problem and how to manage it most effectively. This is reflected in the success of the many self-help groups of fellow sufferers that have developed both inside and outside the women's movement, where individuals help each other to deal with the health problems they have in common *(8)*. It is especially important for health planners to tap this experiential knowledge from women, for two reasons.

First, men have created most medical knowledge, so that when men speak about specifically female conditions, they by definition do not really know anything about the subjective aspects of these conditions. For example, men may downgrade the importance of such conditions as thrush or cystitis, which are not life-threatening but may be extremely important for a woman's perception of herself and her sexuality. Women's experiences of illness may also be different from men's, even when they suffer from the same disease, since society often treats sick men and sick women differently. It is essential that women's knowledge be incorporated into strategies for health promotion.

Second, and most important, women provide most of the care giving in society, and this has given them substantial practical knowledge about such normal procedures as pregnancy and child-birth, and the changes of childhood, adolescence, and aging (9, 10). Women have also developed valuable skills in caring for chronically ill people and in enabling people who will never be fully healthy in the normally accepted sense to live as well and as happily as possible, given their disabilities. Effective promotion policies must incorporate these devalued skills and often denigrated "folk knowledge". At the same time, however, this knowledge and the responsibility that goes with it must be more widely diffused in society, moving particularly from women to men. Otherwise women's skills may be increasingly recognized and exploited but women will not achieve any greater status or reward for their care giving and nurturing activities. Indeed, such a pragmatic recognition of women's skills could simply add to their existing burden of work, thereby limiting rather than promoting their health. It is therefore important that women's own experience, knowledge and skills become a valued part of the information base of health promotion policies, without ignoring the implications this might have for women's health.

In constructing new sources of information on women's health, official statistics and other measures to assess health status must be improved. Official medical statistics are deficient, particularly because they measure sickness rather than positive health. They are especially inadequate, however, in assessing the health status of women — a point that has received much less attention (11 – 14).

In many developing countries where statistics are rudimentary, the deaths of female children and even adult women are less likely to be recorded than those of men, and chronic illness is less likely to be reported. Conditions such as nutritional anaemia or chronic pelvic infection may simply be seen as a woman's lot (15). Even in countries where data are collected more systematically, knowledge about women's health is still insufficient. Many women do not work outside the home or do so only part time, and this effectively excludes them from statistics on absence from work because of illness or on industrial injury compensation. Nevertheless, women's labours can certainly cause ill health. Exhaustion and depression are both likely consequences of child care and housework, especially on a low budget, but are unlikely to be recorded in any statistics. Domestic violence may be an even more immediate threat to women's health at home, but the few cases that are reported are recorded as crime rather than in health statistics. It is therefore important to expand the concept of health hazard to include the other forms of violence and sexual harassment to which women are frequently subjected. Even when married women are working full time outside the home, the effect of work on their health may be obscured because women's occupation is often missing on medical reports or death certificates. Instead, the occupation of the husband is often recorded, making it difficult to link a woman's employment and her health. Official statistics in most countries are still based on an outmoded view of the role of women and of the causes of their ill health.

Similar problems arise in statistics on reproductive hazards. In most countries maternal mortality continues to be emphasized. While this is still a very important indicator in developing countries, in developed countries the risk of dying in childbirth is now extremely small, even among the most impoverished women. Yet maternal mortality continues to be the major focus of official concern. Deaths from legal abortions and contraception, however, have been ignored by most official statistics. One British epidemiologist, Valerie Beral *(16)*, has recently proposed a new measure: the reproductive mortality rate. This would include deaths from complications of contraceptive use and those from pregnancy and abortion, providing a more accurate index of the real reproductive risks women face. The potential value of this measure is obvious; in the United Kingdom, at least, this reproductive mortality rate appears to have risen since 1960 for women aged 35–44 years, largely because of the higher mortality caused by oral contraceptives. Promoting women's health means examining the total price they pay for their reproductive freedom, looking beyond the traditional measures that have preoccupied doctors, and taking into account the wider aspects of women's lives.

It is paradoxical that, in most countries, women now have a longer mean life expectancy than men, yet women use most medical services more than males, and also report more chronic illness and restricted activities *(17)*. Thus statistics that concentrate on mortality are even more inadequate for women than they are for men. This greater incidence of chronic ill health stems in part from women's greater longevity, but the resulting problems of old age have little visibility in official statistics. Robine & Colvez *(18)* stressed the crudity of measures such as life expectancy, pointing out that for women in particular, a surprisingly large part of their longer life was spent in poor health with some degree of disability.

Finally, because health statistics tend to concentrate on the harder, more immediately discernible and easily measurable diseases, they provide little information about mental illness. In most countries, women use more psychiatric services than men *(19,20)*. More women seek help for emotional problems and more are prescribed tranquillizers *(21)*. Yet official statistics help little in understanding this phenomenon. Women who contact the psychiatric services are presented as numbers of cases grouped into conventional psychiatric categories, but almost nothing is known about the subjective experiences behind such labelling — what the symptoms mean to women *(22)*.

Existing evidence about women's health and illness thus has to be interpreted with care. Despite these methodological difficulties, sociologists, psychologists and anthropologists are now beginning to explore the numerous factors influencing women's health, and are moving beyond the narrow medical concern with women's biological characteristics to examine the effect of women's roles as wives, mothers and workers on their experiences of health and illness. These developments are exemplified by current research on three areas of women's lives: reproduction, domestic labour and paid work. All three are important in formulating effective health promotion policies.

Women, Health and Reproduction

The capacity to conceive and give birth is fundamentally important at some stage in the lives of most women. For women involved in heterosexual relationships, the capacity to control their fertility is a central aspect of their autonomy and wellbeing. Nevertheless, both heterosexual and lesbian women may see voluntary motherhood as a vital element in their healthy development. While birth control and

288

childbearing are ultimately biological processes, they are also strongly influenced by social and economic circumstances and by available medical services, and must therefore be considered in the planning of policies to promote women's health (23).

The use of birth control has increased dramatically in most countries since the Second World War, and in the last 20 years new and more effective methods have been developed — oral contraceptives and the intrauterine device (IUD) in particular. Abortion has also been legalized in many countries (24), and sterilization has become an increasingly popular method of birth control for both men and women (25). This increased availability of fertility control has certainly benefited many women, as the more equal spacing of children reduces the health risks of pregnancy for the mother (26). Just as important, women who can choose how many (if any) children to have, when to have them and with whom have much more control over their lives and therefore over their physical and mental health (2,27).

Nevertheless, many women are still unable to obtain these potential benefits of fertility control. In developing countries, few women have access to modern methods (28,29). Even in the developed countries, these services are not equally available to everyone, as regional and class differences in access often persist (30). The services of family planning clinics are not always available to people without money. Many clinics have inconvenient opening hours and are bureaucratic and insensitive in their approach, not taking the needs of individual women seriously (31). Access to safe abortion can pose even greater problems. Induced abortion is now the most common form of birth control in most developing countries. Yet many women have to resort to illegal and unhygienic procedures that may result in permanent physical or psychological damage or even death. Again, even in the developed countries, services may be inadequate. In some countries abortion remains illegal, while in others the removal of legal obstacles has still left financial and moral barriers (32).

The women who have gained access to fertility control have often done so at considerable cost to their health and wellbeing (23,33). Despite their effectiveness, the new methods of birth control have considerable disadvantages (34). The IUD, for example, requires uncomfortable or even painful medical procedures to insert it, while oral contraceptives involve daily medication for otherwise healthy women. Some countries use less invasive techniques for abortion (for instance, vacuum extractions performed on an outpatient basis (35)), but in other countries the norm continues to be more stressful inpatient abortions requiring general anaesthesia (36).

These disadvantages are magnified by the fact that women are using powerful contraceptive methods for much longer periods than ever before. As a result, concern is now growing that women may suffer long-term effects that are not yet evident. The use of an IUD, for instance, has been associated with an increased risk of pelvic infection, leading in rare cases to death or sterility (37). This kind of evidence has sparked criticism of the development and evaluation of birth control methods. As in other fields of medical and scientific activity, contraceptive research continues to be dominated by men — many of them working for private drug companies. This has introduced a serious bias into decisions about which contraceptives should be developed and ultimately marketed (31). In particular, women's interests and feelings are not taken seriously and most of the side effects might not be so easily dismissed if men were the users (38).

The increasing use of oral contraceptives illustrates some of these issues. Oral contraceptives are extremely effective in preventing pregnancy and doctors usually regard them as the most scientific method. In the late 1960s, however, questions were raised about the role of oral contraceptives in causing cancer and circulatory disease. It was revealed that there had been serious deficiencies in the evaluation of most contraceptive drugs. Although their efficacy in preventing conception had been carefully tested, much less effort had been made to assess the wider effect on the user's health. In particular, there had been no research on the effects on women of taking the pill during their entire reproductive lives.

A study of some 46 000 women in the early 1970s in the United Kingdom showed that the risk of dying from circulatory disease was nearly five times greater for women who used oral contraceptives than for women who did not (39). The greatest risk is for women over 35 years of age, women who have taken oral contraceptives for at least five years and women who smoke cigarettes (40). More recent research has also implicated long-term use in an increased risk of breast cancer and cervical cancer (41,42). While the significance of these studies is currently debated, it seems certain that oral contraceptives pose a significant threat to the health of some women. But oral contraceptives affect many more women in less serious but still important ways. The so-called side effects include depression, loss of libido, headaches, nausea and excessive weight gain *(39)*. Significantly, these symptoms have received little attention from researchers or doctors, who often write them off as "all in the mind" or "the price you pay for effective birth control", although 85% of contraceptive users interviewed in Great Britain reported unpleasant side effects from either oral contraceptives or an IUD *(38)*.

In practice, then, new methods of birth control free more women from unwanted pregnancies, but reducing the risks of multiple childbearing has generated new hazards to health. The medical establishment has gained more control over women, medicalizing normal processes in their lives, sometimes to the detriment of their physical and psychological wellbeing *(43)*. Health promotion policies that take women's needs seriously need to provide more appropriate and safer techniques, as well as readily available and sensitive services designed not just to limit pregnancies but to enhance women's freedom of choice.

Similar safety and autonomy issues have been raised in obstetrics. In the developed countries, childbirth is now much safer than it was 100 years ago *(44)*, yet consumer dissatisfaction with doctors is particularly great in this area. Over the last decade, concern has been growing about the direction of care during pregnancy and childbirth, and many lay people and some doctors now agree that current trends in obstetrics are a mixed blessing *(7,45, 46)*.

The place of birth, the participants and the techniques used have all changed to affect profoundly the experiences of both mothers and babies. Two hundred years ago, childbirth was exclusively women's business, taking place in the home and usually attended by female friends and relatives and a midwife. This pattern still prevails in developing countries, but in most developed countries births have been moved out of the home, with 95–100% of babies now being born in hospital. As a result, the subjective experiences and the social relationships involved in giving birth have been significantly altered. Pregnancy and childbirth have been medicalized and treated as abnormal and pathological processes requiring the intervention of an expert to prevent possible disaster. All women are assumed to be at risk and are treated accordingly *(7,47)*.

The techniques employed in the birth process have also changed. While there were few technical developments in obstetrics in the first half of the twentieth century, the active management of labour has developed in the last 20 years *(46)*. The use of new interventionist techniques is flourishing, but they can sometimes be hazardous to health. While induction is of obvious value in a few cases, its widespread use may create new problems for both mother and child. Extensive research connects induction with an increased incidence of premature labour, fetal distress, jaundice and maternal infections *(46)*. Even more alarmingly, perhaps, induction appears to multiply the existing risks by increasing the need for further active intervention including pain relief and operative deliveries.

Lay people have responded broadly to these technological developments. For many women (and their partners), both antenatal care and labour itself have been rendered routine, creating an automated atmosphere for what should be an important and personal experience. Moreover, the organization of hospital care after birth often reinforces these feelings. Inflexible routines can mean the separation of mother and baby, making emotional bonding and breastfeeding more difficult and possibly affecting future family relationships. A highly technological and medicalized childbirth may also contribute to postnatal depression. Doctors usually assume that negative feelings after childbirth are abnormal and a sign of pathology. All mothers are expected to be delighted, and medical explanations have been sought when these positive feelings are not evident. A study *(7)* in England found that 84% of first-time mothers experienced depression, anxiety or other negative feelings in the first weeks after childbirth. Thus, postnatal depression was not unusual in this sample but normal.

Oakley *(7)* points out that a highly controlled and alienating experience during labour may make adjusting to the new role of mother much more difficult. The role of mother itself may be both physically and psychologically stressful. The new mother is often exhausted and in some pain, and has to cope with continual demands from the baby and long periods of broken sleep. These problems are compounded for many women by their lack of experience of looking after babies and their serious anxiety about their capacity to do so. Above all, perhaps, many women become housewives for the first time and experience the associated loss of status, autonomy and independent income. Thus, the experiences of pregnancy and childbirth and their aftermath are often contradictory in their effects; the child gained is sometimes offset by the enormous social, economic and emotional adjustments that women have to make in accepting the conventional role of motherhood *(48, 49)*. These wider factors must be taken into account if policies designed to promote the health of mothers are to achieve the maximum possible success.

Health workers and others must accept the decision of women who want to remain childless. Womanhood should not be equated with motherhood, and for women to achieve a state of positive mental health a variety of options, including childlessness, must remain open. For women who are involuntarily infertile, however, childlessness may be a source of enormous distress (50,51). In the developed countries, techniques such as in vitro fertilization and surrogate motherhood are now receiving significant attention, but serious reservations have been expressed about these new developments (52,53). First, women are not being adequately consulted about how these important new techniques are developed and used. As in other areas of reproductive technology, too many decisions are being made about women's bodies without the real participation of women at either a collective or an individual level. Second, these new developments tend to draw attention away from the basic causes of infertility and attempts to prevent them. Untreated gynaecological disease, pelvic infection from using an IUD, and exposure to certain industrial chemicals can all cause infertility. Yet few countries have developed programmes to prevent this devastating loss for many women (54).

Health Hazards of Housework

The home is usually perceived as a place of rest and recovery from the stresses and strains of the world outside. For most men and older children this is reasonably accurate but, for women, home is also a workplace for most of their waking (and sometimes their sleeping) hours. Women perform millions of hours of domestic work every day, but most of it is invisible and goes largely unacknowledged. Very little is known about this labour or the conditions under which it is performed, yet it clearly affects women's health.

Housework comprises the tasks performed for all members of the household, particularly shopping, cooking, cleaning and washing. Despite the increased availability of domestic appliances, housework can still be physically demanding, sometimes causing accidents or contact with many largely unregulated household chemicals (55,56). A housewife may also be at risk from hazards from her partner's place of work, such as the contamination of clothes by asbestos fibres or radiation. As mentioned earlier, one cause of cervical cancer may be substances to which men are occupationally exposed, which are then passed on to women during sexual intercourse (5). Thus, the home is not necessarily a haven free from the chemical hazards of the workplace. More research is needed to identify these dangers and more effective regulation to control them.

Childcare is an important part of women's domestic work. The content and intensity of this work vary over a woman's life cycle and some never do it at all. The vast majority of women become mothers, however, and this usually means that they are responsible for feeding, clothing, nurturing and socializing children until they are able to fend for themselves. This can be immensely rewarding, but it can also be very physically and emotionally demanding (57,58). Moreover, a woman's role as a care giver is not confined to children but may include others, usually relatives, who are sick, disabled or otherwise dependent. For some women, this may offer significant satisfaction, but it can also block their participation in the labour force or in leisure activities, often imposing a major strain on their wellbeing (9,59,60).

It is a significant consideration in family mental health that most women are also responsible for what has been called emotional housework. Women must deal with the stresses and strains of other family members and hold together both individuals and the group when emotional wellbeing or stability are threatened. It is mainly women who are responsible for satisfying their families' needs, nurturing and caring for them, and compensating for their pains and frustrations (61–64). These responsibilities inevitably multiply as family members find more of their needs unmet in societies in which jobs are scarce and many services are either impersonal, inhuman or nonexistent. The present division of labour between the sexes often means that no one takes the responsibility to care for women's emotional needs and to provide support and nurture. As a result, promoting women's mental health can be a complex and difficult task.

A majority of housewives surveyed in England considered the main advantage of their job to be negative: freedom from the constraints of paid work (65). They avoided the need to clock on or to obey the orders of a supervisor. Nevertheless, few housewives liked the actual tasks involved, most of which were described as monotonous, repetitive, boring and fragmented, and the results of the tasks were only noticed by others when they had not been carried out. Many of the interviewees also mentioned the lack of respect and social worth accorded to housewives. Absence of pay and lack of status were clearly interconnected, making it difficult for the women to generate a positive sense of themselves or their capacities. In addition, many felt that the isolation and the absence of adult relationships made it difficult to achieve a positive self-image as an adult person. Not surprisingly, both clinical experience and community research have shown that many housewives experience intense frustration, which is usually expressed in feelings of emptiness, sadness and worthlessness (66,67). These feelings often go unrecognized but, when they reach a certain stage, they may be brought to the attention of a doctor and labelled depression.

The strains of domestic work and childcare are, of course, greatest under conditions of poverty. Many women face a constant struggle to make ends meet on a low income, since they are primarily responsible for managing the family budget. These women are also most affected by inferior housing and are likely to get an unequal share of food and other resources within the family (68–70). The health of single mothers is especially threatened, since so many have low incomes. The continuing wage differentials between men and women make it difficult for most women to get reasonably paid jobs. This problem is compounded by the lack of jobs with suitable hours and the scarcity of childcare, which can force women back on to state benefits. As a result, most single mothers have to cope with poverty as well as the physical and mental exhaustion of raising children entirely alone. Many women find it difficult to sustain their health and wellbeing under such conditions.

Many women return to a low income in old age. Women's greater life expectancy means that an increasing number are still alive when their partners die and many have few means of material or social support (71). For older women, the aging process is compounded by loss of fertility, of the youthfulness that society values so highly in women, and of children, friends and partners. Older women's sexuality is also consistently ignored as they become less socially visible after the menopause. Doctors have tried to treat menopausal symptoms — another illustration of the medicalization of women's lives (72,73). Nevertheless, the effect of the social and economic aspects of aging on women's health has hardly been explored, despite the great increase in the proportion of older women in the population. Research and action are both urgently needed if the health of this group of women with great needs is to be successfully promoted (74).

Is Paid Work Good for Women's Health?

More women are employed outside the home than ever before. In most of the developed countries women comprise between 30% and 40% of the labour force, and these numbers are rising throughout the world. An increasing number of women are married, and many have young children. This has raised questions about the effect of paid work on women's health and wellbeing and, in recent years, there has been more research on this issue (75–80).

These new research initiatives suggest that paid work can have both damaging and beneficial effects. The balance will vary depending on other aspects of a woman's life: whether she is alone or with a partner, whether she has children, her income and her educational level. These issues can be explored by examining the ways paid work can promote women's health.

Many researchers have emphasized the protective effect for health of being employed compared with being a full-time housewife (66). Employment outside the home can provide self-esteem, companionship and a wide network of social contacts. As poverty is a significant cause of ill health, paid work can also be essential to a woman's material health and wellbeing, and can promote her independence and autonomy within the family. Very few studies have translated rates of labour force participation into patterns of physical health and illness, but one important study in the United Kingdom shows the beneficial effects of paid work on the incidence of both acute and chronic morbidity, as measured by self-reported symptoms and visits to a general practitioner (81). Married women with children who took paid work had better physical health than housewives. Despite these obvious advantages, paid work can potentially damage women's health.

Many more women are now working in industry, contacting for the first time hazards some men (and a few women) have been facing for decades (82). Although women rarely enter the most hazardous industries, such as coal mining, many are still threatened by hazardous chemicals, dust, fumes and other toxic substances in the workplace. There is little evidence of the number of women exposed to particular substances, but the overall figures are substantial.

Women commonly work in the textile industry, for instance; there are about 160 000 female textile workers in the United Kingdom alone. Yet this work can be extremely dangerous to health, causing several lung diseases. Textile workers are also at risk from the

296

chemicals used in processing and dyeing the cloth. Formaldehyde, a suspected carcinogen, is widely used, as are other chemicals that are likely to induce allergies and industrial dermatitis. Women in the electronics industry are also being exposed to new hazards (83). The industry has an image of cleanliness and safety, but many dangerous chemicals are used by its predominantly female labour force. Organic solvents such as xylene and trichloroethylene are used extensively and cause many health problems. As women continue to move into technologically advanced industries, they will be exposed (along with male colleagues) to still more potentially hazardous substances; but in most countries, health and safety legislation does not guarantee their wellbeing (84).

Occupational hazards threaten the unborn children of employed women (85). Certain chemicals such as lead are a serious hazard to reproduction and the exposure of women is subject to legal controls. Nevertheless, not enough is known about the risks of thousands of other chemicals already in use. Studies in Finland, for instance, have shown that women working in certain sectors of the plastics, electronics and pharmaceutical industries all have an increased rate of miscarriage, but the reason is not known (86). In most countries, when a woman gives birth to a stillborn or deformed child her job is not recorded and the effects of these dangerous chemicals are thus difficult to trace. Existing protective legislation is not effective in enabling women to avoid these risks and needs to be re-evaluated to promote effectively the health of female employees and their children (23).

Caring for the sick is traditionally a female occupation, but paradoxically it can damage the health of the care giver, illustrating many of the problems discussed previously. Thousands of nurses suffer serious back injuries every year by lifting heavy patients without the equipment that would probably be available in a factory. They are also at risk from toxic chemicals. Antibiotics, detergents, disinfectants and sterilizing fluids can all be hazardous. The drugs used to treat cancer can be especially dangerous unless adequate precautions are taken, and overexposure to radiation or to anaesthetic gases can cause miscarriages and birth defects. Nevertheless, hospitals are usually assumed to be healthy places and safety precautions are often limited.

Nursing can also be psychologically stressful, partly because of the inevitable strain of caring for sick people, but also because of the work conditions in many hospitals (87). Hospitals are often under-staffed, so that work is speeded up and nurses feel unable to care properly for patients. In some countries, nurses have low pay and little status but are expected to take on substantial responsibility. Stress and anxiety can result, and one symptom of this is the high rates of smoking among nurses (88). Perhaps contrary to popular imagination, a study in the United States found that nurses had more mental health problems than most other occupational groups (89).

There are similar hazards to health in the office, another tradition-ally female workplace (90). Chemical hazards abound, including solvents, correcting and cleaning fluids, and badly ventilated photo-copying machines. The new technology designed to save labour in the office has also been criticized for its effects on health (91, 92). The operators of visual display units experience eye problems, nausea and headaches after continuous periods of work. Many women are also stressed by their position in the office hierarchy. Most are restricted to dead-end jobs with little independence and low pay. Many com-plain that they are treated as inferior — as children, whatever their age. A significant number also report sexual harassment by male col-leagues, a demeaning experience that often leads to symptoms of stress and a general deterioration in wellbeing (93, 94).

Working women's entry into the labour market often harms their physical and psychological health. Too many women are still in poorly paid jobs with high demands, low status and little control over their working environment. Many are in positions that underuse their skills and a large number are doing shiftwork. All these factors increase their dissatisfaction with work, which can be a significant source of disease (89, 95).

People who have direct responsibility for other people suffer more stress than people who only manipulate inanimate objects. As many women have care giving jobs or responsibilities, they suffer more stress. In service jobs dealing directly with the public, such as flight attendants, a particular strain is generated by always having to be nice to people. Again, more women than men are in these roles and suffer more somatic complaints and more frequent accidents (96).

Perhaps most important, women who take paid work do not usually swap one job for another; they take on the double burden of housework and paid employment. Most employed women spend between 20 and 40 hours per week on housework, and most countries have not significantly moved towards a more equal division of household tasks between men and women as women take on more paid employment. Not surprisingly, the strain of trying to juggle two sets of responsibilities can lead to physical exhaustion and loss of wellbeing. In a study at an electronics factory in Finland, 50% of married women workers reported frequent tiredness, 49% suffered from headaches and 47% from mental stress and anxiety (97).

There is therefore no simple answer to the question of what effect paid work has on the health of married women. On the one hand, it can provide much-needed material resources, greater financial independence and important social contacts. On the other hand, it can expose women to serious hazards, threaten their reproductive capacity and impose both mental and physical strain. Moreover, it is clear that the effect of paid work is very different depending on a woman's circumstances — whether she is living alone or with a partner, whether she has children, and the nature of the job itself. Not surprisingly, mothers of young children who work full time suffer more stress than mothers who work part time (81, 98). Health promotion policies for working women need to take account of all three roles: housewife, mother and employee. The effects on health of each role have to be looked at separately and the potential conflicts and contradictions between them must be examined. Detailed analysis becomes even more urgent as married women in general and mothers of young children in particular increasingly enter the labour force.

One obvious result of these developments has been women's increased use of various forms of chemical relief to suppress their feelings. Women use more psychotropic drugs than men. Studies in many countries have shown that women are about twice as likely as men to receive prescriptions for tranquillizers or antidepressants (21, 99–101). While these drugs can be useful in situations of acute distress, concern is now growing about their long-term use. They can lead to both physical and psychological addiction, but most women are unaware of the hazards, assuming that doctors would not prescribe something that could damage their health. Above all, tranquillizers do not solve women's problems, but simply provide relief from some of the more acute symptoms.

The prevalence of both cigarette smoking and alcohol consumption is rising among women in many parts of the world. Alcohol abuse is difficult to define and extremely difficult to measure, since women are much more likely than men to drink at home and alone (102). Nevertheless, indices such as cirrhosis of the liver, offences for drunkenness, admission to psychiatric hospitals for alcoholism and increasing use of alcohol counselling services all suggest that female drinking has increased recently in many countries *(103,104)*. Some of this apparent increase may, of course, be attributable to the reduced stigma attached to women who drink, which makes it easier for them to admit their problems. Most studies suggest, however, that there has been a real increase, not just in women's social drinking, but in problem drinking that may threaten their health and wellbeing. Relatively little is known about the particular effects of alcohol on women, but research suggests that women may be more susceptible than men to liver damage and to other alcohol-related diseases.

Tobacco consumption is easier to measure than alcohol consumption, and in most countries the number of women smokers has increased significantly since the Second World War. In Great Britain, for instance, the gap has narrowed rapidly as more men than women have quit smoking, and more young girls are starting. About 36% of men and 32% of women are now regular smokers, and for women the prevalence is high at both ends of the social scale *(88)*. At the same time, the number of cigarettes smoked per person has risen more among female than male smokers. Between 1972 and 1980, per capita consumption by men rose by about 3%, but the comparable figure for women was 15%. Even in the developing countries, where women have historically had very low smoking rates, more women smoke more as they grapple with the pressure of rapid social and economic change *(105)*. Few researchers have examined the particular problems of women smokers, but the available evidence suggests that women find it much harder than men to give up smoking, as the habit appears to be more deeply embedded in their daily lives *(88,106)*. Not surprisingly, the increasing percentage of women smokers is gradually affecting morbidity and mortality statistics. The incidence of both heart disease and lung cancer is now rising among women in a number of countries, and smoking has been implicated as a significant cause in both diseases.

Implications of Current Research for Promoting Women's Health

The changes in the lives of women over the past century have been complex and contradictory, affecting their health in many different ways. Overall life expectancy has improved, but this has not meant equality of life chances for all women. The twentieth century has brought many emancipatory benefits to women, including relief from certain types of illness, but these benefits have sometimes been obtained at the cost of new physical and mental health problems. Entering the labour market, for instance, has brought some women new freedom and greater financial independence but also exposure to new hazards, a great increase in workload and a double burden of responsibilities. Effective policies to promote women's health (like that of men) cannot be narrowly confined to the medical sphere but need to address all aspects of women's lives. Ultimately, this involves quite profound changes in the way society is organized but, in the meantime, the most immediate priorities for women's health can be identified in relation to medical services and to local and central government policies.

Health care services are extremely important to women as users, as care givers and as workers. Nevertheless, these services currently do little to promote women's health. In most countries more resources need to be spent on community services, especially since the release of many long-term institutional inpatients has put added pressure on individual women. Such a reallocation of funds would improve the health of women both as users and as care givers. Community and hospital services also need to serve women's needs and desires better. To promote women's health, maternity and fertility control services should enable users to maximize their control over what should be normal processes in their lives. This necessitates increased access and consistent respect for the sexual identity, cultural values and material circumstances of women.

Prevention is an essential element in all effective health promotion policies. Screening for breast cancer and cervical cancer saves women's lives and prevents chronic illness, but most countries have not yet realized its potential. Better training for health workers, more laboratory facilities, and an effective call and recall system are needed to ensure that the services reach all women who need them. These services and other less technical preventive services can often best be provided in "well woman" centres where a general check-up, advice and counselling can be provided by various female health workers in a friendly and informal setting. Many community-based health projects initiated by lay women also need more support (107). Funding women-only therapy and self-help groups is especially important. These groups have proved especially successful when

301

women wish to change some aspect of their behaviour but have been unable to do so alone. The value of group support in such endeavours has been recognized for a long time through groups such as Alcoholics Anonymous, but the implications of gender in such activities have only relatively recently begun to be recognized. Women's therapy groups have grown rapidly with smoking, alcohol and food being common topics. These women-only support groups have been much more effective in helping their members to give up smoking, for example, than traditional mixed groups (88). Groups of this kind must be part of any health promotion policy. Indeed, official health services must recognize single-sex groups as a valid thera- peutic approach so that many more women who want to lead healthier lives but cannot find a supportive environment to help them can achieve this. These support networks can be created not just to deal with particular problems but also to help women in their day-to-day task of caring for themselves and others.

It is essential that equal opportunity employment policies be pursued within the health services to ensure that these services are responsive to women's needs. Such policies increase the representa- tion of women at all levels of the health labour force (108). When health services are under national or local state control, women should be better represented on the decision-making committees, so that women's views as users, care givers and workers can be better presented.

Women need more appropriate services, but they must be able to control their health by obtaining more and better information, and not just any information will do. Positive health information must reflect women's experiences of health and illness and take into account the particular conditions of the women receiving the information. A feminist approach to health education is now developing around the world, and the insights of this development need to be incorporated into official practice. It must be recognized that people are best able to develop many aspects of their knowledge and understanding by working collectively. This is especially true in health, where consciousness-raising and sharing experiences make women both more knowledgeable and more confident about acting on their own behalf. Whenever possible, information designed to promote health should be presented to a group and the implications discussed collec- tively. Education and community organizing of this kind is important because, at its best, it enables women to change themselves and also

302

empowers them to change the world that may have disabled them in the first place. The wider spheres of action that women need to take up must be identified if they are to promote their health.

Women have an essential role in regulating health hazards. The opportunities for such action are infinite. Over the past 20 or 30 years some of the drugs and devices given to women have not been adequately tested and their long-term hazards have not been effectively monitored. Women clearly need to press for more effective regulatory procedures in medicine, but for now they need to carry out this task as effectively as possible themselves. This applies to health workers in particular, but women who have had bad experiences from which they want to protect others must also actively cooperate. The recent campaign against the injectable contraceptive Depo Provera in Great Britain, the United States and elsewhere has demonstrated the importance of activities of this kind *(109)*.

In public health, occupational health and safety have traditionally been seen as problems for males. Women are assumed to be either safe at home or working in nonhazardous jobs. In fact, not only are women increasingly being exposed to traditionally male hazards but typically female jobs have their own hazards. If women had not regularly monitored their work environment, this evidence would probably not have come to light. Similarly, in groups monitoring community health hazards, women are usually the most frequent and active participants. Nevertheless, men dominate the various institutions in different countries that control medical practice, determine research priorities, regulate working conditions and ensure a healthy environment. These institutions reflect the policies of society in limiting women from entering positions of public authority. Women need to be equally represented in public health organizations, to ensure that health promotion policies genuinely reflect the interests of women.

Wider political and legislative changes are essential in ensuring the promotion of women's health. At a local level, housing policies need to respond to the needs of women, since cost, design and location can all significantly affect women's health. Public transport policies also need to respond to women's needs. Women depend more than men on public transport for basic mobility, and access can be a special problem for older women, for women with young children and for women with disabilities. The resulting inability to move around can cause isolation in both urban and rural environments, sometimes resulting in mental health problems. Adequate community care services are also essential to provide appropriate help to women with physical or mental disabilities who could then manage alone. Women who care for others need more material and emotional support. Women who care for chronically ill and disabled people need respite care for these dependants to enable women to maintain their own health and autonomy. Adequate preschool child care and after-school arrangements for older children are also needed if women are to compete equally with men in the labour market.

At central government level, increased expenditure on appropriate health and social services will benefit women disproportionately, since they use more of these services and are the major care givers for people for whom the formal system takes no responsibility. Economic policies are also crucial; effective equal pay legislation is needed to enable women to obtain a reasonable wage. For the millions of women who do not want or cannot obtain paid work, social security benefits need to be high enough to achieve a healthy standard of living. Benefits for caregivers are especially important, and need to be paid regardless of sex or marital status. In most countries, more comprehensive legislation and more effective mechanisms for ensuring its implementation are also needed to remedy discrimination based on race and sex. All these policies are important, but women will only realize their potential for health when all aspects of their work are socially valued and supported, and they achieve autonomy and self-determination in their domestic, productive, reproductive and sexual lives.

References

1. **Doyal, L**. Women, health and the sexual division of labour: a case study of the women's health movement in Britain. *International journal of health services*, **13**(3): 373–387 (1983).
2. **Ruzek, S.B**. *The women's health movement: feminist alternatives to medical control*. New York, Praeger, 1978.
3. **Ettorre, B**. Women and drunken sociology: developing a feminist analysis. *Women studies international forum*, **9**(5): 515–520 (1986).
4. **Thom, B**. A process approach to women's use of alcohol services. *British journal of addiction*, **79**: 377–382 (1984).

5. **Robinson, J.** Cervical cancer: a feminist critique. *London times health supplement*, 27 November 1981, p. 12.

6. **Robinson, J.** Cancer of the cervix: occupational risks of husbands and wives and possible preventive strategies. *In*: Jordan, J. et al., ed. *Preclinical neoplasia of the cervix*. London, Royal College of Obstetricians and Gynaecologists, 1982.

7. **Oakley, A**. *Women confined: towards a sociology of childbirth*. Oxford, Martin Robertson, 1980.

8. **Hatch, S. & Kickbusch, I., ed**. *Self-help and health in Europe: new approaches in health care*. Copenhagen, WHO Regional Office for Europe, 1983.

9. **Finch, J. & Groves, D**. *A labour of love: women, work and caring*. London, Routledge & Kegan Paul, 1983.

10. **Graham, H**. *Women, health and the family*. Brighton, Harvester, 1984.

11. **MacFarlane, A**. Women and health: official statistics on women and aspects of health and illness. *UK Equal Opportunities Commission research bulletin*, **4**: 43–77 (1981).

12. **Muller, C**. Women and health statistics: areas of deficient data collection and integration. *Women and health*, **4**(1): 37–59 (1979).

13. **Oakley, A. & Oakley, R**. Sexism in official statistics. *In*: Irvine, J. et al., ed. *Demystifying social statistics*. London, Pluto Press, 1979.

14. *Improving concepts and methods for statistics and indicators on women*. New York, United Nations, 1983 (Studies in Methods, Series F, No. 33).

15. WHO Technical Report Series, No. 580, 1975 (*Control of nutritional anaemia with special reference to iron deficiency:* report of an IAEA/USAID/WHO Joint Meeting).

16. **Beral, V**. Reproductive mortality. *British medical journal*, **2**: 632–634 (1979).

17. **Waldron, I**. Why do women live longer than men? *Social science and medicine*, **10**: 349–362 (1976).

18. **Robine, J.M. & Colvez, A**. Life expectancy free of disability and its components: new indicators for measuring population health needs. *Population*, **39**: 27–46 (1984).

19. **Howell, E. & Bayes, M**. *Women and mental health*. New York, Basic Books, 1981.

20. **Briscoe, M**. Sex differences in psychological well-being. *Psychological medicine*, Monograph Supplement No. 1, 1982.

21. **Gabe, J. & Williams, P**. *Tranquillisers: social, psychological and clinical perspectives*. London, Tavistock, 1986.

22. **Smith, D.E**. The statistics on mental illness: what they will not tell us about women and why. *In*: Smith, D.E. & David, S.J., ed. *Women look at psychiatry*. Vancouver, Press Gang, 1975.

23. **Petchesky, R.P**. *Abortion and woman's choice: the state, sexuality and reproductive freedom*. London, Verso, 1986.

24. **Francome, C**. *Abortion freedom: a worldwide movement*. London, Allen & Unwin, 1984.

25. **Kessel, E. & Mumford, S.D**. Potential demand for voluntary sterilization in the 1980s: the compelling need for a non-surgical method. *Fertility and sterility*, **37**(6): 725–733 (1982).

26. *Towards a better future: maternal and child health*. Geneva, World Health Organization, 1980.

27. **Homans, H**. *The sexual politics of reproduction*. London, Gower Press, 1985.

28. **Michaelson, K.L., ed**. *And the poor get children: radical perspectives on population dynamics*. New York, Monthly Review Press, 1981.

29. **Minces, J**. *The house of obedience: women in Arab society*. London, Zed Press, 1982.

30. **Doyal, L**. Women and the NHS: the carers and the careless. *In*: Lewin, E. & Oleson, V., ed. *Women, health and healing*. London, Tavistock, 1985.

31. **Roberts, H**. Male hegemony in family planning. *In*: Roberts, H., ed. *Women, health and reproduction*. London, Routledge & Kegan Paul, 1981.

32. **Lovenduski, J. & Outshoorn, J**. *The new politics of abortion*. London. Sage, 1986.

33. **Gordon, L**. *Woman's body woman's right: a social history of birth control in America*. Harmondsworth, Penguin Books, 1977.

34. **Shapiro, R**. *Contraception: a practical and political guide*. London, Virago, 1987.

35. **Andolsek, L. et al**. The safety of local anesthesia and outpatient treatment: a controlled study of induced abortion by vacuum aspiration. *Studies in family planning*, **8**(5): 118–124 (1977).

36. **Tietze, C.** *Induced abortion: a world review*, 4th ed. New York, Population Council, 1981.

37. **Smith, P.A. et al.** Deaths associated with intrauterine contraceptive devices in the UK between 1973 and 1983. *British medical journal*, **287**: 1537–1538 (1983).

38. **Pollock, S.** Refusing to take women seriously: "side effects" and the politics of contraception. *In*: Arditti, R. et al., ed. *Test tube women: what future for motherhood*. London, Pandora Press, 1984.

39. **Royal College of General Practitioners.** *Oral contraceptives and health*. London, Pitman Medical, 1974.

40. **Beral, V.** Cardiovascular disease, mortality trends and oral contraceptive use in young women. *Lancet*, **2**: 1047–1051 (1976).

41. **Pike, M. et al.** Breast cancer in young women and use of oral contraceptives: possible modifying effect of formulation and age at use. *Lancet*, **2**: 926–930 (1983).

42. **Vessey, M.P. et al.** Neoplasia of the cervix uteri and contraception: a possible adverse effect of the pill. *Lancet*, **2**: 930–934 (1983).

43. **Riesman, C.K.** Women and medicalization: a new perspective. *Social policy*, Summer, pp. 3–18 (1983).

44. **Kirk, M.** *Demographic and social change in Europe 1975–2000*. Liverpool, Liverpool University Press, 1981.

45. **Cartwright, A.** *The dignity of labour? A study of childbearing and induction*. London, Tavistock, 1979.

46. **Chard, T. & Richards, M., ed.** *Benefits and hazards of the new obstetrics*. London, SIM and Heinemann Medical, 1977.

47. **McKinlay, J.B.** The sick-role: illness and pregnancy. *Social science and medicine*, **6**: 561–572 (1972).

48. **Badinter, E.** *The myth of motherhood*. London, Souvenir Press, 1982.

49. **Rich, A.** *Of woman born: motherhood*. London, Virago, 1977.

50. **Greer, G.** *Sex and destiny: the politics of human fertility*. London, Secker & Warburg, 1984.

51. **Pfeffer, N. & Woollett, A.** *The experience of infertility*. London, Virago, 1983.

52. **Arditti, R. et al., ed.** *Test tube women: what future for motherhood*. London, Pandora Press, 1984.

53. **Stanworth, M., ed.** *Reproductive technologies*. Cambridge, Polity Press, 1987.

54. **Doyal, L**. Infertility: a life sentence? *In*: Stanworth, M., ed. *Reproductive technologies*. Cambridge, Polity Press, 1987.

55. **Dowie, M. et al**. The illusion of safety. *Mother Jones*, June, pp. 38–48 (1982).

56. **Rosenberg, H**. The home is the workplace: hazards, stress and pollutants in the household. *In*: Chavkin, W., ed. *Double exposure: women's health hazards on the job and at home*. New York, Monthly Review Press, 1984.

57. **Graham, H. & McKee, C**. *The first months of motherhood*. London, Health Education Council, 1980 (Research Monograph, No. 3).

58. **Richman, N**. Depression in mothers of young children. *Journal of child psychology and psychiatry*, **17**: 75–78 (1976).

59. **Bayley, M**. *Mental handicap and community care*. London, Routledge & Kegan Paul, 1973.

60. *Who cares for the carers? Opportunities for those caring for the elderly and handicapped*. Manchester, Equal Opportunities Commission, 1982.

61. **Balbo, L**. The servicing work of women and the capitalist state. *Political power and social theory*, **3**: 251–270 (1982).

62. **Kickbusch, I**. A hard day's night: women, reproduction and service society. *In*: Rendel, M., ed. *Women, power and political systems*. London, Croom Helm, 1981.

63. **Prokop, U**. Production and the context of women's daily life. *New German critique*, **13**: 18–33 (1978).

64. **Vedder-Shults, N**. Hearts starve as well as bodies: Ulrike Prokop's production and the context of women's daily life. *New German critique*, **13**: 5–17 (1978).

65. **Oakley, A**. *The sociology of housework*. Oxford, Martin Robertson, 1974.

66. **Brown, G.W. & Harris, T**. *Social origins of depression: a study of psychiatric disorders in women*. London, Tavistock, 1978.

67. **Nairne, K. & Smith G**. *Dealing with depression*. London, Women's Press, 1984.

68. **Land, H**. Poverty and gender: the distribution of resources within the family. *In*: Brown, M., ed. *The structure of disadvantage*. London, Heinemann, 1983.

69. **Pahl, J**. Patterns of money management within marriage. *Journal of social policy*, **9**(3): 313–335 (1980).

70. **Piachaud, D**. Patterns of income and expenditure within families. *Journal of social policy*, **11**(4): 469–482 (1982).

71. **Peace, S.M**. *An international perspective on the status of older women*. Washington, DC, International Federation on Aging, 1981.

72. **Kaufert, P**. Myth and the menopause. *Sociology of health and illness*, **4**(2): 141–166 (1982).

73. **McCrae, F**. The politics of menopause: the discovery of a deficiency disease. *Social problems*, **31**(1): 111–123 (1983).

74. **Harrison, J**. Women and aging: experience and implications. *Aging and society*, **3**(2): 209–235 (1983).

75. **Nathanson, C.A**. Illness and the feminine role: a theoretical review. *Social science and medicine*, **9**: 57–62 (1975).

76. **Verbrugge, L.M**. Sex differentials in morbidity and mortality in the United States. *Social biology*, **23**: 275–296 (1976).

77. **Verbrugge, L.M**. Marital status and health. *Journal of marriage and the family*, **7**: 267–285 (1979).

78. **Verbrugge, L.M**. Recent trends in sex mortality differentials in the US. *Women and health*, **5**: 17–37 (1980).

79. **Waldron, I**. Employment and women's health: an analysis of causal relationships. *International journal of health services*, **10**(3): 435–454 (1980).

80. **Waldron, I**. Sex differences in illness incidence, prognosis and mortality: issues and evidence. *Social science and medicine*, **17**: 1107–1123 (1983).

81. **Arber, S. et al**. Paid employment and women's health: a benefit or a source of role strain? *Sociology of health and illness*, **7**(3): 375–400 (1985).

82. *Women and occupational health risks*: report on a WHO meeting. Copenhagen, WHO Regional Office for Europe, 1983 (EURO Reports and Studies No. 76).

83. **Baker, R. & Woodrow, S**. The clean, light image of the electronic industry: miracle or mirage? *In*: Chavkin, W., ed. *Double exposure: women's health hazards on the job and at home*. New York, Monthly Review Press, 1984.

84. **Chavkin, W., ed**. *Double exposure: women's health hazards on the job and at home*. New York, Monthly Review Press, 1984.

85. **Sullivan, F.M. & Barlow, S.M**. *Reproductive hazards of industrial chemicals*. London, Academic Press, 1982.

86. **Hemmintzi, K. et al.** *Occupational hazards and reproduction.* Washington, DC, Hemisphere, 1982.
87. **Coleman, L. & Dickinson, C.** The risks of healing: the hazards of the nursing profession. *In*: Chavkin, W., ed. *Double exposure: women's health hazards on the job and at home.* New York, Monthly Review Press, 1984.
88. **Jacobson, B.** *Beating the ladykillers: women and smoking.* London, Pluto Press, 1986.
89. **Colligan, M.J. et al.** Occupational incidence rates of mental health disorders. *Journal of human stress*, **3**: 34–39 (1977).
90. **Craig, M.** *The office worker's survival handbook.* London, British Society for Social Responsibility in Science, 1981.
91. **Huws, U.** *A woman's guide to the new technology.* London, Pluto Press, 1982.
92. **de Matteo, B.** *Terminal shock: the health hazards of video display terminals.* Toronto, NC Press, 1985.
93. **Hadjifotiou, N.** *Women and harassment at work.* London, Pluto Press, 1983.
94. **Crull, P.** Sexual harassment and women's health. *In*: Chavkin, W., ed. *Double exposure: women's health hazards on the job and at home.* New York, Monthly Review Press, 1984.
95. **Karasek, R.** Job demands, job decision latitude and mental strain: implications for job redesign. *Administrative science quarterly*, **24**: 235–238 (1979).
96. **Hochschild, A.** *The managed heart: commercialization of human feeling.* Berkeley, University of California Press, 1983.
97. **Honkasalo, M.-L.** Dead end — views on career development and life situation of women in the electronics industry. *Economic and industrial democracy*, **3**(4): 445–465 (1982).
98. **Liff, S.** Mental health of women factory workers. *Journal of occupational behaviour*, **2**: 139–146 (1981).
99. **Christensen, D.B. & Bush, P.J.** Drug prescribing: patterns, problems and proposals. *Social science and medicine*, **15A**: 343–355 (1981).
100. **Cooperstock, R.** A review of women's psychological drug use. *In*: Howell, E. & Bayes, M. *Women and mental health.* New York, Basic Books, 1981.
101. **Cooperstock, R. & Parmele, P.** Research on psychotropic drug use: a review of findings and methods. *Social science and medicine*, **16**: 1179–1196 (1982).

102. **Celentano, D.D. et al**. Substance abuse by women: a review of epidemiologic literature. *Journal of chronic diseases*, **33**: 383–394 (1980).

103. **Camberwell Council on Alcoholism**. *Women and alcohol*. London, Tavistock, 1980.

104. **McConville, B**. *Women under the influence*. London, Virago, 1983.

105. **Muller, M**. *Tobacco and the third world: tomorrow's epidemic*. London, War on Want, 1978.

106. **Graham H**. Health promotion and women's smoking. *Health promotion*, **3**(4): 371–382 (1988).

107. **Kenner, C**. *No time for women*. London, Pandora Press, 1985.

108. **Sedley, A**. Equal opportunities in the National Health Service. *Equal opportunities review*, March/April, pp. 10–17 (1987).

109. **Coordinating Group on Depo Provera**. *Submission to the UK public hearing on Depo Provera*. London, Women's Health Information Centre, 1983.

14

Unemployment as a stressor: findings and implications of a recent study[a]

David Dooley & Ralph Catalano

This chapter explores job loss and related events as risk factors for illness. These phenomena have become of increasing interest to health professionals in developed countries, as economic restructuring has displaced redundant workers. The pathogenic effect of displacement is explained by the stress model and is elaborated on by describing the results of recent research conducted by the authors. The implications for health promotion of this and similar research are also discussed.

The relationship between economic change and mental disorder has been measured in the aggregate (for example, the relationship between rates of unemployment and suicide) at least since the last century *(1)*. The depression of the 1930s stimulated research on individuals that seemed to confirm the adverse effects of unemployment *(2)*. In this chapter, we view the relationship between unemployment and mental health from the perspective of the stress model. After characterizing the literature and framing it in terms of a chain of hypothetical causal links, we illustrate the model with a summary of a recent survey that combined aggregate- and individual-level measures of economic stress.

---

[a] The authors acknowledge the suport of this research by a grant from the US National Institute of Mental Health.

Economic Events in the Stress Model

Terms of the model

A stressor is an event that potentially induces stress, and stress is the subjective experience of being unable to cope with this event. Stress is typically experienced as unpleasant distress that, if intense or prolonged, may result in measurable symptoms of psychological or physical ill health.

A cognitive element in this model pertains to the way a stressor becomes an actual cause of stress rather than a potential one. Typically, stress models implicate the cognitive act of appraising the stressor and one's coping resources. This requirement of cognition explains why events induce stress for some people but not for others. Some events are not usually considered stressors because they do not induce stress in most people: for example, being glanced at by a stranger. One can find people with disordered appraisal processes, however, such as paranoid schizophrenics, for whom being glanced at by a stranger could initiate a stress loop (3). Other events are regarded as stressors because they are believed to induce stress in most people. Unemployment is generally considered a stressor.

Unemployment as a rubric

The present concept of unemployment is a relatively modern idea (4). Many labourers under feudalism and earlier modes of production would be stunned by the notions that work could be exchanged for money and that an employer could disemploy a person, cutting off both the work and the flow of money. The economic recessions of the past century have necessitated a re-evaluation of the meaning of work, employment and unemployment (2). Loss of income is a tangible consequence of losing a job but the study of unemployment transcends the study of poverty because employment serves important psychological functions. Jahoda (2), for example, reminds one of the Freudian aphorism that work is the strongest tie to reality, implying that unemployment weakens one's grip on reality. Other aspects of the jobless environment have been identified as psychologically threatening. Warr (5) discusses nine such components. Considerable literature, dating from the depression of the 1930s, covers the social psychology of unemployment (6).

Unemployment both arouses interest and poses research difficulties because it is not a simple event. Unemployment is a general label for a complex of events, of which losing a job is only one. For example, one need not lose a job to be unemployed. People who have been occupying other roles (housewife, student) and who enter the job market and do not find work are also unemployed.

Beyond joblessness, many events connected with employment and finances can induce stress and are related conceptually and operationally to indicators of unemployment. Disemployed workers are not the only workers who experience these events. When the unemployment rate rises to 10% in a major recession, 90% of the workforce is still employed. Nevertheless, these employed workers may experience stressful working conditions or anticipate stressful job changes. People not in the workforce experience other events related to unemployment. A principal wage-earner who loses a job, or fears losing it, may behave in ways that function as stressors (economic or noneconomic) for other family members.

A broad range of economic and noneconomic events affect unemployed and employed workers and their dependants. Economic events can be conceptualized and measured both at the personal level (a particular individual loses a job) and at the aggregate level (the prevailing unemployment rate). The aggregate level represents a salient aspect of the social environment in which personal economic and noneconomic events are experienced and appraised. Although most studies of stressful events treat an event as a variable with unknown external causes, this study examines the sequence of events (from the aggregate economy to personal unemployment and from economic events to noneconomic events). Most studies focus on the person experiencing the event: this study looks at other significant people in the environment.

Background

The questions
Studies of unemployment as a stressor can be grouped under two main questions. First, is unemployment (broadly defined) stressful and what is the impact of this stress? This suggests a series of direct and indirect hypothetical links between changes in the economy and subsequent stressful life events, symptoms of stress, and outcomes such as suicide or seeking help. Second, what are the mechanisms and process by which stressful events and their moderators influence

outcomes? This deals primarily with one of the above-noted causal links, the mechanism by which stressors (events) lead or do not lead to symptoms of distress.

This chapter does not comprehensively treat the topic of economic stress. Such an overview would not only exceed the limits of this work but would also repeat several appearing in recent years (7).

The literature on the impact and process of the stress caused by unemployment is first reviewed and then summarized in a conceptual model. This model is then illustrated by a recent (1978–1982) large-scale survey that included the deepest point of the worst recession in the United States since the depression of the 1930s.

Analysis of impact

The assertion that the economy influences wellbeing finds empirical support in two different kinds of research. Research based on the correlation of aggregate measures of the economy and aggregate measures of disorder was begun earlier and is more frequently cited in the media and in policy discussions. Although such correlations can be conducted over spatial units (such as between countries for a given year), the longitudinal correlation over temporal units (such as years for a given country) is preferred for drawing causal inference. Although this approach is traceable to the last century (1) improved econometric techniques have revived interest in this method in the past 20 years (8).

Dozens of such mental health studies have been conducted using archival measures such as suicides or admissions to psychiatric hospitals. Typically, unemployment appears to affect adversely the indicators of pathology, but the interpretation of such findings is limited by several features. First, the complicated statistical controls required by such designs have spawned many technical criticisms (9–11). Second, the units of analysis, both geographical and temporal, are so coarse that it is difficult to translate them into meaningful economic or psychological terms. For example, countries consist of many smaller economic units that do not necessarily behave uniformly. The year is the most common unit of time-series analysis, reflecting more that archival data are available in annual form than any psychological theory that might link current behaviour to economic conditions a year or more ago. Finally, even if the statistical debates and problems with the units of analysis were resolved, the aggregate results can be interpreted at the individual

316

level only by risking the ecological fallacy: a link between the rates of unemployment and suicide cannot support the conclusion that any particular person committed suicide because of losing a job *(12)*.

The aggregate time-series analysis has mainly stimulated interest in the "black box" of individual-level mechanisms that accounts for the overarching association between the economy and social indicators of pathology. It is implicit in the presentation of such time-series findings that some kind of stress process links aggregate unemployment and aggregate mental disorder. A different research approach measuring the impact of economic events on the wellbeing of individual people has emerged to test such a stress hypothesis. There are several variants: following up workers who have lost their jobs in comparison with continuously employed counterparts *(13)*; following up workers who are about to lose their jobs (sometimes identified by announcements of plant closures) *(14)*; and following up people who are experiencing other kinds of economic transition (such as young people leaving school and about to enter the workforce) *(15)*.

This type of research on the individual has also typically reported that unemployment adversely affects wellbeing. The magnitude of such effects is usually small, however, especially in contrast to the large effects reported in the aggregate literature. Moreover, the individual-level research has limitations. It ignores the prevailing economic climate, a potentially important contextual variable that is usually assumed to cause personal economic events, but its relationship to the incidence of subsequent job loss is almost never measured. The aggregate economy may moderate the impact of such events, possibly through appraisal processes. Remedying this omission and yet retaining the benefits of the individual-level approach requires a cross-level strategy that simultaneously measures individual events and their economic context. Such a cross-level method is illustrated later in this chapter.

Process analyses
Unlike the analysis of the impact of unemployment noted above, the study of the psychological mechanisms by which job events are linked to symptoms of distress is necessarily limited to individual-level designs. In addition to the longitudinal individual-level designs noted above, process research can also be advanced by cross-sectional studies. For example, within a sample of unemployed workers, some people show more disorder than others. The aspects of

317

the people and their environments that determine high and low reactivity to the same stressor provide clues to the nature of vulnerability. Unfortunately, such cross-sectional designs can only suggest causality, since a prior level of disorder could account for both the present level of disorder and its correlates (such as length of unemployment).

Such individual-level studies are so numerous that only a few examples are noted here, but together they point to several potential moderators of the impact of unemployment. Most of these moderators can be interpreted using the cognitive stress model: the stress felt by an unemployed person should be positively correlated with the perceived importance of the needs being threatened and negatively correlated with the perceived resources or alternatives available to meet the needs previously supplied by the employment. Time structure is one psychological need commonly thought to be affected by unemployment. Swinburne (16) reported that how well unemployed people adapted to losing their jobs depended on how well they were able to fill their time. One factor that would be expected to influence the way unemployed people fill their time is whether there are other socially approved activities. Brinkman (17) reported that people who lost their jobs were better off if they enjoyed attractive and legitimate alternative social roles. It is not clear to what extent such alternative roles are beneficial because they structure time, provide approved social status or supply nurture. Recent research also indicates the importance of the level of psychological involvement in the job in determining a person's response to unemployment. Unemployed people who had more personal investment in their work were worse off than unemployed people for whom a job was just the source of a pay-packet (18–20). In summary, individual-level research has provided evidence consistent with the cognitive stress model as applied to unemployment, but this work is still in the exploratory stage.

Summary model
Time-series research has provided the overarching connection between aggregate economic conditions and aggregate indicators of pathology without specifying the individual-level causal pathways between them. The literature on stress caused by unemployment can be organized by a model consisting of seven hypothetical links that connect aggregate economic change and sever pathological outcomes. The first link connects the aggregate economy with personal

318

economic events; this is generally assumed to be valid but is rarely tested. This link represents one of the advantages of studying unemployment as a stressor. Unlike most other stressful life events, unemployment can be traced back to policy choices and therefore offers greater opportunity for prediction and prevention. Also largely ignored is the possible second link between the aggregate economy and personal symptoms, controlling for personal job loss (for example, people who are not likely to lose their jobs or are not in the workforce may nevertheless worry about possible future events). A third seldom studied link involves the interaction between the aggregate economy and personal economic events in provoking symptoms.

Individual-level research has concentrated on a fourth link between personal economic events and symptoms. Having found support for the impact of events on symptoms, individual-level research increasingly tries to study the moderation of this link by personal resources and attributes (such as personal involvement in the job or social support). One seldom studied facet of this link is the interaction of events. Job and financial events are not the only ones implicated in producing stress, but little is known about the way they affect noneconomic events either within individual people or between people (such as stress among unemployed workers affecting their spouses or children).

Individual-level research usually stops with the measurement of symptoms of disorder. More severe outcomes such as suicide (or suicidal ideation) and entering hospital (or seeking other help for emotional problems) are so rare that they usually do not appear in small sample studies. Implicit in the research model, however, is a fifth link between symptoms and the kinds of severe outcome that are ultimately counted in aggregate social indicators. Although some of these types of behaviour may be independent of the socioeconomic context, others may be influenced in ways not explained by the previous stress links. For example, hospital admission rates depend not only on the demand for services (seeking help) but also on the supply of services, which may be influenced by the fiscal choices of governments and agencies dealing with economic (revenue) fluctuations. At the level of households, hospital admission may result not because new symptoms are provoked (link 4), but because the household is less able to provide care in the home for a chronically disordered member (that is, the discovery of existing pathology)

(21, 22). As a result, other possible links may be hypothesized. Changes in the aggregate economy may lead directly to increases in such outcomes as hospital admission, controlling for intervening personal events and symptoms (link 6). Alternatively, life events may lead directly to such outcomes, controlling for intervening symptom changes (link 7).

These seven pathways describe a model that is difficult to test simultaneously in a single data set. Most studies assume or ignore one or more of the hypothesized links, to focus on just one or two. A recent study that attempted to measure each construct from aggregate economic conditions through personal life events, moderators, and symptoms to individual- and aggregate-level outcomes, illustrates more concretely each of these links.

Los Angeles Stressor Project

Summary of design
The project was a cross-level study that planned to address all seven links in the model. This study monitored an economically meaningful geographic unit in the United States over time at both the aggregate and individual levels for both economic events and health outcomes.

Additional details can be found in the references accompanying these results. Briefly, the design was a random-digit-dialing telephone trend survey: a series of 16 cross-sectional samples (about 500 respondents per sample) drawn from the same population at intervals of three months. The population consisted of all English- or Spanish-speaking adults living in residences in Los Angeles County, California (where over 90% of all households have telephones). This large metropolitan community is also a meaningful economic unit (called a standard metropolitan statistical area) for which economic and health statistics are routinely gathered each month. The main interview was cross-sectional within each of the 16 samples, and there was also a small panel component. Three months after each of the first 15 interview periods, 40 respondents were reinterviewed. More than 8000 respondents were interviewed once (during one of the 16 interview periods) and more than 600 of these were interviewed a second time.

The principal survey items included a variety of life events, symptoms of disorder, and potential moderators (such as social support). Economic and noneconomic life events were separately

320

rated as desirable or undesirable. The principal symptom scale consisted of 25 items adapted for telephone survey from the Psychiatric Epidemiology Research Instrument (PERI) *(23)*. PERI measures general emotional demoralization rather than identifying cases with specific diagnoses. To approximate clinical case identification, the cut-off point for severe disorder was the top 20% of the sample in the PERI symptom score. A second symptom measure, Center for Epidemiologic Studies-Depression (CES-D), was used in the second interviews because it reflected very recent (past week) mood *(24)*.

Economic indicators at the aggregate level were based on archival records characterizing the workforce and economy of Los Angeles during the two months before the interview and the month of the interview. In addition to the unemployment rate, many other measures were developed, including ones representing change *per se* (economic activity, whether favourable or unfavourable) to reflect Durkheim's approach to anomy and employment change in specific industries. Each respondent could be characterized in both individual-level terms (personal events and symptoms) and in terms of the local economic climate at the time of the interview.

The ability to generalize the results of a study is limited by the representativeness of its sample with respect to place and time. Los Angeles was selected because it represents a large, ethnically diverse, metropolitan community similar to many others in the United States. It has a diverse economy that does not rely on a single industry that might be vulnerable to extreme peaks and troughs such as oil, steel or cars. Any such prospective study risks insufficient variation in the chief independent variable (too much economic stability) and thus the study fails to represent any serious economic difficulties. In fact, the period of this study, 1978–1982, included the worst economic recession in 50 years. The unemployment rate in Los Angeles closely paralleled that of the United States as a whole in this period, rising to more than 10% in 1982. Although it did not experience the catastrophic economic conditions of such communities as Youngstown, Ohio, Los Angeles provided a more representative sample of the economic experience of the United States during the time period studied.

Findings
This section summarizes the key findings relevant to the seven hypothetical links offered earlier.

1. *How do changes in the aggregate economy affect personal life events?* The incidence of life events may be nearly random for individuals within a community in any given period. If the current understanding and measurement of social processes are even approximately correct, however, this incidence must be related over time to such variables as the economy. When the unemployment rate increases, for example, the incidence of undesirable economic life events would be expected to increase. This link is obvious and crucial but has rarely been tested.

As expected, an archival measure of structural economic change (shifts in the relative size of the economic sector without regard to total increase or decrease in jobs) was positively associated with the probability of experiencing surveyed life events that have desirable or uncertain valence *(25)*. Surprisingly, the unemployment rate was not associated in a simple way with the incidence of undesirable economic events. The likelihood of experiencing one or more such events varied positively with unemployment only for the group of medium socioeconomic status *(26)*. Respondents of lower socioeconomic status were more likely to experience such events than respondents of higher socioeconomic status, but this likelihood did not decrease with decreases in the unemployment rate, at least in the range experienced during 1978–1982 (quarterly mean unemployment ranged from 4.8% to 8.6%). Conversely, respondents of higher socioeconomic status were less likely to experience undesirable economic events and seemed immune to a worsening economic climate.

This complex finding is important in the interpretation of subsequent findings linking undesirable economic life events to increased symptoms and adverse outcomes, because the implicit indirect effect (from unemployment rate to life event to outcome) holds true only for the subgroup of medium socioeconomic status. More generally, aggregate economic change in an entire community can be experienced quite differently by groups within that community. This conclusion echoes the earlier findings of Brenner *(8)*, who reported that the incidence of admission to mental hospitals rose more with rising unemployment for the people who had more to lose during economic recession. One practical consequence of this finding is that the use of macroeconomic intervention to improve the general welfare becomes complicated.

322

2. *How do changes in the economic climate affect surveyed symptoms, controlling for possible intervening life events?* One health outcome studied early in this project was physical health change (recent illness or injury). The first 12 samples of the project showed that such health events were not related directly to the aggregate economic measures after controlling for other events (that is, there was no direct cross-level effect).

Nevertheless, in the full data set, psychological symptoms according to PERI were directly related to the aggregate unemployment rate, even after controlling for the personal experience of unemployment and other life events. Individuals interviewed in the quarters in which the unemployment rate was at least 7.4% were 35% more likely to fall in the symptom range corresponding to clinical disorder than those interviewed in quarters where the unemployment rate was below 7.4% *(27)*. Similar to link 1, this cross-level association between the aggregate economy and individual-level symptoms is rarely tested. Nevertheless, this finding invites future exploration of the way stress might be transmitted cognitively (for example, people reading headlines reporting an economic recession) rather than behaviourally (personally experiencing an economic event).

3. *Is there an interaction effect on symptoms between personal economic life events and community economic climate?* Although the perception of the aggregate economy would seem likely to moderate people's appraisal of job events, this interaction has seldom been studied. Cohn *(28)* reported an interaction that suggested that job loss was more stressful when the unemployment rate was relatively low. One interpretation of this finding is that, in assigning blame for an unpleasant event, people assess how frequently the event occurs in the local environment. If many other people are unemployed, it is easier to blame the economy than if few are unemployed. Brown *(29)* also found a negative interaction between aggregate and individual unemployment, but interpreted the finding differently: the adverse effect of increasing unemployment was being felt more by the employed than the unemployed. In the absence of the necessary indicators, the mechanisms for such a phenomenon might be: reduced job security, tangible decreases in the quality of working conditions (increased job-related stressors other than loss of job), decreased freedom to move to other jobs or power to bargain for improvements in the present job.

The Los Angeles stressor project, however, provided no evidence of an interaction between aggregate unemployment and personal unemployment. The effect of unemployment did not seem to depend on the economic climate (30).

4. *Do adverse economic life events affect symptoms at the individual level?* One methodological problem that is often overlooked in answering this question is that more than one type of event may be experienced by the respondent, and this may confound the relationship between the economic events and the symptoms. Suppose a worker experiences a noneconomic event (such as a divorce) that leads both to increased depression and to losing a job. The observed association of loss of job and depression does not indicate a causal connection of the type hypothesized. Because measures of a variety of economic and noneconomic events were available, noneconomic events were routinely controlled for in testing the association between economic events and symptoms. Neverthess, as expected, undesirable economic events and adverse health changes (recent illness or injury) were positively associated (25).

Also as expected, the personal experience of unemployment (as well as other types of less catastrophic economic event) was positively associated with symptoms. Students and homemakers who desired work were more than five times as likely to have clinical symptoms as employed people. People who had recently lost jobs but had become re-employed by the time of the interview had a threefold increased risk of symptoms. Thus, the aggregate economy appeared to have both direct (link 2) and indirect (via life events for people of medium socioeconomic status) effects.

The apparently large effects of personal unemployment are subject to the rival explanation of reverse causation (prior symptoms causing both the unemployment and the subsequent symptoms). In one analysis of the data on the panel, undesirable life events (combined economic and noneconomic) were still significantly related to depression at second interview (according to CES-D) despite controlling for symptoms at first interview. The panel results indicated, however, that in the 16 main samples a substantial part of the cross-sectional association between events and symptoms could be accounted for by prior symptoms (26). In the panel analysis restricted to members of the workforce and after controlling for both first-interview symptoms and undesirable nonjob events, only two kinds of unemployment experience were significantly associated with

324

second interview depression (according to CES-D). People who were unemployed at both interviews showed a relative decrease in symptoms. People who were unemployed at the first interview but re-employed at the second interview reported a relative increase in symptoms (27). Such unexpected findings seem to indicate an adjustment or plateau effect in long-term unemployment and a secondary stress effect caused by re-entering the workplace after a period of unemployment. The literature on this subject is growing; one recent review (7) listed almost 20 studies on the effect of unemployment on symptoms. Some of these studies have found that unemployment has relatively small effects but that there are interesting cognitive or anticipation effects. For example, Levi et al. (31) found that the psychological wellbeing of unemployed workers reached the lowest point in the period between the announcement of plant closure and actual closure, and increased after actual unemployment. In contrast, other recent findings indicate that unemployment has stronger and more lasting adverse effects (13, 32).

5. *Are elevated symptoms associated with indicators of more severe outcomes such as seeking help or suicidal ideation?* Seeking help was measured by a question asking whether the subject had considered seeking help in the past three months for an emotional problem and, if so, whether actual help had been sought. Based on the first 12 samples, seeking help was positively associated, as expected, with psychological symptoms (according to PERI) (33). In another analysis, the symptom variable was the strongest correlate of suicidal ideation (34). Although these findings are not surprising, they do support another intervening link in the chain that extends back from symptoms to life events (link 4) and from events to the aggregate economy (link 1).

6. *Does the aggregate economy affect such outcomes as seeking help or suicidal ideation, controlling for intervening symptoms and life events?* This link would indicate that such outcomes could be triggered by the economy even in people not experiencing job events and in people in whom new symptoms were not provoked. One analysis of the first 12 samples showed an overarching relationship between change *per se* (absolute change) in the aggregate economy and the number of people seeking help (33). Nevertheless, this relationship was curvilinear (U-shaped) and should be replicated before this interpretation is confirmed.

In a follow-up analysis based on all 16 samples, a sector-specific measure of job security was derived from archival data and linked to each respondent based on sector of employment. Workers in declining industries felt more insecure in their employment, which in turn was associated with a greater likelihood of seeking help, even after controlling for other events and symptoms *(35)*. In addition to the indirect effect of this aggregate measure of objective job security (via perceived job security), objective job security also interacted with symptoms to affect the seeking of help. Highly symptomatic respondents were more likely to seek help when the economy was contracting than when it was expanding, controlling for life events.

Economic stress and suicide are most often studied using aggregate time-series analysis, and most often a strong positive relationship is found over time between rates of unemployment and suicide. We conducted a traditional aggregate time-series analysis of completed suicide and a cross-level analysis using survey measures of suicidal ideation on the same community for the same time period *(34)*. The replication of the overarching, aggregate time-series analysis found support for the hypothesized positive effect of unemployment rate only on the suicide rate among females and the age group 50–64 years. An unexpected positive correlation between rates of employment and suicide was found for people aged 35–49 years. In short, the study was both consistent and inconsistent with previous studies that used the aggregate-only method.

In the individual-level analysis, after controlling for symptoms, aggregate economic conditions did not directly affect suicidal ideation (no support for link 6), but people long-term or voluntarily unemployed reported less suicidal ideation in periods in which total service sector employment was expanding. Thus, to the extent that the aggregate economy and personal economic events influence suicidal ideation, they appear to do so primarily indirectly via symptoms (link 5).

7. *Do economic life events affect such outcomes as seeking help and suicidal ideation, controlling for symptoms?* Seeking help was positively correlated with undesirable job and financial events, controlling for symptoms *(33)*. The findings for links 6 and 7 are relatively isolated in the literature on economic stress and should be interpreted cautiously, pending replication. Taken together, these results describe a complex model in which multiple direct and

326

indirect paths lead from changes in the local economic climate to various kinds of mental and physical distress.

Process findings

Given the real, if modest, impact of economic stressors, the question becomes one of process. Although the Los Angeles stressor project was not primarily designed to explore the cognitive aspects of how economic stress is created, several studies have examined the way events interact and the way various factors do or do not moderate the effects of events.

One area of interest is the varying impact of different kinds of event and the links between events, both within and between people. Valence is a major qualitative dimension of life events — desirable (positive) or undesirable (negative). There are different views on the way event valence operates. The earliest view held that change *per se* is stressful, regardless of the valence. Subsequently, empirical findings reflected more adverse effects for negative events than for positive events, leading many researchers to drop desirable events from their analyses. Interest in this topic has been revived by the recent finding that positive events can buffer the adverse effects of negative events *(36)*.

Positive job events seem to buffer negative job events *(30)*, but this effect was complicated by sex (stronger for females than for males) and did not survive the panel analysis (controlling for first interview symptoms). Interestingly, desirable job events appeared to affect symptoms adversely in the main (cross-sectional) analysis, in contrast to the usual findings that only undesirable events affect symptoms. Nevertheless, after controlling for first-interview symptoms, the stressful effect of desirable events disappeared and desirable nonjob events produced a favourable main effect. These mixed findings have led us to investigate further the nature of event valence.

Most previous research on event valence contrasted negative and positive events in the aggregate by using the sums of events of each type as scores. The large sample size used in the Los Angeles stressor project allowed more precise analysis based on specific pairs of events that are identical in content but opposite in presumed desirability (such as moving to a better versus a worse residence). The results suggest that negative events produce more stress than positive events.[a] This finding reinforces the perception of the complexity of apparently simple events. Desirable events appear to produce some potentially stressful demands for adaptation (such as the physical and mental demands of moving to a different residence, even a more desirable one). These demands may be partially offset or even reversed by the desirable features of the event (such as increased salary accompanying a promotion), accounting for the asymmetry between undesirable and desirable events and for the capacity of positive events to buffer negative events.

Another complicating feature of life events is that they do not appear in isolation. At the simplest level, this implies that analysis of the impact of selected events (such as job loss) must control for other potentially confounding kinds of event (such as divorce). The studies summarized above routinely included such controls, but they may be too conservative if, for example, the effects attributed to noneconomic events are indirectly caused by economic events (by a causal chain from economic events to noneconomic events to symptom outcome). To test this possibility, events were disaggregated by type (economic versus noneconomic) and timing (less than versus more than three months). The findings suggested that non-Latino white men who experience undesirable economic events are at increased risk of subsequent undesirable noneconomic events, and non-Latino white women who experience undesirable noneconomic events are at increased risk of subsequent undesirable economic events (37). At least for men, this implies that analysis of the impact of unemployment underestimates the total effect of economic events on stress, because the indirect effect of economic events on other kinds of stressor is typically omitted.

Just as events can occur in causal chains within individuals, it seems intuitively likely that events generate interpersonal consequences. It has been noted since the depression of the 1930s and replicated more recently (38,39) that spouses and families of people who lose their jobs feel the adverse effects of unemployment. The effects on respondent spouses of the job events of principal wage earners were assessed (40). Not only did these undesirable job events adversely affect the respondents' symptoms, but the symptoms were equal in magnitude to the adverse effect of the respondents' own

---

[a] **Rook, K.S**. *Positive vs. negative valence of life events*. Unpublished data, 1988.

328

undesirable nonjob events. Since most of those who were not principal wage earners were women, all female respondents were analysed, comparing those who were principal wage earners with those who were not. The adverse effect of job stressors was just as great when the events were experienced indirectly (by the principal wage earner spouse of the respondent) as when they were personally experienced by the respondent.

The stress model emphasizes the importance of the balance between the perceived demand for adaptation and the resources perceived to be available for adapting. The demographic characteristics of the person undergoing life change potentially condition these perceptions. For example, sex appears to influence how positive life events moderate the effect of negative life events. Even after controlling for first-interview symptoms, undesirable nonjob events appeared to affect women more adversely than men (30).

Ethnicity is another demographic factor of interest. Because Los Angeles is ethnically diverse, it was possible to test for racial and cultural differences in the impact of economic stressors on wellbeing. In different tests of this hypothesis, using different statistical methods, different economic indicators and different subsets of the survey sample, little evidence was found for effects of race or cultural background (30,41). Some analyses showed effects but, after controlling for sex, age, socioeconomic status, other life events and potential moderator variables, no interactions indicated differing reactivity to aggregate or personal economic conditions by race or cultural background.

Finally, the effect of age was studied in three different types of analysis. Age is usually included as a control variable. After controlling for the effects of first-interview symptoms, older respondents reported fewer symptoms at second interview, but they did not appear to be more or less sensitive to life events than their younger counterparts (30). Despite these negative findings, the meaning of major life events may still be conditioned by the appropriateness of the events for particular ages.

The impact of an event may depend on the social norms for the timing of events over the life span. Age norms for selected events were generated in two ways: *de facto* age means within the sample and prescriptive norms were estimated using a separate survey (42). According to the social clock hypothesis (43), events occurring at an atypical age, either too early or too late, are expected to be more stressful than those occurring at a typical age. In partial support of this hypothesis, being behind the *de facto* schedule in the timing of desirable events was associated with more emotional distress than being on schedule. Nevertheless, contrary to this hypothesis, the early occurrence of undesirable events was associated with fewer symptoms than being on schedule.

Age might also be implicated in the stress process because different coping responses may be used during the various stages of life. This can be explored using data on financial stress and two types of coping style, including cognitive ones (focusing on the positive aspects of one's life, maintaining an optimistic attitude and merely waiting for circumstances to improve) and behavioural ones (cutting back on expenses, borrowing money and improving one's job skills). Controlling for first-interview symptoms, coping styles differed by age group (18–34, 35–59 and ≥ 60 years). Younger workers were more likely to cut back on expenses, and older workers were less likely to seek to improve their job skills. Although different coping styles affected symptoms of depression at second interview, none of the coping methods moderated (interacted with) economic stress.[a]

Social support may also moderate the adverse effects of economic and noneconomic events. The evidence supported only the beneficial main effects of social support, as people with more job and nonjob social support reported fewer symptoms, and the main effect for nonjob social support survived the control for first-interview symptoms. In general, the Los Angeles stressor project provided little evidence that such psychosocial resources as coping skills or social support moderated the effects of job events *(30)*.

Implications

Research on the stress model
Most studies of economic stress, including the Los Angeles stressor project, have assumed some variant of the social and psychological model linking life change to decreases in wellbeing. Few such studies, however, were primarily designed to test or elaborate this model. The unemployment experience is a promising arena for such empirical development not only because of its social significance but also because of its intrinsic complexity.

---

[a] **Rook, K.S**. *Age differences in coping with stressful life events.* Unpublished data, 1988.

330

One of these complicating factors is that the personal experiences of job and financial events are not a simple function of the aggregate economy and that the aggregate economy has an independent impact, even on people currently employed. It follows that future studies of economic stress should take into account the socioeconomic climate: both objective climate, as measured by archival records, and subjective climate, as measured by the perceptions of the subjects of the study.

The complexity of the experience of unemployment also derives from the many different functions employment can have. Losing a job can imply personal financial catastrophe, a crushing loss of social status or the disappearance of orderly social roles and timed activities. As our work has indicated, economic events can trigger other events within and between people. Detailing the causal sequence of these events in the pertinent social system (usually the family) and the meaning attributed to each event by each person requires more fine-tuned research tools than are typically applied in studying the stress caused by unemployment.

Application to Health Promotion

Researchers have focused on reducing the adverse effects on health and behaviour of economic recession *(44,45)*. Prevention has been conceptually classified into proactive strategies that control exposure to stressors, and reactive strategies that increase the ability of people to cope with stressors.

Proactive strategies
Proactive strategies cut the link between the stressor and its effects early in the causal sequence, thus stopping a variety of possible direct and indirect processes with a single intervention. Proactive prevention can be further categorized into programmes that work from the top down, using government power to reduce economic stressors, or from the bottom up, giving individual people greater power over the institutions that employ them. Such top-down efforts as reducing unemployment rates should especially benefit people whose anxiety is affected by perceived community unemployment (link 2) and those affected personally (indirect effect via links 1 and 4). Bottom-up proactive prevention, in contrast, is more narrowly targeted at workers immediately threatened by personal job loss.

331

Specific examples of top-down proactive prevention suggested in the literature or debated in the political arena include using government resources to keep markets stable *(46)* or making a declining region attractive to capital investment *(30)*. It has been argued that the health and behavioural costs of displacing redundant labour should be included in cost–benefit analyses that precede the choice of economic programmes *(47)*. Such human cost-accounting would supposedly demonstrate that keeping people employed is often a more rational economic choice than displacing them, given the direct and indirect costs of providing services to those who may become ill because of loss of job or income. This argument has historically been based on two beliefs. The first was that research would continue to support the intuition that economic recession unambiguously destroys the health of the population. The second was that political institutions would care about the adverse effects of economic recession because the public sector would assume much of the cost of services for those affected. Both assumptions now seem naïve.

The research described above suggests that, at least in the United States, the economy affects health and the demand for health services in complex ways. Not all groups are equally likely to experience the stress of economic recession when a community loses part of its economic base. For example, respondents of medium socioeconomic status were the most likely group to experience personal undesirable economic events during economic downturns. The effect of economic stressors also varies by sex and age. Moreover, the strength of the effects is not as great as might be expected given such aggregate-level findings as Brenner's *(48)*. Even assuming that such survey-based methods underestimate the number of people who are casualties of economic downturns (for example, by failing to contact those who move, lose their homes or disconnect their telephones), it seems more likely that such people were symptomatic even before losing their jobs, which revealed rather than provoked disorder. Audits of these effects, therefore, are not likely to produce cost estimates that will mobilize top-down proactive prevention to stimulate local economies *(49)*. In fact, evidence shows that stimulating the economy may increase injuries resulting from work and transport accidents *(50)*.

The complexity of the effects of economic recession makes top-down proactive prevention politically problematic. The people who are hurt may not be equivalent in numbers or power to those whose status does not change or even improves. A policy option that allows firms or cooperatives to lay off workers, for example, may be resisted by people whose jobs are at risk because they fear the effects on their health of losing income and work-related benefits. People with financial assets that are threatened by inflation, however, may not resist this policy because they will be spared the stress of reduced economic security and its sequelae. Other people may advocate this policy because they believe it will spare them and future workers the stress of an even greater economic recession that will result if productivity is not increased by laying off workers.

The second assumption that sparked interest in top-down proactive prevention was that the public sector would have to assume the costs of caring for the victims of economic recession and would, therefore, want to keep the number of such victims to a minimum. The governments of most countries, however, have shown greater interest in increasing productivity than in protecting redundant labour. The health and social service programmes of most developed countries have been reduced instead of expanded *(51)*. The implication is that redundant workers in most industrialized countries will have to bear a growing proportion of the economic, physiological and behavioural costs of unemployment.

As top-down proactive prevention is not imminent in the industrialized world, bottom-up strategies pursued by people who are most hurt by economic recession should be expected. Indeed, these are already emerging in North America and in Europe. In the United States, this movement comprises primarily associations of workers that use their resources to purchase facilities that might be marginally profitable, although not sufficiently so to warrant the continued interest of large firms *(52, 53)*. Communities can also purchase these facilities *(54)*. Local governments have become very aggressive in pursuing private investment to keep communities from suffering economic decline *(55)*. In western Europe, workers join local governments to pressure national governments to pursue policies that are more proactive than those offered by the national parties *(56)*. Groups of workers in eastern Europe have attempted to alter the centralized economic planning of several countries, apparently because these systems have not responded well enough to workers' needs for economic security.[a] These bottom-up strategies to avoid economic

---

[a] *Vulnerability among long-term unemployed: longitudinal approaches*: report on a WHO meeting. Copenhagen, WHO Regional Office for Europe, 1986 (unpublished document ICP/HSR 801m02).

stressors assume that the given locale or group has been left out of a larger, more prosperous economy. Although this happens frequently, international recessions such as that in 1980–1982 leave very little opportunity for less productive organizations to survive without some form of public subsidy. Bottom-up proactive prevention may, therefore, be most effective when its goals are political as well as economic.

Reactive strategies

Unlike proactive strategies, reactive prevention seeks to preclude the adverse effects of economic recession by increasing the ability of individual people to cope with stressors. Such efforts are based on the so-called process literature, which studies how stress links (such as link 4) can be moderated. This type of intervention ranges from programmes to supplement income to training programmes that supposedly give workers the skills needed not only to find new work but also to cope better with the stress of losing a job and with reduced income (57). The income-supplement programmes are almost all funded by the public sector and vary greatly between countries in the amount and duration of supplement (51). The training programmes vary in their sponsorship and content. The best available inventory of these programmes in the United States (58) suggests that programmes are typically sponsored by a combination of private groups (often trade unions) and state governments. Although no similar inventory of programmes is available for western Europe, the best known programmes also appear to have both public and private sponsors (56).

The most innovative element of training programmes is that intended to enable workers to cope better with economic stressors. Social scientists have suggested how the content of these programmes could reflect what is known of stress inoculation (45,59). At least one programme has followed these recommendations (58) and has been evaluated. The training improved workers' ability to cope with the stress of losing a job and of searching for new employment (60). It is not known how much of the success was attributable to the stress inoculation in the programme, compared with job training and the general benefit of group support.

Training to improve coping skills is potentially controversial. The implicit goal of such training is to enable workers to absorb stressors without experiencing stress. This would allow policy-makers to restructure economies faster without having to bear the

334

political costs that arise from concern over displaced workers. This type of stress inoculation has been characterized as exploitation, as workers are expected to become callous to their own feelings, to serve the needs of the people who benefit most from economic restructuring *(56)*. The argument logically depends on who benefits most from restructuring; this leads to the long-standing debate on whether private or public ownership of capital best serves the general welfare.

References

1. **Durkheim, E.** *Suicide.* New York, Free Press, 1951.
2. **Jahoda, M**. *Employment and unemployment: a socio-psychological analysis.* Cambridge, Cambridge University Press, 1982.
3. **Fisher, S**. *Stress and the perception of control.* London, Lawrence Erlbaum, 1984.
4. **Garraty, J.A**. *Unemployment in history: economic thoughts and public policy.* New York, Harper & Row, 1978.
5. **Warr, P.B**. *Work, unemployment, and mental health.* New York, Oxford University Press, 1987.
6. **Kelvin, P. & Jarrett, J.E**. *Unemployment: its social psychological effects.* Cambridge, Cambridge University Press, 1985.
7. **Dooley, D. & Catalano, R**. Do economic variables generate psychological problems? Different methods, different answers. *In*: MacFadyen, A.J. & MacFadyen, H.W., ed. *Economic psychology: intersections in theory and application.* Amsterdam, North-Holland, 1986, pp. 503–546.
8. **Brenner, M.H**. *Mental illness and the economy.* Cambridge, MA, Harvard University Press, 1973.
9. **Catalano, R**. Contending with rival hypotheses in correlation of aggregate time-series (CATS): an overview for community psychologists. *American journal of community psychology,* **9**: 667–679 (1981).
10. **Cohen, L.E. & Felson, M**. On estimating the social costs of national economic policy: a critical examination of the Brenner study. *Social indicators research,* **6**: 251–259 (1979).
11. **Gravelle, H.S.E. et al**. Mortality and unemployment: a critique of Brenner's time-series analyses. *Lancet,* **2**: 675–679 (1981).

12. **Robinson, W.S**. Ecological correlations and the behavior of individuals. *American sociological review*, **15**: 352–357 (1950).

13. **Warr, P.B. & Jackson, P.R**. Factors influencing the psychological impact of prolonged unemployment and or re-employment. *Psychological medicine*, **15**: 795–807 (1985).

14. **Cobb, S. & Kasl, S.V**. *Termination: the consequences of job loss*. Cincinnati, OH, National Institute for Occupational Safety and Health, Behavioral and Motivational Factors Research, 1977 (Report No. 76–1261).

15. **Tiggeman, M. & Winefield, A.H**. The effect of unemployment on the mood, self-esteem, locus of control, and depressive affect of school leavers. *Journal of occupational psychology*, **57**: 33–42 (1984).

16. **Swinburne, P**. The psychological impact of unemployment on managers and professional staff. *Journal of occupational psychology*, **54**: 47–64 (1981).

17. **Brinkman, C**. Health problems and psycho-social strains of unemployed: a summary of recent empirical research in the Federal Republic of Germany. *In*: John, J. et al., ed. *Influence of economic instability on health*. Berlin (West), Springer Verlag, 1983, pp. 263–285.

18. **Feather, N.T. & Bond, M.J**. Time structure and purposeful activity among employed and unemployed university graduates. *Journal of occupational psychology*, **56**: 241–254 (1983).

19. **Frolich, D**. Economic deprivation, work orientation and health: conceptual ideas and some empirical findings. *In*: John, J. et al., ed. *Influence of economic instability on health*. Berlin (West), Springer Verlag, 1983, pp. 293–320.

20. **Stafford, E.M. et al**. Employment, work involvement and mental health in less qualified young people. *Journal of occupational psychology*, **53**: 291–304 (1980).

21. **Catalano, R. et al**. Economic predictors of admissions to mental health facilities in a nonmetropolitan community. *Journal of health and social behavior*, **22**: 284–297 (1981).

22. **Catalano, R. et al**. Economic antecedents of help seeking: re-formulation of time-series tests. *Journal of health and social behavior*, **26**: 151–152, (1985).

23. **Dohrenwend, B.P. et al**. Nonspecific psychological distress and other dimensions of psychopathology. *Archives of general psychiatry*, **37**: 1229–1236 (1980).

24. **Radloff, I.S**. The CES-D scale: a self-report depression scale for research in the general population. *Applied psychological measurement*, **1**: 385–401 (1977).

25. **Catalano, R. & Dooley, D**. The health effects of economic instability: a test of the economic stress hypothesis. *Journal of health and social behavior*, **24**: 46–60 (1983).

26. **Dooley, D. & Catalano, R**. The epidemiology of economic stress. *American journal of community psychology*, **12**: 387–409 (1984).

27. **Dooley, D. et al**. Personal and aggregate unemployment and psychological symptoms. *Journal of social issues*, **44**: 107–123 (1988).

28. **Cohn, R.M**. The effect of employment status change on self attitudes. *Social psychology*, **41**: 81–93 (1978).

29. **Brown, R.L**. *Mental health and the economy: a disaggregated analysis*. Thesis, Ann Arbor, MI, University of Michigan, 1982.

30. **Dooley, D. et al**. Job and non-job stressors and their moderators. *Journal of occupational psychology*, **60**: 115–132 (1987).

31. **Levi, L. et al**. The psychological, social, and biochemical impacts of unemployment in Sweden. *International journal of mental health*, **13**: 18–34 (1984).

32. **Kessler, R.C. et al**. Unemployment and health in a community sample. *Journal of health and social behavior*, **28**: 51–59 (1987).

33. **Dooley, D. & Catalano, R**. Why the economy predicts help seeking: a test of competing explanations. *Journal of health and social behavior*, **25**: 160–175 (1984).

34. **Dooley, D. et al**. Economic stress and suicide: Multilevel analyses. *Suicide and life-threatening behavior*, **19**: 321–351 (1989).

35. **Catalano, R. et al**. Labor markets and help-seeking: a test of the employment security hypothesis. *Journal of health and social behavior*, **27**: 277–287 (1986).

36. **Cohen, S. & Hoberman, H.M**. Positive events and social supports as buffers of life change stress. *Journal of applied social psychology*, **13**: 99–125 (1983).

37. **Catalano, R. et al**. A test of reciprocal risk between undesirable economic and noneconomic life events. *American journal of community psychology*, **15**: 633–651 (1987).

38. **Grayson, J.P**. The closure of a factory and its impact on health. *International journal of health services*, **15**: 69–93 (1985).

39. **Liem, R. & Rayman, P**. Health and social costs of unemployment: research and policy considerations. *American psychologist*, **37**: 1116–1123 (1982).

40. **Rook, K.S. et al**. Stress transmission: the effects of husbands' job stressors on the emotional health of their wives. *Journal of marriage and the family*, **53**: 165–177 (1991).

41. **Dooley, D. & Catalano, R**. Economic change and primary prevention: ethnicity effects. *In*: Hough, R.H. et al, ed. *Psychiatric epidemiology and prevention: the possibilities*. Los Angeles, Neuropsychiatric Institute, University of California, Los Angeles, 1986, pp. 207–230.

42. **Rook, K.S. et al**. The timing of major life events: effect of departing from the social clock. *American journal of community psychology*, **17**: 233–258 (1989).

43. **Elder, G.H**. Age differentiation and the life course. *Annual review of sociology*, **1**: 165–190 (1975).

44. **Aboud, A., ed**. *Plant closing legislation*. Ithaca, NY, Cornell University Press, 1984.

45. **Catalano, R. & Dooley, D**. Economic change in primary prevention. *In*: Price, R.H. et al., ed. *Prevention in community mental health: research, policy and practice*. Beverly Hills, CA, Sage, 1980, pp. 21–40.

46. **Solo, R**. Industrial policy. *Journal of economic issues*, **18**: 697–714 (1984).

47. **Dooley, D. & Catalano, R**. Money and mental disorder: toward behavioral cost accounting for primary prevention. *American journal of community psychology*, **5**: 217–227 (1977).

48. **Brenner, M.H**. *Estimating the social costs of national economic policy*. Report to the Congressional Research Service of the Library of Congress and Joint Economic Committee of Congress. Washington, DC, US Government Printing Office, 1976 (Paper No. 5).

49. **Buss, T. & Redburn, F**. *Mass unemployment and mental health*. Beverly Hills, CA, Sage, 1983.

50. **Catalano, R. & Serxner, S**. Time series designs of potential interest to epidemiologists. *American journal of epidemiology*, **126**: 724–731 (1987).

51. European countries seek ways to get unemployed into job training programs. *Los Angeles times*, 30 March 1988, Part IV, p.2.

52. **Bellas, C.J**. *Industrial democracy and the worker owner firm*. New York, Praeger, 1972.

53. **Whyte, W.F**. The emergence of employee-owned firms in the United States. *Executive*, **3**: 22–24 (1977).

54. **Beck-Rex, M**. Youngstown: can this steel city forge a comeback? *Planning*, **44**: 12–15 (1978).

55. **Catalano, R**. Local economies and healthy communities. *In*: Duhl, L., ed. *Urban conditions II*, Beverly Hills, CA, Sage, in press.

56. **Keiselbach, T. & Svensson, P.-G**. Health and social policy responses to unemployment in Europe. *Journal of social issues*, **44**: 173–191 (1988).

57. **Hansen, G**. Services to workers facing plant shutdowns: California and Canada. *International journal of manpower*, **7**: 35–52 (1986).

58. *Unemployment and mental health: a report on research resources for technical assistance*. Washington, DC, National Institute of Mental Health, 1985.

59. **Manuso, J**. Coping with job abolishment. *Journal of occupational medicine*, **19**: 598–602 (1977).

60. **Beasalell, V.B**. *Finding a job*. Berkeley, Ten-Speed Press, 1982.

15

Health promotion among the elderly

Kathryn Dean & Bjørn E. Holstein

Framework and Orientation

Many people, especially people classified as elderly, might question why old people are receiving special consideration in a book on health promotion. Professionals often treat old people as a vulnerable group. As older people, especially those seen by professionals, are more likely to have chronic health problems and diseases that have been statistically correlated with certain risk factors, elderly people have become associated with ill health.

The implicit assumption (often made explicit) behind this vulnerability is that disease, deterioration and ill health are inevitably determined by chronological aging. In recent years, considerable opposition has arisen to terminology that implies that pathology and incompetence automatically accompany aging. This labelling process arises more from cultural values *(1)* and misinterpretation of findings from cross-sectional research investigations than from valid documentation of the factors and processes that often result in deteriorating health in advancing age *(2)*.

This discussion focuses on health and functioning rather than vulnerability, risk or disease. An important reason to emphasize health is that the vast majority of elderly people in developed countries are in good health, functioning as active and independent members of the community *(3)*.

Another reason to emphasize health is related to the concept and application of health promotion. The concept of health promotion guides approaches to research, policy and programme development, ultimately determining the strategies selected to promote the health of aging populations. Our definition of health promotion focuses on the health potential of individuals and communities rather than on preventing specific disorders. In Nutbeam's (4) health promotion glossary, health promotion is defined as a unifying concept, a process enabling individuals and communities to increase control over the determinants of health and recognizing "the basic need for change in both the ways and conditions of living in order to promote health".

Important issues are involved in promoting and preserving re-maining health and functioning in a population group that ultimately faces a biologically determined decrease in health reserve and func-tional capacity. The concept of ultimate decline, however, must be carefully and cautiously used because there is considerable interindi-vidual variation in health and function even at very advanced ages. Studies assessing the health of elderly populations indicate that there is considerable variation in health status (5). A majority of old people have one or more chronic ailments, but a significant minority have no health problem or complaint. Most of those with chronic health problems manage their lives without help and with only minor restrictions in functional capacity.

At the other end of the health spectrum there is a large minority — about a quarter of people over 70 years of age — that has severe problems in managing daily life, and half of the people in this group are so incapacitated that they depend on help for basic daily activities (6,7).

The health gap seems to increase with increasing age. Differences in health status among old people are not only greater than the differences in children and young adults, but this phenomenon seems to increase steadily with increasing age. The differences in health status also seem to be different in different cohorts (5). Disease is not some fixed component of aging and little is known about the potential for healthy aging. This suggests the fundamental importance of a life-long perspective in promoting the health of populations. Can effec-tive health promotion for elderly people be initiated only among young people? This might be the best long-term solution to protect health, but it does not diminish the need for appropriate health promotion among existing elderly populations. Indeed, health

promotion becomes increasingly important with increasing age because of the need to protect remaining psychological and biological
reserves.

The discussion and examples presented will thus consider health
promotion from the perspective of protecting and enhancing the
remaining health potential of people who are already old. We have
looked at prototype programmes that address human living
conditions and the forces that are shaping and changing them, and
which emphasize the physiological, emotional, cognitive and interpersonal aspects of health. The examination of programmes for
elderly people considers themes that are part of the new thinking on
health promotion: emphasis on positive health, on community (or
consumer) participation, and on intersectoral action.

Strategies for Health Promotion in Elderly Populations

Three main health promotion strategies will be discussed. These do
not, of course, represent the entire range of strategies to promote the
health of the elderly or even the most important ones. The health of
the elderly is based on the health of the population of which they are
a segment. Therefore, the health of old people is mainly determined
by the quality of the environment and the living conditions of the
society in which they live. Aging does, however, change circumstances. The three strategies deal with some specific aspects of health
maintenance, where changes in social situation and functional
capacity lead to the need for specialized approaches. The three
strategies are: maintaining and increasing functional capacity, maintaining or improving self-care, and stimulating social networks.

The three approaches are inherently interrelated. Actually, they
are aspects of each other, as maintaining functional capacity is a core
component of self-care, and stimulating social networks is an essential element in maintaining functional capacity. Nevertheless, for
purposes of elaboration, health promotion will be examined using
these three categories.

The differences in health status in the elderly population also
indicate a need for a wide range of health promotion activities.
Activities beneficial for healthy elderly people are not necessarily
suited for impaired elderly people and vice versa. As it is necessary to
implement health promotion programmes and services for
individuals, regardless of their health status, activities will be

343

described that promote health in three distinct life situations: healthy elderly people, elderly people with special needs and impaired or chronically ill elderly people.

The purpose of this classification is to identify important aspects of the social situation and social role of elderly people that influence the need for health promotion. The three strategies and the three life situations form a matrix (Fig. 1) that may stimulate thinking about the variability necessary in health promotion programmes. Examples are not provided for each cell of the matrix as the matrix is a heuristic instrument for developing health promotion programmes for elderly people. Although, most of the examples provided are from Scandinavia, health promotion programmes are not widely accepted in the Scandinavian countries. On the contrary, such programmes are far more frequent in many other countries.

Maintaining functional capacity

The aging process is complicated and the individual manifestations of aging are immensely varied. Those who design health promotion

Fig. 1. Matrix of different health promotion approaches in the elderly

| | | **Strategies** | | |
		Maintaining functional capacity	Maintaining or improving self-care	Stimulating social networks
Life situations	Healthy elderly people	Exercise programmes	Self-care education programme (SAGE)	Professional home-visiting project
	Elderly people with special needs	Needs or resources fit for acutely ill elderly people	Confidant, control, comparison project	Self-help intervention for widows
	Impaired or chronically ill elderly people	24-hour domiciliary care	Project to reorient housing and support services for the elderly	Activation of networks of institutionalized elderly people

initiatives for elderly people have to know how human functions change with age.

Social responsibility, experience and artistic performance can potentially increase with age. Glucose tolerance, memory and coping responses to threat and strain remain practically unchanged. Most physiological functions deteriorate with age, although at different rates (8,9).

Perhaps the most important characteristic of the aging process is the constant loss of biological reserve capacity, which is the difference between the maximum biological capacity and the capacity required to maintain independent daily living. This loss may be delayed by sufficient self-care and a healthy lifestyle, but the loss of maximal heart rhythm and lung capacity and of eye lens adaptability are inevitable. Such deterioration is not necessarily important in the daily life of people who are generally healthy and have no special needs for fitness and activity.

In case of illness, however, reserve capacity is of central importance. Recovery from illness requires reserve capacity. The less reserve capacity one has, the less successful is one's recovery from illness. One of the important functions of health promotion among elderly people, then, is to maintain or expand the biological reserve capacity of individuals.

Health and functioning have psychological, social and physical aspects. Researchers are only beginning to document and understand the extent to which these aspects are interdependent. The capacity for social and mental action does not necessarily deteriorate significantly in later life. Nevertheless, both stress and malfunctioning social environments can have negative effects on psychological and social functioning.

Self-reported declines in memory and energy level among older people are related to the internalization of cultural stereotypes (10). The expectation of decline and deterioration may lead to less active approaches to coping with such age-related changes as retirement and loss of loved ones. Passive approaches to coping may be more prevalent among old people (11,12) but the evidence is not clear and some authors take the opposite position (13,14).

Extensive literature now documents the relationships between the social environment and health and longevity (11,15). The mechanisms involved in these relationships have not been described or understood, but social interaction and obtaining the appropriate

345

type and amount of social support when needed are essential aspects of maintaining health.

Thus effective health promotion policies and community intervention among elderly people need to direct concerted attention towards maintaining and expanding functional capacity. Social and psychological functioning need clear focus and priority along with the activities of daily living. Enhancing psychological and social functioning may be the best way to protect physical capacity.

Programmes that are directed towards enhancing functional capacity include exercise programmes, intervention in risk situations and 24-hour domiciliary care.

Exercise programmes

There are many exercise programmes and sports programmes for older people. The programmes vary considerably in content and organization, but they are based on the assumption that physical exercise makes good sense for elderly people. The evidence is still unclear on the importance of physical exercise in preventing heart disease in this age group, although most experts believe that it has a positive effect *(16)*. There seems to be more consensus on other evidence of the impact of physical exercise in old age: it increases lung function, oxygen uptake, muscle strength, general vitality and general wellbeing *(17)*.

Physical exercise delays or prevents the age-related bone loss in females that often leads to fractures *(16,18)*. Physical exercise programmes are common, but they are a limited approach to protecting functional capacity. Attending physical exercise classes may provide some protection for general functional ability, but the programmes are based on the risk-factor approach to prevention and are not directed towards the whole person. Programme development has been relatively limited.

Maintaining functional capacity during illness

The importance of maintaining functional capacity among elderly people experiencing such critical incidents as acute illness is illustrated by a model project from Holbæk, Denmark *(19)*. The project developed from an attempt to identify risk groups, stimulate the people in these risk groups and enhance general health and functioning. The first step in identifying risk groups was to conduct a prospective survey, to identify the characteristics of groups with increased risk of losing functional capacity (such as people in institutions).

346

It was possible to identify risk factors but this was not very helpful for health care professionals. First, the vast majority of the people in the risk group already had frequent contact with their family doctor and received home help services or home nursing, and thus were under the continual surveillance of professionals. Second, the information obtained is difficult to use in the clinical setting.

Relevant and effective health promotion actions have not been identified for individual members of a given group for which there is some generalized information on, for example, the increased risk of being admitted to hospital within the next two years. What, if anything, can general practitioners or other health care professionals do with such information when most of the risk group will not be admitted to hospital during the next two years *(20)*?

The next attempt was to identify elderly people in risk situations, defined as episodes of acute illness and after discharge from hospital. The objective of the intervention programme was to prevent avoidable social breakdown and avoidable readmission to hospital among people over 70 years of age. The method used was a programme to maintain functional capacity during an episode of acute illness or the recovery period immediately after discharge from hospital. Maintaining functional capacity during an illness episode often requires formal help and this should be given according to need, but should be reduced as quickly as possible, stimulating people to take over these functions when possible.

By carefully monitoring the community, a total of 470 individuals were identified as being either acutely ill at home or recently discharged from hospital. The vast majority of these people were in frequent contact with the health and social services, especially their general practitioner (68% of the acutely ill and 56% of the newly discharged reported contact within the last month) and the home help services (82% of the acutely ill and 56% of the newly discharged received regular home help).

These 470 people were visited at home by a community nurse either during the episode of acute illness or the first or second day after discharge from hospital. The nurse interviewed these people, assessed the situation and offered to help with their unmet needs *(19)*.

Among the 206 just discharged from hospital, 55% needed help of some kind, such as home help, nursing care, contact with the general practitioner, other contacts or equipment; 8% received too much help and 26% received too little or the wrong kind of help. The nurse evaluated the help that was given as being harmful to functional capacity in 13% of these cases.

Of the 264 people who were acutely ill at home, 61% had unmet needs; 3% of these people received too much help and 40% too little help. The nurse evaluated the help that was given as being harmful to functional capacity in 24% of these cases.

Consequently, the community social services department tried to meet the unmet needs and alter the inappropriate help. The nurse visited these people two weeks later and reassessed the situation. In most cases the help provided had been adjusted to fit the needs better. In most cases the health status of the person had improved and the social situation had become more stable.

The project was carried out without randomization or a control group, and no conclusive evidence about the effectiveness of the programme is therefore available. Nevertheless, the professionals involved in the project felt that avoidable acute social breakdown and avoidable readmissions were significantly reduced. Consequently, the home care was reorganized to provide acute home care permanently.

Twenty-four-hour domiciliary care
Most municipalities in Denmark have introduced 24-hour domiciliary care during the last ten years. This service is organized in different ways in different municipalities, but it usually includes the opportunity for impaired elderly people to be visited by home nurses and home helpers day and night. Most municipalities restrict this service to elderly people already referred to the system, but a few have organized access for everybody in need regardless of prior referral.

The aim of this service is primarily to establish an alternative to institutionalized care for impaired elderly people and other elderly people unable to manage daily tasks without help. It was hoped that establishing 24-hour domiciliary care would reduce the cost of care for the elderly and increase the health and quality of life of impaired elderly people in the community.

Several municipalities have studied and carefully evaluated 24-hour domiciliary care. Data in Næstved, a municipality of 45 000 inhabitants, are shown in Fig. 2 and Table 1. The 24-hour service was introduced in 1982. The staffing in the evening is two nurses and nine home helpers, and at night one nurse and nine home helpers. Fig. 2 illustrates the number of visits per hour, and Table 1

348

shows the reasons for over 55 000 visits to 595 clients included in the service during the first year of operation. (Some visits had several reasons.) Most of the clients (88%) were referred to domiciliary care in the daytime prior to inclusion in the 24-hour service.

The service was carefully evaluated by interview studies and analyses using health economics. The vast majority of the clients reported that they would have been unable to stay in their homes without this service, and most of them wanted to do so even though they could have been referred to and admitted to a nursing home.

The 24-hour service reduced the demand for nursing home beds by 50–60 beds. The demand for hospital-based nursing care was reduced by about 3000 bed-days a year. The total savings in public expenditure for care were estimated to be about US $700 000 a year without harmful effects *(21)*.

Improving self-care behaviour
The maintenance of functional ability cannot be separated from effective self-care. Functional maintenance, or living life fully at

Fig. 2.   Visits per hour in an average evening and night, Næstved, Denmark, 1982–1983

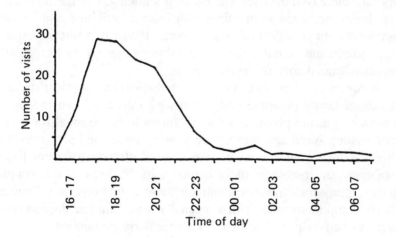

Table 1. Main reasons for 54 040 planned and 1729 acute visits during the first year of the 24-hour domiciliary care service in Næstved (1983), as a percentage of the total number of evening and night visits

	Planned visits (%)	Acute visits (%)
Observation	32	20
Administering medicine (including injection)	38	12
Changing clothes	29	7
Serving dinner	20	1
Helping into or out of bed	23	8
Colostomy and personal hygiene	22	7
Helping with visits to the lavatory	13	7
Conversation about illness	4	7
Care of ulcers and bedsores	17	4

given levels of fitness, is an important aspect of self-care, but we will focus on more conscious health-directed behaviour in daily life and in changing life situations.

There is today a strong belief, and some moderate evidence to support it, that improving health-related habits is helpful for people who are already old. They should stop smoking, change their diet, exercise more, engage in stimulating social activities and expose themselves to intellectual stimulation. Physical exercise, social participation and intellectual stimulation seem to be especially important ingredients of healthy aging.

A conscious effort to enhance psychological and physical strength to expand health potential and resistance to disease is an individual approach to health promotion that continues to be essential for health maintenance in old age. Nevertheless, many forces and processes that affect health in old age arise from cultural attitudes or from living conditions and problems more common in the lives of old people. Active approaches towards changing these conditions or enhancing effective coping despite them are equally important health-promoting forms of self-help and self-care within elderly populations.

The active self-care of chronic conditions is another area of great potential within elderly populations. Old people tend to accept disabilities as inevitable and irreversible, seeking palliation rather than health-promoting action and corrective treatment (2,11,22). At the same time, most old people have one or more chronic health problems. Approaches that stress self-care or self-management for the care of chronic conditions have grown rapidly in type and number. Many of these approaches rely on learning as much as possible about the chronic condition or disease, normalizing this condition to the greatest extent possible within the person's life situation, and building health potential. Many of the programmes are professionally initiated as community education programmes for the self-care of a specific condition (23) or self-help or peer-counselling strategies incorporating self-care of a condition.[a]

Self-care of chronic conditions requires effective interaction with professional care (24,25). The safe use of medicines is becoming especially important for old people as medicine prescription continues to rise. Elderly people increasingly get prescriptions renewed without face-to-face contact, even though they are less likely to be aware of side effects and are more vulnerable to the harmful effects of medicine (26,27). Older people also report that they have greater confidence that medical care can preserve health (11), and older people are less likely than younger people to question medical advice (24). Health promotion programmes for elderly people need to focus on effective interaction with professional care.

Self-care programmes directed towards healthy elderly people
This example illustrates programmes directed towards improving health-enhancing self-care in populations of healthy old people. We have not identified formal programmes of this type in Scandinavia. This type of programme appears to be more developed in the United States.

The prototypical example of activated elderly people who are working to change the cultural attitudes and living conditions that negatively affect the health and wellbeing of old people is the Gray Panthers. This grassroots organization uses an approach emphasizing community action in changing the conditions necessary for healthy lifestyles. Elderly people identify their own problems, find meaningful solutions and work to achieve them.

Senior actualization and growth exploration (SAGE) is an individually oriented programme directed towards improving

---

[a] **Bremer Schulte, M**. *Counselling by and for chronically ill and handicapped persons*. Paper presented at the Second International Congress on Patient Counselling and Education, The Hague, 1979.

351

psychological and physical strength to increase the health potential and resistance of healthy elderly people. Developed by a group of lay and professional people, this approach consciously avoids any premise that elderly people are vulnerable in developing its programme and activities. The programme combines a wide range of activities focused on physical, psychological and social development and change *(28)*. Group sessions and individual exercises seek to improve physical condition, strengthen self-image, develop awareness of the full range of capabilities, and reduce the use of palliative treatments, especially psychotropic drugs.

A randomized control study of the SAGE programme found that the programme had significant effects on self-esteem, psychological distress, anxiety about illness, and coping with marital problems, but not on medication, behaviour or reported health status. The experimental group gained self-esteem, experienced reduced symptoms of psychological distress and anxiety about health, and coped more effectively with marital problems compared with the control group. Significant changes in health and medication use patterns may not occur in a nine-month study period. Reduced psychological distress and anxiety about health would probably ultimately lead to reduced use of psychotropic drugs.

Another approach to lay health activation in the United States is self-care education programmes *(29)*. One such programme for people over 60 years of age was evaluated in a controlled trial *(30)*. The test group participated in a thirteen-session educational intervention, while the control group heard only one two-hour lecture demonstration. The educational programme involved training in assessing illness (acute illness, chronic conditions and emergencies), the use of medicines, physical fitness, nutrition, emotional wellbeing and the appropriate use of health and human resources, including coordination of health and welfare needs. Improved health knowledge, skills performance and confidence in health matters resulted. The intervention also stimulated healthier behaviour and reports of improved quality of life. A re-examination of the participants after one year found that the improvements had been sustained.

Activating lonely elderly people
An intervention study was directed towards lonely elderly people seeking a community service in Stockholm *(31)*; 108 people on a

waiting list for a day care centre who rated themselves as lonely were randomly divided into an intervention group and a control group.

The intervention group was exposed to a special group-meeting programme to reduce loneliness, using the confidant, control, comparison method. The approach is based on the view that regular club activities and group meetings where elderly people convene reduce social isolation but not loneliness. The reduction of loneliness requires the activation of the individual. Other features of the programme were the following.

First, participants were ecouraged to develop at least one real confidant among the group members, a more intense social contact than is usually obtained in such club activity. To promote such confidant relations, the participants were given challenging and meaningful tasks such as planning negotiations with local politicians on improving the living conditions of elderly people in the community.

Second, participants were to experience a situation that increased their feeling of control over their lives. In practice, negotiating with local politicians and top community civil servants about improvements for the elderly in the community comprised the programme.

Third, one psychological rationale for the programme was that loneliness is partly caused by lack of meaningful and real social comparison. The group meetings prior to the negotiations with local politicians gave the participants an impression of their own strengths and those of the other participants.

The results were quite remarkable. The people in the intervention group experienced significantly less loneliness, had more social contacts, felt that life was more meaningful, had higher self-esteem, had greater willingness to trust, had lower blood pressure (systolic and diastolic), participated more in organized activities and more often took a holiday trip, compared with the situation prior to the implementation of the programme. The control group showed no significant changes in these areas.

Activating self-care among chronically impaired elderly people
An innovative community experiment by a Danish municipality reorganized and reoriented residential arrangements and support services to strengthen the autonomy and improve the self-care skills of impaired elderly people *(32)*. The project was planned and carried out by an interdisciplinary nursing team with representatives of the

353

home help, home nursing, public health nursing and nursing home services. The project emphasized self-care and was based on the intersectorality and reorientation of health services associated with the health for all strategy of the World Health Organization (33).

The objectives of this community-based project included increased flexibility in delivering services, an improved relationship between needs and services, and ensuring equal rights for the elderly no matter where they live. Three main techniques were used.

First, the previous distinction between nursing home staff and domiciliary care staff was eliminated. All staff now work under one administration, sharing tasks and responsibilities for elderly people needing care no matter where they live (private home, sheltered housing, nursing home). Second, the nursing home was changed from a formally managed institution to a cluster of private residences. The residents were no longer institutionalized although they lived in the same location. They could lock their doors; they received their old-age pensions without reduction and had to pay rent and services like all other citizens. Third, 24-hour domiciliary care was introduced, making it possible to provide nursing home services in ordinary private residences.

These changes transformed this nursing home from a physical facility to a source for the delivery of services according to need. Appropriate services are provided for the people who live in the former nursing home (a house) and all other elderly people no matter where they live. The people living in the former nursing home can cancel the services they do not want or need. This change has created an autonomous role and social situation for the people living there. They manage their affairs to the extent of their capacity, actively making decisions on health and care.

The project has been carefully evaluated. A questionnaire-based survey has demonstrated that the vast majority of elderly people are greatly satisfied with the new arrangement. Self-care behaviour has clearly improved. The residents of the former nursing home use significantly less medicine, and the number of hospital bed-days decreased during the first year of their new status as non-institutionalized. Finally, the mood, social participation and functional capacity of these people has improved.

Stimulating social networks

Satisfying social interaction is a vital aspect of the quality of life. Supportive social networks are apparently also vital aspects of maintaining health, and therefore are a strategic area for health promotion. There is a correlation between social network factors and health factors: although the mechanisms are still not known, the strengthening of network support and social interactions in elderly populations can clearly enhance wellbeing and the quality of life. Experimental intervention to improve social network functioning also seems to improve health. A few carefully evaluated projects have demonstrated that social network or support interventions improve health.

The Rødovre intervention programme

In Rødovre, a suburb of Copenhagen, 600 people aged 75 years or older were randomized into an intervention group and a control group. The members of the intervention group were visited by a doctor or a community nurse (the same visitor every time) every three months. The visits were relaxed and unstructured and provided the opportunity to discuss the problems and the pleasures of health-related matters, daily activities and social and personal issues. The visitor tried to establish an easy and trusting relationship, and thus serve as a social network resource. The visitors did not carry out treatment or nursing care, but referred these people to the health and social services available in the community.

The effect was remarkable. The intervention group had 33% fewer hospital admissions and hospital days (4884 bed-days) than the control group (6442 bed-days) and fewer emergency doctor calls. The numbers of contacts with general practitioners were identical in the intervention group and the control group. Mortality and admission to nursing homes dropped significantly in the intervention group compared with the control group (Table 2). About 25% more home help was provided to the intervention group than to the control group. Table 3 shows the numbers of people receiving various social services during the study.

The results have received significant attention. This kind of intervention can potentially generate positive health in elderly people. Interestingly, the control group received considerably more medical treatment than the intervention group, but ended up with poorer health and higher mortality than the intervention group.

These results provide no firm conclusions. The concept of social support, however, is a likely explanation. The health visitors became important resource people and an important part of the social support network of elderly people. Moreover the additional delivery of home

355

Table 2. Number of deaths and mortality rate (%) in each group
in six periods of six months

Six-month period	Deaths			
	Intervention group		Control group	
	N	%	N	%
1	14	4.9	14	4.9
2	9	3.3	8	2.9
3	9	3.4	12	4.6
4	10	4.0	15	6.0
5	7	2.9	17	7.2
6	7	3.0	9	4.2
Total	56	3.6	75	4.2

help in the intervention group strengthened the social network of these people and reduced unmet needs for help.

There were no differences between the control group and the intervention group during the first 18 months. The differences appeared after about 18 months, and seemed to increase during the second 18 months. There seems to be a long latency period from the introduction of a social support resource until health is affected (34). A follow-up study was conducted after the programme ended and this showed that the desirable effects of the programme lasted for several months. After a year or two the differences between the groups disappeared (35).

Table 3. Number of people in each group receiving various
social services over three years

Social services	Number of recipients	
	Intervention group	Control group
Admission to hospital	168	181
Home nurse	116	106
Home help	46	29
Supplies or equipment	101	65
Modification of home	40	25
Payment for dentures, glasses, hearing aid, shoes	99	88
Meals on wheels	28	29
Occupational and physical therapy	41	47
Home day care	12	13

In Oslo, a similar experiment carried out in an elderly population in the inner city obtained quite similar results *(36)*.

Self-help intervention for widows
Widowhood and retirement frequently cause great distress in elderly populations. These events are fundamental intrusions in the social networks of elderly people. Given the evidence on the implications for health of social support *(11)*, programmes to facilitate coping with and adjustment to these stressful situations are priority areas for health promotion among elderly people.

Self-help and mutual aid are especially well suited to these situations. We have not been able to identify an example of this cell of the matrix in Scandinavia, but there is an example in Canada. A controlled study of a self-help intervention programme for widows found that peer support from another widow during the post-bereavement phase of adaptation was beneficial *(37)*.

The members of the intervention group received a letter from one of six women who had adjusted well to their own bereavement. These widows had participated in a training seminar that examined problems of bereavement, supportive counselling and the resources available in the community. The support was available to the new widows as long as they needed it, first in the form of individual support, and later, small mutual-aid groups.

The intervention group passed more rapidly and successfully through phases of intrapersonal and interpersonal adaptation to resolve the overall distress. This study provides evidence that mutual aid is effective among people who understand a given problem from personal experience.

Nursing homes
Several institutions for impaired elderly people (nursing homes) have been used as laboratory settings for model projects attempting to maintain or improve functional capacity and social network contacts among the residents. Improvements in daily functioning and activity and in social network contacts can be achieved regardless of physical capacity. The key mechanism seems to be the attitudes and work principles of the staff.

A conscious and active attempt to involve relatives in the management and daily life of the nursing home has been associated with improved physical and psychological functioning of the residents *(38)*. Admission to a nursing home has several undesirable side

357

effects: lost of autonomy and independence, loss of previous social network contacts, and increasing pseudo-dementia. Admission also affects relatives by introducing feelings of guilt, anger, embarrassment and fear.

Eleven nursing homes tried to improve the social relations between the residents, staff and relatives. Each nursing home had to find and implement one or more techniques to improve social relations. Nine techniques were developed, most of which were minor changes in the daily life of the institution. The combined effect of these techniques, however, can introduce quite a change in social relations. Each nursing home used a different mixture of these techniques:

— meetings for relatives and residents to discuss matters of importance to the residents and the institution;
— formalized relatives' council with specified management tasks;
— systematic admission interview with relatives to make explicit decisions on sharing tasks and responsibilities; the interview resulted in a formal (written) agreement to make each party's expectations visible;
— questionnaire-based inventory of resource people and activities offered by the relatives to the institution; this inventory facilitated the identification of relatives to take part in various activities at the institution;
— systematic family consultations: meetings between staff and all significant family and social network members to discuss the role of the family openly;
— education of relatives based on group consultations, in which relatives of several residents exchanged their feelings and experiences and gained insight into the social and psychological situation of the residents;
— newsletter for relatives, edited by residents or staff;
— delivering services from the institution to relatives: child care for grandchildren, lending tools, tableware and kitchen equipment, baking biscuits for family parties; and
— educating the staff to begin and maintain relaxed and open social interaction with relatives.

Although all these activities were minor changes in the management of the nursing home, the inverview-based evaluation revealed that the overall programme was perceived as being very successful. Tense relationships in the resident-relative-staff triangle tended to disappear, and all three parties felt relieved by the visibility and open discussions of expectations and responsibilities. The residents reported an improved level of activity and quality of life *(38,39)*.

Another study *(40,41)* reports that physical and psychological functioning and social network contacts are most likely to be maintained in nursing homes in which:

— the staff has extensive knowledge of the past history and present interests and resources of the residents;
— the staff has many informal contacts with the residents in situations where staff member and resident are in a balanced (non-hierarchical) situation, such as drinking coffee in the resident's private room; and
— the staff has positive expectations about the residents' own resources and allows the residents to perform more activities than is normal in institutions for impaired elderly people.

These examples show that the traditional way of running institutions for impaired elderly people (sociologists would use the term total institutions) seems to be counter-productive to maintaining functional capacity and social contacts. Moreover, it seems to be possible to improve the functional levels of people considered to be incapable of taking care of themselves. The best approach seems to be a caring programme in which management stresses the importance of symmetrical social relations between staff and residents and of catalysing the residents to higher levels of activity instead of passively receiving care.

Conclusions

The examples cited do not exhaust the range of types of health promotion programme for elderly people, nor are they necessarily the best examples. They illustrate the potential for protecting and expanding remaining functioning at all levels of health status and the beneficial effects of a range of strategies built into projects designed for the special circumstances of subgroups.

While some prototype projects have been identified that suggest impressive gains from health promotion programmes, it appears that such programmes are still relatively rare. The Member States of the

European Region of WHO have adopted 38 concrete targets for health for all *(33)*. Many countries have used them as a basis for statements on national health policy. These developments have not yet been translated into the range and number of projects that are needed to achieve the targets for health for all. Health promotion projects for healthy elderly people and for those coping with special problems especially need priority in health policy.

References

1. **Johnson, M.** Age as a labelling phenomenon. *In*: Dean, K. et al., ed. *Self-care and health in old age*. London, Croom Helm, 1986, pp. 12–34.
2. **Riley, M.W. & Bond, K.** Age strata in social systems. *In*: Binstock, R. & Shanas, E., ed. *Handbook of aging and the social sciences*. New York, Van Nostrand Reinhold, 1985.
3. **Dean, K. et al., ed.** *Self-care and health in old age*. London, Croom Helm, 1986.
4. **Nutbeam, D.** Health promotion glossary. *Health promotion*, **1**(1): 113–127 (1986).
5. **Svanborg, A. et al.** *Epidemiological studies on social and medical conditions of the elderly*: report on a survey. Copenhagen, WHO Regional Office for Europe, 1982 (EURO Reports and Studies No. 62).
6. **Heikkinen, E. et al., ed.** *The elderly in eleven countries: a sociomedical survey*. Copenhagen, WHO Regional Office for Europe, 1983 (Public Health in Europe No. 21).
7. **Platz, M.** *De ældres levevilkår 1977* [Conditions of life for the elderly 1977]. Copenhagen, Socialforskningsinstituttet, 1981.
8. **Fromholt, P.** Psykologi — ældes mennesket psykologisk set [Psychology - do people grow old psychologically]? *In*: Viiddik, A., ed. *Aldringens mange facetter* [The many facets of aging]. Aarhus, Dansk Gerontologisk Selskab, 1983, pp. 51–68.
9. **Heikkinen, E.** Den normale aldring [Normal aging]. *In*: Magnussen, G. et al., ed. *Den normale aldring. II. Biologi og fysiologi* [Normal aging. II. Biology and physiology]. Copenhagen, Månedsskrift for praktisk lægegerning, 1982.
10. **Fiske, M.** Tasks and crises of the second half of life: the interrelationship of commitment, coping and adaption. *In*: Birren, J. & Sloane, R., ed. *Handbook of mental health and aging*. Englewood Cliffs, NJ, Prentice-Hall, 1980, pp. 337–373.

11. **Dean, K**. Social support and health: pathways of influence. *Health promotion*, **1**(2): 133–150 (1986).
12. **Pfeiffer, E**. Psycho-pathology and social pathology. *In*: Birren, J.E. & Schaie, K.W., ed. *Handbook of the psychology of aging*. New York, Van Nostrand Reinhold, 1977, pp. 650–671.
13. **Neugarten, B**. Personality and aging. *In*: Birren, J.E. & Schaie, K.W., ed. *Handbook of the psychology of aging*. New York, Van Nostrand Reinhold, 1977, pp. 626–649.
14. **Vaillant, G.E**. *Adaption to life*. Boston, Little, Brown & Co., 1977.
15. **Cohen, S. & Syme, S.L**. *Social support and health*. New York, Academic Press, 1985.
16. **Kane, R.L. et al**. Prevention and the elderly: risk factors. *Health services research*, **19**(6): 945–1006 (1985).
17. **Hodgson, J.L. & Buskirk, E.R**. Effects of environmental factors and life patterns on life span. *In*: Dannon, D. et al., ed. *Aging: a challenge to science and society. Vol. 1. Biology*. Oxford, Oxford University Press, 1981.
18. **Mosekilde, L**. Knoglestyrken med alderen — hvordan bevares den [Bone strength in aging - how is it maintained]? *Gerontologi og samfund*, **3**(3): 36–37 (1987).
19. **Almind, G. et al**. *Syge gamle mennesker i eget hjem* [Ill elderly people in their own homes]. Copenhagen, FADL, 1987.
20. **Almind, G**. Risk factors in eighty-plus year olds living at home: an investigation of a Danish community. *International journal of aging and human development*, **21**: 227–234 (1985).
21. **Hansen, E.B. & Werborg, R**. *Døgnhjemmeplejen i Næstved. II. Virkninger og økonomi* [24-hour domiciliary care in Næstved. II. Effects and finances]. Copenhagen, AKF, 1984.
22. **Dean, K. et al., ed**. Self-care of common illness in Denmark. *Medical care*, **21**: 1012–1016 (1983).
23. **Lorig, K. & Holman, H**. Long-term outcomes of an arthritis self-management study: effects of reinforcement efforts. *Social science and medicine*, **29**: 221–224 (1989).
24. **Haug, M.R**. Doctor-patient relationships and their impact on elderly self-care. *In*: Dean, K. et al., ed. *Self-care and health in old age*. London, Croom Helm, 1986, pp. 230–250.
25. **Kane, R.L. & Kane, R.A**. Self-care and health care: inseparable but equal for the wellbeing of the old. *In*: Dean, K. et al., ed. *Self-care and health in old age*. London, Croom Helm, 1986, pp. 251–283.

26. **Anderson, R. & Cartwright, A**. The use of medicines by older people. *In*: Dean, K. et al., ed. *Self-care and health in old age*. London, Croom Helm, 1986, pp. 167–203.

27. **Eve, S.B**. Self-medication among older adults in the United States. *In*: Dean, K. et al., ed. *Self-care and health in old age*. London, Croom Helm, 1986, pp. 204–229.

28. **Lieberman, M.A. & Gourash, N**. Effects of change groups on the elderly. *In*: Lieberman, M.A. et al., ed. *Self-help groups for coping with crisis*. London, Jossey-Bass, 1979, pp. 387–405.

29. **De Friese, G. et al**. From activated patient to pacified activist: a study of the self-care movement in the United States. *Social science and medicine*, **29**: 195–204 (1989).

30. **Nelson, E.C. et al**. Medical self-care education for elders: a controlled trial to evaluate impact. *American journal of public health*, **74**: 1357–1362 (1984).

31. **Anderson, L**. *Aging and loneliness*. Stockholm, Department of Psychosocial Environmental Medicine, Karolinska Institute, 1984.

32. **Wagner, L**. *Skævinge-projektet — en model for fremtidens primære sundhedstjeneste* [The Skævinge project — a model for the primary health care service of the future]. Copenhagen, Forlaget Kommune Information, 1988.

33. *Targets for health for all*. Copenhagen, WHO Regional Office for Europe, 1985 (European Health for All Series No. 1).

34. **Hendriksen, C. et al**. Consequences of assessment and intervention among elderly people: a three year randomised controlled trial. *British medical journal*, **289**: 1522–1524 (1984).

35. **Hendriksen, C**. Konsekvenserne af forebyggende hjemmebesøg til ældre: en follow up undersøgelse 2,5 år efter afslutningen af en intervention [Consequences of prophylactic home visits to elderly people: a follow-up investigation 2.5 years after the conclusion of an intervention procedure]. *Ugeskrift for læger*, **149**: 2097–2100 (1987).

36. **Rø, O. et al**. *Eldreomsorgens nye liv — et eksperiment med styrket innsats i primærtjenesten i Oslo* [New way of caring for the elderly — an experiment with intensified effort in the primary sector in Oslo]. Oslo, Gruppen for Helsetjeneste-forskning, 1983 (Rapport nr. 6).

37. **Vachon, M. et al**. A controlled study of self-help intervention for widows. *American journal of psychiatry*, **137**: 1380–1384 (1980).

38. **Ramian, K**. *Projekt pårørende. Familien på plejehjem* [Project next of kin. The family at the nursing home]. Part 1. Aarhus, Jydsk Teknologisk Institut, 1979.

39. **Ramian, K**. *Projekt pårørende. Familien på plejehjem* [Project next of kin. The family at the nursing home]. Part 2. Aarhus, Jydsk Teknologisk Institut, 1980.

40. **Korremann, G. et al., ed**. *Bedre plejehjem — hvordan* [Better nursing homes — how]. Copenhagen, AKF, 1985.

41. **Meldgaard, K. & Andersen, B.R**. *Mere liv på plejehjemmene* [More life in the nursing homes]. Copenhagen, AKF, 1985.

16

Health promotion
for chronically ill people

Bernhard Badura[a]

Millions of people in developed countries have to live with chronic illness. Because of changes in the pattern of disease, increased life expectancy and declining birth rates, the number of chronically ill people will increase dramatically in the future. Health promotion for chronically ill people is therefore on the top of the agenda of health policy-makers, and is a major concern for health professionals, patients and lay networks. Although the health care system is crucial in treating chronically ill people, the Ottawa Charter for Health Promotion *(1)* clearly suggests that health promotion goes far beyond somatic health, the activities of the medical profession and clinical settings. According to the Ottawa Charter, health promotion is based on a holistic concept of health, emphasizing not only the physical but also the psychological and social dimensions of wellbeing. Health promotion is based on a socioecological perspective of health, emphasizing the interdependence between humans and their social and physical environment. Some of these ideas had already been expressed in an earlier WHO definition of recovery as "the sum of activities required to ensure patients the best possible physical,

[a] The author would like to thank Gary Kaufhold, Harald Lehmann, Holger Pfaff, Thomas Schott, Millard Waltz and Charles Jodd for their help in preparing this chapter.

mental and social conditions so that they may, by their own efforts, resume as normal a place as possible in the life of the community".[a]

What are the main problems and experiences of chronically ill people? What are the mechanisms and outcomes of the process of recovery? What are the main conditions and determinants of this process? These are some of the most important questions that have to be answered to clarify the meaning and practical implications of health promotion in this area.

The vulnerability of ill people to further physical damage, psychological complications and even premature death substantially depends on the social conditions of the recovery process and the social consequences of the illness. The risk of long-term psychological and physical problems increases if people who suffer from chronic disease have to cope in a hostile or frustrating environment, or if the social consequences of the disease, such as increased marital problems or losing one's job, are distressful. If, however, people feel adequately supported by their doctor, spouse or other significant members of their social network, and if they feel good about the rest of their life situation, the risk of further physical and psychological complications will be diminished, with positive consequences for morale and a return to normal life.

Relevant Research

Substantial scientific information is available on chronically ill people. Nevertheless, there have been few comprehensive studies of the course of a disease that relate outcomes such as case mortality, repeat episodes, exacerbation, length of recovery, and the quality of life to a well-defined and conceptually integrated set of physical, psychological, social and behavioural variables (2). In a review of recovery from coronary heart disease, Doehrman (3) placed the available knowledge into the following categories: advocacy articles on rehabilitation programmes, the role of service providers or specific treatment components, clinical studies on people and their relatives during rehabilitation, and empirical research on different determinants and outcomes of the rehabilitation process. Cohen &

---

[a] *Rehabilitation of patients with cardiovascular diseases*: report on a seminar. Copenhagen, WHO Regional Office for Europe, 1969 (unpublished document EURO 0381).

366

Lazarus *(4)* distinguished between descriptive accounts of coping with chronic disease, research on possible causal mechanisms linking different independent variables with different types of outcome, and intervention studies that try to evaluate medical or psychosocial treatment procedures. Although the amount of interdisciplinary research has grown during the past decade, most of the knowledge is still either medical or psychosocial.

The implications of health policy, the influence of the labour market and the social security system, and other macroeconomic or macrosociological issues are very rarely discussed. In medicine, rehabilitation is an adjunct of cardiology, oncology or other subdisciplines. Most research and professional activities concentrate on somatic problems of the acute phase of illness. Psychologists (such as Mages & Mendelsohn *(5)*) are interested in (short-term) psychological consequences and in coping behaviour. Sociologists (such as Croog & Levine *(6)*) are interested in the role of the family and more recently, with very promising results, in the protective influence of social integration and social support *(7–9)*. Interdisciplinary research on chronic disease raises serious conceptual, methodological and measurement problems. Researchers need a more comprehensive theory and longitudinal studies in the future to monitor carefully the long-term influence of physical status, medical treatment, psychological factors, and family and work situation on recovery and the quality of life *(2,10–13)*.

At present perhaps the most subtle theory has been generated by social psychologist Richard Lazarus and colleagues. According to Lazarus, the major issues for research are mechanisms of psychosocial causation and exacerbation of any given illness, the causative role of stress and coping, the psychosocial similarities and differences of diverse types of illness, and factors that can ameliorate the negative consequences of illness *(14)*.[a] The Lazarus approach to coping is microanalytical and focuses on describing thoughts and actions and their social context and on transactional measurement of coping processes. Coping is defined as "cognitive and behavioural efforts to manage specific external and/or internal demands that are appraised as taxing or exceeding the resources of the person" *(14)*. To meet the needs of a socioecological and holistic perspective on

---

[a] **Lazarus, R.S.** *Coping with the stress of illness.* Copenhagen, WHO Regional Office for Europe, 1987 (unpublished document ICP/HSR 630).

health, this approach has to be expanded in two directions: the psychobiology of stress and attachment (Ursin, Chapter 7) and the sociology of social relations and social support (Williams & House, Chapter 6).

Health Promotion through Social Relations and Interpersonal Processes: Cancer

Social relationships and interpersonal processes can be detrimental or beneficial to health. They can weaken people's ability to cope with the stress of illness or can enable better coping. Sometimes even the same significant others (such as doctor or spouse) or the same group (family or self-help group) can have both positive and negative effects on health, depending on the situation, the stage of the recovery process and the social behaviour of the patients themselves.

Wortman & Dunkel-Schetter *(15)* focused on the effect of cancer on patients' interpersonal relationships, and on the effect of these relationships on patients' coping with their negative emotions. Several studies demonstrate that people who have cancer "appear to experience considerable difficulty in their interpersonal relationships as a function of their disease". Wortman & Dunkel-Schetter assume that one reason for these difficulties is that healthy people feel uneasy in the presence of a cancer victim. Healthy people share negative feelings about this illness; at the same time they believe that they should interact with cancer patients positively, optimistically and cheerfully. This discrepancy between actual feelings and perceived rules about feelings may contribute to the avoidance of people with cancer, or at least to avoidance of open communication and to discrepant behaviour towards them. According to this view, the specific image of cancer elicits feedback from the social environment that is inconsistent, confusing and ultimately destructive in a situation in which the patient needs exactly the opposite: integration, clarification and support. Wortman & Dunkel-Schetter propose that the nonverbal behaviour associated with encounters with people with cancer be systematically investigated. This interactionist perspective is part of mainstream sociology and social psychology.

Charles H. Cooley and George H. Mead assume that the self is a reflection of reactions, signals and verbal statements of significant others, and therefore is an important determinant of wellbeing. If rejection and devaluation by others is an important cause of

368

devaluation of self *(16)*, the opposite should also be true. Substantial evidence now available suggests that there is a positive relationship between the quality of the social relationships of people with cancer and their ability to cope with the illness *(5,15,17–19)*.

Health care professionals are in a unique position to promote the health of people with cancer and their families, by providing adequate information about the physical state of the patient and about feelings related to cancer and its treatment, by counselling and, perhaps most importantly, by providing opportunities for open communication and discussion of the experiences, needs and problems of people with cancer and their relatives. An essential aspect of this approach to health promotion is that the psychosocial problems raised by cancer "are problems of adaptation rather than psychopathology" *(5)*.

Clearly, the problems and experiences of people with cancer and other chronically ill people go beyond physical state and medical treatment, and involve the social, cognitive and emotional aspects of family life, work situation and the public image of the disease. Unfortunately, almost nothing is known about the role of work in adapting to cancer, about how men cope with cancer (most of the research is on women), or about how the labour market and social security system of a country affect the prospects and the quality of life of cancer survivors. The analysis of health services, social epidemiology and policy analysis are powerful scientific instruments that have not yet been sufficiently used to promote health. In the future, the microanalysis of cancer and other chronic conditions should benefit from and be supplemented by a macroanalytical approach.

A Socioecological Perspective on Recovery from Myocardial Infarction

The psychosocial aspects of cancer were used to demonstrate the importance of the social environment in health promotion. Significant others and social networks, as well as cultural values and social institutions, are crucial in hindering or promoting the coping process of chronically ill people. The literature on heart disease mostly equates health promotion with the control of risk factors through behavioural change on the part of people with heart disease or members of high-risk groups *(20)*. The behavioural change of health care professionals and institutional change are only rarely discussed. A socioecological approach can be used to demonstrate the effect of

369

the social environment on long-term recovery from heart disease, and to draw conclusions from that evidence about where and how to introduce health promotion interventions: among individuals, among small groups or social networks, or in the medical care system and the social security system. The data presented are from the Oldenburg longitudinal study (OLS), in which I have been a principal investigator since 1979.

In the OLS, a social epidemiological design has been used to learn how people adapt to a serious, life-threatening disease. Almost 1000 males (up to the age of 60 years) suffering from a first myocardial infarction were surveyed using written questionnaires five times in five years: in the hospital about four weeks after onset (T_1) after six months (T_2), after one year (T_3), and again after 3.5 years (T_4) and 4.5 years (T_5). A representative sample of 213 hospitals in the Federal Republic of Germany was used.

Questionnaires were sent to the hospital physician, the subject, his spouse and his general practitioner. The available data included biomedical data and data on medical treatment, the social security system, personality variables, family situation and work situation. Fig. 1 provides the main variables (in the boxes) and hypotheses (indicated by arrows) of this socioecological model of coping and long-term adaptation. According to this model, people suffering from myocardial infarction are usually confronted by three different types of (potential) stressor: chronic stressors such as marital discord or chronic job stress that might even have contributed to the onset of the illness; the acute, time-limited stressor of the illness experience itself or of (unexpected) early retirement; and chronic stressors initiated by the illness such as perceived permanent disability and illness-related discrimination, disadvantages and losses.

The coping process at the core of this model has cognitive (world cognition, self-cognition), emotional (anxiety, depression, positive affect, self-esteem) and behavioural aspects (type A behaviour pattern). Coping *(14, 21)* is crucial to the whole process of recovery because it relates the social context to psychological processes, and psychological processes to physiology and behaviour. Nevertheless, the main epidemiological objective of the OLS was to conceptualize, operationalize and measure the effect of social support from the doctor, spouse, work colleagues and others on the process of recovery. It was expected that different sources and types of support would either reduce the level of stress of people with heart disease or

370

enable them to cope with it better. For a detailed description of the design, the conceptualization and the main results of the OLS, see Badura et al. *(22)*.

Fig. 1. A socioecological model of coping with chronic disease

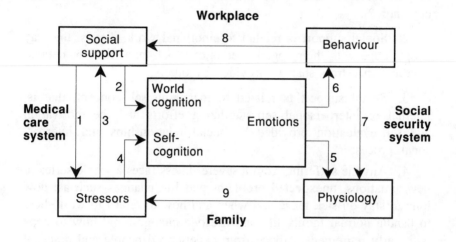

In the OLS, social support is conceptualized as a very ordinary phenomenon, important to everybody's wellbeing and not only to people confronted with a serious life event. Wellbeing involves continual reciprocal interaction between social, environmental, cognitive emotional and behavioural influences *(23)*. Conceptual differences between sociologists (for example, symbolic interactionists) and psychologists (for example, cognitive phenomenologists such as Lazarus or cognitive learning theorists such as Bandura) on the sources of wellbeing are a matter of emphasis and not substance. Psychologists are used to focusing on cognition and emotions as intrapersonal processes. Sociologists, however, stress the interpersonal and social origin of cognition and emotions *(24,25)*. In the OLS, social support is defined as properties of social networks, social relations and interpersonal processes that are experienced as valuable, helpful, comfortable or delightful.

The most important pathways relating social to psychological processes involve four aspects of internal or behavioural coping efforts.

1. Reality construction refers to cognitive activities such as the definition (appraisal) of a situation, the interpretation of a message or an event, and the perception of oneself and of available resources within situations. In times of crisis, significant others (such as a doctor or spouse) are crucial in reducing painful uncertainties (Am I able to survive?) and in redefining situations (Will life make sense any more?).

2. Social support is related to emotional work, that is, the way people cope with their negative emotions such as anxiety or depression and the stress-sharing provided by others.

3. Social support is related to managing self-concept, that is, internal or interpersonal self-stabilizing efforts and the motivation and self-evaluation provided by social relationships and interpersonal processes.

4. Anyone suffering from a severe illness faces a whole series of new situations, unexpected problems and life changes such as: how long to stay on sick leave and when and how to return to work, how to handle normal family life and lifestyle changes, and how to cope with early retirement. Advice from experienced people and practical help from the social environment can determine whether people successfully adapt to new situations and unexpected life changes. Doctors, social workers, the spouse, other members of the family, friends or members of a self-help group are the most appropriate candidates to support patients in practical problem-solving.

People play a significant role in creating and promoting (and weakening or even destroying) their social networks in behaviour in daily interactions. At the same time, people depend on these relationships to cope with the problems and difficulties of everyday life. In crisis situations, people are even more susceptible to external influence and may depend even more desperately on orientation, care and stimulation from the social environment. The OLS distinguishes between the following three empirical correlates of social support: (objective) network properties, interpersonal provisions, and (subjective) network cognition (Table 1 provides examples of sources and measures of social support in the OLS). The main aspects of social relations and interpersonal processes are:

— either to prevent cognitive disorientation or to enable people to regain a sense of coherence (26);

— to help to overcome negative emotions and to promote positive ones;

— to keep or to regain a self-concept that is realistic, stable and positive;

— to adapt successfully to new situations and unexpected life changes.

The main psychosocial process and outcome variables of the OLS were: cognitive appraisal of the illness (a twelve-item scale on how subjects perceive and assess the illness experience and its consequences; we developed and tested this scale); negative and positive affect (developed by Bradburn (27)); anxiety and depression (as used by Pearlin and Schooler (28)); self-derogation and self-worth (developed by Rosenberg (29)); sense of mastery (developed by Pearlin et al. (21)). For all the other indicators mentioned and further elaboration see Badura et al. (22).

Table 1. Sources and measures of social support in the Oldenburg longitudinal study

Measures	Sources		
	Medical system	Spouse, family	Workplace
Network properties (objective)	Participation in supervised heart groups	Marital status Number of children Number of confiding relationships with relatives	Number of acquaintances Number of friends Number of confiding relationships Social isolation
Interpersonal processes (perceived)	Medical counselling and advice Psychosocial provisions of heart groups	Support by spouse: − emotional − social − practical help Joint activities Support by children	Social support from confidants Practical help Informal communication: − frequency − availability
Network cognition (subjective)	Quality of medical counselling and advice	Quality of marital relationship Adequacy of marital relationship Adequacy of relations with children	Group cohesion Supportive culture Adequacy of relationships with workmates

Effect of the medical care system on recovery

Experts agree on the health-promoting function of early mobilization for people surviving a heart attack. The Gothenburg model recommends walking around the room on the seventh or eighth day after the heart attack *(30)*. Table 2 shows the findings of the OLS on early mobilization in the Federal Republic of Germany. Only 25% of heart attack survivors surveyed in the Federal Republic of Germany received early mobilization, as defined in the Gothenburg model. Surprisingly, not only the patients' physical state influenced the time of early mobilization in our sample, but also the type of hospital. The smaller the hospital, the later the heart attack survivors began early mobilization. Twenty per cent of the subjects reported that they had not been mobilized early at all.

Table 2. Time elapsed before early mobilization
of OLS subjects (N = 998)

Time elapsed	OLS subjects mobilized (%)
0 – 8 days	25.1
9 –12 days	21.7
13 –16 days	25.4
17 – 20 days	11.0
> 20 days	16.8

On average, the people surveyed spent 32 days in the community hospital, about twice as long as in countries such as the United Kingdom or the United States. As early as 1973, people with acute myocardial infarction in the United Kingdom spent only 15 days in hospital. According to Wenger et al. *(13)*, people experiencing a mild infarction in the United States are kept in hospital for only 7–14 days. In the Federal Republic of Germany, however, about half the people with mild infarction spend more than four weeks in hospital, and most of these people are referred afterwards to special rehabilitation clinics where they spend another four to six weeks. Again, the size of the hospital significantly influences the amount of time people spend there. The smaller the hospital, the longer people stay. This pattern remains largely the same after controlling for physical state. Table 3 presents the results of a multivariate analysis of days spent in hospital. Contrary to expectations, the variance explained is not significantly increased by factors such as age or the severity of the

Table 3. OLS: stepwise regression on time spent in the acute hospital

Variables	R^2	Increment of variance	F-value
Severity of illness (objective data)	0.08	0.08	7.4
Severity of illness (clinical assessment)	0.10	0.02	4.3
Type of hospital	0.12	0.02	8.6
Age of the patient	0.12	0.00	0.0
Length of intensive care	0.19	0.07	46.8
Time of early mobilization	0.35	0.16	185.9

illness, but it is increased by factors such as time of early mobilization. The smaller the hospital, the more conservative its treatment procedures seem to be, and the longer people have to stay there. People with mild infarction are apparently used in the Federal Republic to fill beds and thus conceal an oversupply of hospital services. This is not only financially counterproductive, but also harmful to people's wellbeing. The longer people stay in hospital, the more they worry about another infarction, their future in general and death.

The counselling behaviour of physicians demonstrates the discrepancy between people's needs and the activities of the medical services. From the point of view of health promotion, this fact is especially disturbing. Comprehensive counselling with consistent and understandable advice is one of the most powerful instruments to improve the health of chronically ill people. Table 4 shows some of the main issues, the information needed, and the information actually provided by doctors. Medical doctors concentrate on issues such as smoking and medication, but when their patients have psychological or social problems they are less able, or inclined, to comply with these information needs. As about one quarter of our sample reported increased feelings of uncertainty caused by receiving inconsistent information, the urgent necessity of behavioural change by physicians becomes even more obvious. People with heart disease, like most chronically ill people, need accurate information about their physical condition. They need sympathetic treatment. They need advice about the practical (for example, sexual) problems with which the illness confronts them. They need help in seeking or avoiding early retirement, and other advice as well.

Table 4. OLS: percentage of information needs expressed by people with heart disease (N = 998) versus percentage of information actually received from the hospital physician

Topic	Patient needs (%)	Physician behaviour (%)
Illness and drugs	97	92
Weight control and diet	85	70
Smoking and alcohol	76	87
Sexual behaviour	74	19
Physical function	95	80
Psychological problems with family and work	88	59
Return to work	92	63
Early retirement	68	23
Supervised heart groups	70	25

The social context of the ill person plays an important role in health promotion, disease prevention, and recovery from serious illness. One issue the OLS has addressed, therefore, is what physicians do about the social network of ill people. To what extent do physicians comply with people's desire to include important members of their social network in the therapeutic process? Spouses play an important role in the social network of married people, as a source of social support or of serious stress. Including the spouses is important to help them cope with their own negative emotions and uncertainties, and to enable them adequately to support the ill spouse and reduce interpersonal problems within the marriage. A majority of the people with heart disease surveyed wanted their spouses to be included (Table 5). There were other significant people that ill people wanted to include and inform. The needs go far beyond what is actually provided. In networking and in counselling, the compliance of medical personnel is very low.

Physical exercise and informal gatherings in physician-supervised groups are becoming more popular among cardiologists, general practitioners and (former) heart disease patients in the Federal Republic of Germany. Although physicians are paid for initiating or running these groups, however, only 10% of our subjects were informed of their existence. People who joined these groups benefited from them (Table 6). Participants felt less threatened by the illness, reported that they coped better with it and were better off psychologically than nonparticipants. After having spent on average

376

more than four weeks in hospital, 86% of those surveyed were referred to a special rehabilitation clinic, where they spent another four to six weeks. This emphasis on the clinical setting means that people with heart disease are away from their normal home life for about ten weeks or more. The majority of the OLS subjects were not able to influence the time, location or dates of this second phase of hospitalization. More than 50% of those surveyed found this prolonged separation from their families and homes to be stressful.

Table 5. OLS: physician compliance with subjects' desire to include significant others in the therapeutic process

Significant others	Subjects who expressed that desire		Compliance of physicians	
	N	(%)	N	(%)
Spouse	420	(76%)	230	(55%)
Adult children	120	(32%)	16	(13%)
Employer or supervisor	104	(26%)	11	(11%)
Company physician	137	(36%)	24	(18%)

Table 6. OLS: differences in outcome variables between subjects (N = 608) participating and not participating in physician-supervised group activities

Outcome variables	Median of participating subjects	Median of nonparticipating subjects	t-test
Cognitive appraisal of illness	47.2	50.8	$P < 0.002$
Coping with illness symptoms	51.8	49.4	$P < 0.008$
Subjective assessment of health status	53.0	49.9	$P < 0.001$
Depression	46.9	50.5	$P < 0.001$
Anxiety	47.4	51.0	$P < 0.004$
Positive affect	53.1	49.6	$P < 0.004$
Self-worth	52.4	49.5	$P < 0.012$

Note. Median = 50.

The influence of the social security system

The system of social security and welfare institutions in the Federal Republic of Germany is the result of incremental growth for more than 100 years. There is no central planning and no coherent health policy. Even the most rudimentary centralized decision-making is lacking in this excessively complex system of health and welfare institutions that consumes almost one third of the gross national product. Cardiac rehabilitation falls under the jurisdiction of six different institutions, of which the most important are the pension funds. These institutions conflict on matters of jurisdiction and money, which often exposes people to bureaucratic procedures. For example, to determine which institution has to provide the ill person's income during rehabilitation, the person has to go to a special medical department of a particular institution and undergo different diagnostic procedures. This department also decides whether the patient has to go back to work or face early retirement. This is added to the treatment in hospital, in the rehabilitation clinics and from the general practitioner. Most of those surveyed were subject to these bureaucratic procedures. The data suggest that these procedures were a source of psychological distress, as they increased anxiety, depression and other psychological problems in the people surveyed.

Stress and support in marriage

The next element studied was cognitive processes and emotional reactions. How do perceptions of health influence adaptation after a heart attack? How are cognition and emotions related to the family situation of people with heart disease? One way of looking at the influence of perception and cognition is to consider their effects over a fixed period of time. Table 7 presents the results of a standard multiple regression analysis of Bradburn morale measures at T_3 on indicators of perceived recovery at T_2. The data suggest that health perceptions were related to wellbeing, and subjective rather than objective measures of health and recovery better predicted psychological adaptation.

Table 8 examines the same outcome from a somewhat different perspective. How does perceived social functioning influence psychological adaptation after myocardial infarction? The data show that cognitive appraisal of the illness, perceived disabilities in the family roles and returning to work are more strongly related to negative emotions than is objective health.

378

Table 7. OLS: standard multiple regression analysis of Bradburn morale measures at T_3 on indicators of perceived recovery at T_2 and medical status at T_1

Predictors	Negative affect	Positive affect
Doing well or poorly	0.27	− 0.12
Self-definition as sick and disabled	0.23	− 0.15
Cardiac symptoms	0.14	− 0.18
Medical status	NS	NS
R^2	0.27	0.14

Note. $P < 0.01$ for all variables; $N = 604$; NS = not significant.

Table 8. OLS: standard multiple regression analysis of Bradburn negative affect at T_3 on cognitive appraisal of the illness and perceptions of health at T_2

Predictors	Standardized regression coefficients
Primary appraisal (high stress of illness)	0.41 ($P < 0.01$)
Disability in family role	0.27 ($P < 0.01$)
Disability in sexual role	0.07 ($P < 0.05$)
Return to work	− 0.14 ($P < 0.01$)
Disability in work role	0.09 ($P < 0.05$)
Cardiac symptoms	0.08 ($P < 0.05$)
Medical status	NS
Adjusted R^2	0.36

Note. $N = 604$; NS = not significant.

Table 9 examines potential causal explanations. How do social factors such as stress within the family or social support from the spouse influence the cognitive appraisal of the illness and psychological wellbeing? The data strongly support some of our general hypotheses about the coping process after a serious life event. The social context affects how ill people define their situation and, consequently, affects the whole process of cognitive and emotional adaptation. Marital problems and the lack of emotional integration in

Table 9. OLS: association of cognitive appraisal of the illness and negative affect at T_3 with measures of social context in the family

Contextual variables	Cognitive appraisal	Negative affect
Marital status (married or unmarried)	NS	0.21
Marital conflict T_2	0.35	0.52
Marital conflict T_3	0.37	0.50
Marital role strain T_1	0.24	0.49
Marital role strain T_3	0.26	0.68
Emotional support T_2	− 0.24	− 0.45
Adequacy of support T_2	− 0.24	− 0.52
Sense of reliable alliance with spouse:		
— at T_2	− 0.18	− 0.39
— at T_3	− 0.32	− 0.34

Note. Gamma coefficients used; N = 604; NS = not significant.

the family appear to handicap people in coping with the stress of illness, as reflected in cognitive appraisal. Marital conflict as part of chronic role strains appears to cause low morale. In addition, a lack of gratification of socioemotional needs seems to have a negative effect. In a life crisis such as myocardial infarction, inadequate social support appears to affect subjective wellbeing negatively. This may be caused by the close relationship between supportive interaction and the quality of the marital bond; or not being loved and esteemed or not being able to count on others in a crisis may be very pervasive environmental stressors. The standard regression analysis shown in Table 10 suggests the same conclusions.

In sociological (31) and in psychological (23) theory the self-concept, or the way people perceive themselves, is an important determinant of behaviour. Fig. 2 shows how the quality of the marital relationship influenced the sense of mastery or self-efficacy during the first year after myocardial infarction. For this part of the analysis our sample was divided into three groups.

In group I, both the ill person and his spouse said that they had a good marital relationship. In group III, at least one partner reported being dissatisfied with the marital relationship. Group II included all the remaining subjects, the residual category of "normal" marriages.

Table 10. OLS: standard regression analysis of
Bradburn morale measures at T_3 on measures of social context

Predictors	Negative affect	Positive affect
Quality of marriage (good or poor)	0.23 ($P < 0.01$)	NS
Marital conflict	0.31 ($P < 0.01$)	-0.13 ($P < 0.01$)
Negative appraisal of wife	0.11 ($P < 0.05$)	NS
Sexual rapport	-0.25 ($P < 0.01$)	0.16 ($P < 0.01$)
Disability in sexual role	0.11 ($P < 0.05$)	-0.15 ($P < 0.01$)
Emotional support	-0.08 ($P < 0.05$)	0.29 ($P < 0.01$)
Adjusted R^2	0.33	0.11

Note. N = 604; NS = not significant.

Fig. 2. OLS: effect of quality of marital relationship on sense of mastery during the first year after myocardial infarction

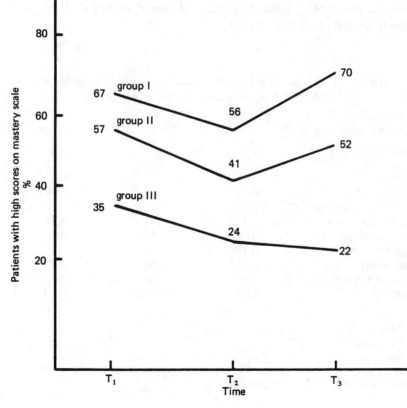

Emotionally close and normal marriages seemed to protect the person's sense of mastery or self-efficacy from the psychological effect of the heart attack and provided a supportive context for recovery. In marriages characterized by a low level of social support and a high level of stress, the coping resources of the individual may become exhausted, leading to demoralization and a low sense of self-worth and self-efficacy.

The interplay of type A behaviour, stress and support
The type A behaviour pattern is one of the best known and well established psychosocial risk factors. How does the type A behaviour pattern influence recovery from heart disease? How do people who tend to be aggressive, ambitious and autonomous cope with a serious life event? Are they more or less effective at coping than type B people? The OLS type A subjects found it much more difficult to adapt themselves to this new situation than type B subjects. Type A subjects seemed to be more threatened by the heart attack and suffered from more anxiety and depression. The psychological well-being of the type A subjects steadily declined during the first year after heart attack (Table 11).

Table 11. OLS: Pearson correlations *(r)* between type A behaviour and selected outcome variables

Outcome variables	Correlations		
	T_1	T_2	T_3
Anxiety	0.11^a	0.15^b	0.21^b
Depression	0.11^a	0.21^b	0.19^b
Cognitive appraisal of illness	0.21^b	0.21^b	0.24^b
Positive affect	NS	NS	NS
Negative affect	0.15^b	0.19^b	0.18^b
Self-worth	0.13^a	NS	NS
Self-derogation	NS	NS	NS
Mastery	-0.09^c	-0.13^b	-0.14^b

[a] $P < 0.01$.
[b] $P < 0.001$.
[c] $P < 0.05$.

Note. N = 560; NS = not significant.

382

To explain this rather significant development, we examined the social network of the type A subjects and asked their spouses to comment on marital relationships. The data are revealing, and may be relevant to future rehabilitation programmes. The coping style of the type A males had a negative effect on their marriage (Table 12). The spouses of the type A subjects agreed more often with negative statements about the marital relationship and less often with positive ones than spouses of the type B subjects. The OLS suggests the following three conclusions. Type B males are better copers than type A males. The social support provided by the spouse positively influences the wellbeing of type B males. Type A males do not benefit from spousal support. Indeed, social support offered to type A people is sometimes negative for their wellbeing. One reason may be that explicit help threatens the sense of control of type A people. Being offered help may connote being deprived of dominance or autonomy, which may result in increased uncertainty and helplessness.

Influence of work status on recovery

One year after their heart attacks, only 45% of the blue-collar subjects were working. Social class was one of the best predictors of returning to work, which is perhaps the most important social aspect of recovery from heart attack (Table 13). The physical condition of the subjects appeared to exert no influence on employment status; the important factors were age, social class and psychological wellbeing.

Work status was centrally important for recovery. People who were back at work one year after myocardial infarction were much better off psychologically (and, of course, financially) than people who were still on sick leave or who had had to accept early retirement. People whose future work status was still unclear after one year suffered most from the stress of illness: for example, they scored significantly higher on the anxiety scale and risked becoming chronically depressed. Only 25% of the subjects who retired early welcomed their new status without reservation; 75% of them had been more or less forced to quit their jobs.

These facts should cause concern for two reasons: first, whether people seek early retirement after a heart attack should be a personal decision; second, the social and psychological costs of early retirement appear to be quite high and should therefore be avoided. One of the reasons why those who returned to work were better off psychologically may be that the work environment is not just a source of

Table 12. OLS: correlations between type A behaviour and various aspects of interaction in marriage, according to statements made by wives about their husbands

Statement	Correlation[a]
We do not have enough family life because of my husband's job	0.21[b]
I'm worried about our relationship	0.22[b]
My husband:	
— hardly takes any time for me because of his work	0.22[b]
— is very loving towards me	−0.11[c]
— and I have a good sexual relationship	−0.11[d]
— appreciates my skills and accomplishments	−0.13[d]
— usually wants more from me than he is willing to give	0.12[d]
— keeps on interfering with my business	0.23[b]
— often goes his own way	0.11[c]
— puts himself at the centre of attention too often	0.22[b]
— tries to make me do things his way	0.26[b]
— and I have hardly any interests in common	0.12[d]
— does not accept my friends	0.10[c]
— does not let me decide for myself	0.17[b]
We have seldom had a good laugh together in recent weeks	0.12[d]

[a] Pearson correlation coefficients used; N = 470.
[b] $P < 0.001$.
[c] $P < 0.05$.
[d] $P < 0.01$.

stress; it is also a source of social support and can provide opportunities for using skills and other meaningful activities (Table 14). The degree of social integration, supportive interaction and decision latitude seem to be important resources for coping and directly affect indicators of positive health. Nevertheless it is incorrect to conclude that the working environment is a healthy place for people with heart disease. Stressors such as work overload and problems with supervisors or colleagues may have a noticeable negative effect on wellbeing (Table 15).

Long-term effects
The data strongly suggest that a first myocardial infarction has long-term effects on both the psychological and the social dimensions of our outcome measures. The average anxiety and depression scores in our sample 3.5 years after a heart attack were still significantly higher

Table 13. OLS: work status in relation to social class
one year after myocardial infarction (T_3)

Type of employee	Back at work (%)	Not back at work (%)
Blue-collar workers	45	55
White-collar workers	68	32
Civil servants	63	37
Self-employed	73	27

Note. N = 608; missing values = 22.

than in people surveyed in hospital four weeks after a heart attack. Anxiety was strongly correlated with subjective health 3.5 and 4.5 years after heart attack. These correlations were much higher than those between anxiety and objective health. Emotional support provided by the spouse had no positive long-term effect on anxiety, but stress within marriage was strongly related to this outcome. There was less depression in the patients who reported being happily married and in good health.

At the time of discharge from hospital, there were no differences in objective health between people who later returned to work and people who had to retire early. Both groups showed remarkable differences 4.5 years later on almost all of the outcome variables that measured subjective health and psychological wellbeing. Subjects who returned to work after myocardial infarction seemed to cope much better with the stress of illness than subjects who did not. Among subjects who returned to work, blue-collar workers scored higher than white-collar workers on the scale measuring stress of illness. Subjects who experienced discrimination and stigmatization at work one year after the heart attack reported similar experiences after 3.5 years. The general public seems to equate heart disease with loss of effectiveness and efficiency. These image-related results fit the general disadvantages the blue-collar workers in our sample faced in the labour market after heart attack. Mortality 4.5 years after onset was correlated with social class, delayed mobilization, lack of emotional support by the spouse and living in an urban environment.[a]

_____

[a] **Badura, B. et al**. Unpublished data, 1987.

Table 14. OLS: relationships between social factors at T_2 and outcome variables at T_3

| Social factor | Correlations[a] | | | | | | | | |
	Depression	Anxiety	Self-worth	Self-derogation	Positive affect	Negative affect	Mastery	Cognitive appraisal of illness
Group cohesiveness	-0.21^b	NS	NS	-0.28^b	0.27^a	-0.25^b	0.25^b	-0.13^b
Quality of social relations	-0.18^b	-0.22^b	NS	-0.15^c	NS	-0.31^b	0.16^c	-0.18^b
Illness-related support and care of colleagues	NS	NS	NS	NS	NS	NS	NS	NS
Work-related support	NS	NS	NS	NS	NS	NS	NS	NS
Decision latitude	-0.15^c	-0.17^c	0.23^c	-0.20^b	0.26^b	-0.18^c	0.20^b	-0.18^c

[a] Pearson correlation coefficients used; N = 181.

[b] $P < 0.01$.

[c] $P < 0.05$.

Note. NS = not significant.

386

Table 15. OLS: relationships between selected stressors at work at T_2 and outcome at T_3

Stressor	Correlations[a]						
	Depression	Anxiety	Self-worth	Self-derogation	Negative affect	Mastery	Cognitive appraisal of illness
Work overload	0.20^b	0.16^c	NS	NS	0.22^b	-0.36^b	0.18^b
Problems with boss	0.29^b	0.23^b	-0.17^c	0.28^b	0.28^b	-0.26^b	0.32^b
Problems with colleagues	NS	NS	-0.19^b	0.20^b	0.17^c	-0.14^b	0.14^b

[a] Pearson correlation coefficients used; N = 181.

[b] $P < 0.01$.

[c] $P < 0.05$.

Note. NS = not significant.

387

Health-promoting Action for Chronically Ill People

Everyone experiences illness differently and therefore needs individualized treatment and support. Nevertheless, some common features and issues of chronic illness can be identified and therefore addressed by health promotion programmes.

Comprehensive rehabilitation services
In all developed countries, the medical care systems tend to over-emphasize somatic problems during the acute phase of chronic illness, and tend to neglect psychosocial and practical problems and problems of long-term adaptation. The social context in the hospital, at home and at work is centrally important to recovery. People require adequate medical treatment, but they need more to cooperate effectively during and after acute treatment and to cope with their social, practical and psychological problems. People need adequate consistent and clear information, emotional support and practical help, and opportunities to discuss openly their feelings and uncertainties. Physicians need to know more about a comprehensive and socio-ecological perspective in treating people with cancer, heart disease and other chronic conditions. Mages & Mendelsohn (5) said that: "Training programmes designed to increase the understanding of the psychosocial effects of cancer and to facilitate the early identification of atypical courses and high-risk individuals would be helpful.". More social workers might be needed within the medical care system who are specially trained and experienced in managing the psychosocial and practical problems of chronically ill people in active cooperation with the rest of the rehabilitation team. Kannel (32) pointed out that: "Physicians seldom take the trouble to learn what community resources are available to them to help provide ... comprehensive care for their patients.".

Promoting self-reliance and self-determination
The health care system should not exacerbate the psychological problems of ill people or hinder the process of normalization of people recovering from illness. For heart disease, a new treatment and rehabilitation philosophy of early mobilization has been developed that stresses self-reliance and self-determination as the major objectives of recovery. One well documented implementation of this new philosophy has taken place in the cardiac department at St Vincent's Hospital in Dublin. People with uncomplicated myocardial infarction

are ambulatory in two or three days, discharged in less than ten days, reviewed at an outpatient clinic three weeks after discharge, and encouraged to return to work whether they have blue-collar or white-collar jobs. A long-term exercise programme is negotiated and comprehensive rehabilitation implemented by a team of physicians, nurses, physical therapists and dieticians. Mulcahy *(33)* emphasized the importance of close communication between the attending physician during the first illness and the physicians who are responsible for the patient's rehabilitation. An evaluation of this programme has revealed that 76% of the subjects have returned to work within 100 days. Social and psychological factors predominantly account for failures to return to work *(34,35)*. This programme and its results contrast remarkably with cardiac rehabilitation in the Federal Republic of Germany.

Support the supporters

Social support has two facets. It is a potential source of health (for people receiving it) and a potential source of stress (for people who offer it). The supporters must be supported, especially the supporters of terminally ill people, to avoid the burn-out syndrome *(36)*. Physicians, nurses and lay care givers, who provide emotional and social support every day, often work under severe stress *(37)*. Caring for people with cancer seems to be especially stressful. Primary supporters of chronically ill people should be given more support themselves so that they can provide adequate care to others. Support programmes for the supporters should be developed and applied.

Networking

Health promotion emphasizes the importance of social integration and mutual understanding in coping with the stress of life and illness. Including the family and significant others in the treatment procedures and promoting patient groups in the hospital and self-help groups in the community are important steps in health promotion for chronically ill people. Preventing social isolation and distorted communication between chronically ill people and the rest of the community is perhaps the most urgent health policy priority in the future.

Towards active reintegration

Data from the OLS and from other studies demonstrate the health-promoting potential of work in industrialized societies. Our data

389

suggest that people with heart disease are facing serious problems because of the present labour market. In the future, high unemployment and widespread public prejudices about people with chronic illnesses such as cancer and heart disease might even increase the tendency to keep these people out of the labour market and to discriminate against them in the workplace.

References

1. Ottawa Charter for Health Promotion. *Health promotion*, **1**(4): iii–v (1986).
2. **Kasl, S.V**. Social and psychological factors affecting the course of disease: an epidemiologic perspective. *In*: Mechanic, D., ed. *Handbook of health, health care, and health professionals*. New York, Free Press, 1983, pp. 683–708.
3. **Doehrman, S.R**. Psycho-social aspects of recovery from coronary heart disease: a review. *Social science and medicine*, **11**: 199–218 (1977).
4. **Cohen, F. & Lazarus, R.S**. Coping with the stresses of illness. *In*: Stone, G.C. et al., ed. *Health psychology — a handbook*. San Francisco, Jossey-Bass, 1980, pp. 217–254.
5. **Mages, N.L. & Mendelsohn, G.A**. Effects of cancer on patients' lives: a personological approach. *In*: Stone, G.L. et al., ed. *Health psychology — a handbook*. San Francisco, Jossey-Bass, 1980, pp. 255-284.
6. **Croog, S.H. & Levine, S**. *The heart patient recovers. Social and psychological factors*. New York, Human Sciences Press, 1977.
7. **Badura, B., ed**. *Soziale Unterstützung und chronische Krankheit. Zum Stand sozialepidemiologischer Forschung*. Frankfurt, Suhrkamp, 1981.
8. **Ruberman, W. et al**. Psychosocial influences on mortality after myocardial infarction. *New England journal of medicine*, **311**: 552–559 (1984).
9. **Waltz, M. & Badura, B**. Subjective health, intimacy and perceived self-efficacy after heart attack: predicting life quality 5 years afterwards. *Social indicator research*, **20**: 87–114 (1988).
10. **Lazarus, R.S**. Stress and coping as factors in health and illness. *In*: Cohen, J. et al., ed. *Psychosocial aspects of cancer*. New York, Raven Press, 1982, pp. 163–190.

11. **Moos, R.H., ed**. *Coping with physical illness. Vol. 2. New perspectives*. New York, Plenum Press, 1984.

12. **Moos, R.H. & Tsu, V.D., ed**. *Coping with physical illness*. New York, Plenum Medical Books, 1977.

13. **Wenger, N.K. et al., ed**. *Assessment of quality of life in clinical trials of cardiovascular therapies*. Atlanta, GA, Le Jacq, 1984.

14. **Lazarus, R.S. & Folkman, S**. *Stress, appraisal and coping*. New York, Springer, 1984.

15. **Wortman, C.B. & Dunkel-Schetter, C**. Interpersonal relationships and cancer: a theoretical analysis. *Journal of social issues*, **35**: 120–155 (1979).

16. **Rose, A.M**. A socio-psychological theory of neurosis. *In*: Rose, A.M., ed. *Human behavior and social processes*. Boston, MA, Houghton Mifflin, 1962, pp. 537–549.

17. **Baltrusch, H.J.F. & Waltz, M**. A life span and personological model of host–tumor relationships. *In*: Day, S.B., ed. *Cancer, stress, and death*. New York, Plenum Medical Books, 1986, pp. 261–283.

18. **Schafft, S**. *Psychische und soziale Probleme krebserkrankter Frauen*. Munich, Minerva, 1987.

19. **Wortman, C.B. & Conway, T.L**. The role of social support in adaptation and recovery from physical illness. *In*: Cohen, S. & Syme, S.L., ed. *Social support and health*. New York, Academic Press, 1985, pp. 281–302.

20. **Maddox, G.C**. Modifying the social environment. *In*: Holland, W.W. et al., ed. *Textbook of public health*. Oxford, Oxford University Press, 1984, Vol. I, pp. 19–31.

21. **Pearlin, L.I. et al**. The stress process. *Journal of health and social behavior*, **22**: 337–356 (1981).

22. **Badura, B. et al**. *Leben mit dem Herzinfarkt. Eine sozial-epidemiologische Studie*. Berlin (West), Springer Verlag, 1987.

23. **Bandura, A**. The self system in reciprocal determinism. *American psychology*, **37**: 344–358 (1978).

24. **Berger, P.L. & Luckmann, T**. *The social construction of reality*. New York, Basic Books, 1966.

25. **Hochschild, A.R**. Emotion work, feeling rules and social structure. *American journal of sociology*, **85**: 551–575 (1979).

26. **Antonovsky, A**. *Health, stress and coping*. San Francisco, Jossey-Bass, 1979.

27. **Bradburn, N.M**. *The structure of well-being*. Chicago, Aldine, 1969.

28. **Pearlin, L.I. & Schooler, C**. The structure of coping. *Journal of health and social behavior*, **19**: 2–21 (1978).

29. **Rosenberg, M**. *Society and the adolescent self-image*. Princeton, NJ, Princeton University Press, 1965.

30. **Reindell, H. & Roskamm, H**. *Herzkrankheiten — Pathophysiologie — Diagnostik — Therapie*. Berlin (West), Springer Verlag, 1977.

31. **Rosenberg, M**. *Conceiving the self*. New York, Basic Books, 1979.

32. **Kannel, W.B**. Foreword. *In*: Croog, S.H. & Levine, S. *The heart patient recovers. Social and psychological factors*. New York, Human Sciences Press, 1977, pp. 9–13.

33. **Mulcahy, R**. The rehabilitation of patients with coronary heart disease: a clinician's view. *In*: Stockmeier, U., ed. *Psychological approach to the rehabilitation of coronary patients*. Berlin (West), Springer Verlag, 1976, pp. 52–61.

34. **Hickey, N. & Mulcahy, R**. St Vincent's Hospital rehabilitation program. *Journal of cardiopulmonary rehabilitation*, **5**: 386–388 (1985).

35. **Hlatky, M.A. et al**. Medical, psychological and social correlates of work disability among men with coronary artery disease. *American journal of cardiology*, **58**: 911–915 (1986).

36. **Belle, D**. The stress of caring: women as providers of social support. *In*: Goldberger, L. & Breznitz, S., ed. *Handbook of stress*. New York, Free Press, 1982, pp. 496–505.

37. **Schott, T. et al**. Wives of heart attack patients: the stress of caring. *In*: Anderson, R., ed. *Living with chronic illness*. London, Croom Helm, 1988.

Part V

Community intervention in health promotion

17

Community control of chronic diseases: a review of cardiovascular programmes

Aulikki Nissinen & Pekka Puska

Towards the end of the 1960s and at the beginning of the 1970s, the magnitude of the problem caused by cardiovascular disease became obvious. About one half of all deaths, nearly one third of permanent disability, and a high proportion of the use made of the health services were found to be caused by cardiovascular diseases.[a] An analysis of data from several developed countries showed that the control and prevention of cardiovascular diseases could be expected to have the greatest impact on the longevity of the adult population (1). The high mortality and morbidity of cardiovascular diseases are not a result only of the aging of the population. In many developed countries, about 40% of all deaths in the middle-aged population are caused by cardiovascular diseases. About three quarters of these deaths are caused by coronary heart disease, mainly acute myocardial infarction. The seven countries study (2), which surveyed and followed middle-aged male population samples in different parts of the world, and the acute myocardial infarction registration study coordinated by WHO (3) showed a high prevalence of atherosclerotic circulatory diseases, including an even larger burden of nonfatal cases than fatal cases, and regional differences in the prevalence of cardiovascular diseases.

---

[a] *Methodology of multifactor preventive trials in ischaemic heart disease*: report on a Working Group. Copenhagen, WHO Regional Office for Europe, 1971 (unpublished document EURO 5011 (3)).

The considerable differences in prevalence even between the developed countries have been demonstrated repeatedly by mortality statistics (4,5). This important information was the basis for the idea of launching well conceived comprehensive efforts for population-wide control of cardiovascular diseases in a number of countries, and to invite WHO to coordinate such an activity.

General Principles of the Community Cardiovascular Programmes

A great deal was already known about the precursors and risk factors of cardiovascular diseases when the community programmes of control were launched. Research had proceeded from descriptive epidemiological studies of populations at high and low risk and retrospective studies of patients to prospective follow-up studies; the first major one was the Framingham study in the Unites States (6). Results from another major international prospective study, the seven countries study (2), were available, and a summary of several other prospective studies initiated in the United States in the 1950s and the 1960s was published as the final report of the Pooling Project (7). All these studies indicated that the major factors — smoking, elevated serum cholesterol, and elevated blood pressure — predict most of the subsequent risk of coronary heart disease, independent of other potential factors studied. The results of basic biochemical studies and of a few experimental and quasi-experimental studies on various risk factors such as smoking cessation, cholesterol-lowering diets and treatment of high blood pressure were also available.

By the beginning of the 1970s, these studies had already led to a number of reviews and recommendations by expert groups for further studies or national applications of preventive activities. In 1970, a WHO expert group proposed that preventive trials concentrate on combined intervention for smoking, hypertension, elevated serum cholesterol level, and physical inactivity. In the same year, the Inter-Society Commission for Heart Disease Resources (8) in the United States recommended that primary prevention efforts should attempt to eliminate smoking, change diet to reduce serum cholesterol levels, treat and lower high blood pressure, and place special emphasis on combinations of these risk factors.

The major risk factors have been chosen for most community cardiovascular programmes, but their role has had to be balanced in somewhat different ways in different countries. Several other possible risk factors were also considered, including physical inactivity, obesity, psychosocial stress, diabetes and alcohol abuse.

The intervention strategy used has been a community (or total population or public health) approach, which attempts to modify the general risk-factor profile of a whole population. Although an individual's risk of coronary heart disease increases with the increasing levels of risk factors, it was crucial to realize that individuals at high risk in most of the countries with high rates of cardiovascular disease produce only a small proportion of the disease cases. Many cases arise among people with only moderate risk, but usually in several risk factors at once. Because the people with moderate risk outnumber the few individuals at really high risk, and because the simultaneous presence of several risk factors has a synergistic impact, the number of disease cases in a community can be substantially reduced only if the general risk-factor levels can be modified in this great majority — in practice, the whole population. The clearly greater potential of the community approach versus the high-risk approach in reducing rates of coronary heart disease has been demonstrated by case studies (9,10). These strategies are obviously not mutually exclusive, and most community programmes combine both strategies for maximum impact.

A quasi-experimental study design has been used to evaluate most community cardiovascular disease programmes. One or several communities are chosen where experimental intervention is carried out, and one or several other communities are chosen as reference areas. These communities represent "natural" development. Except for the experimental project activities, the reference community is not deprived of any "naturally" arising development that might occur there.

Community Cardiovascular Programmes in Europe

The comprehensive cardiovascular community control programme (CCCCP), sponsored by the WHO Regional Office for Europe, has been implemented in a number of European countries since 1974. The programmes in different countries have followed the same general principles, but the types of programme and community have varied greatly from country to country (11).

In some countries the intervention areas have been larger (such as North Karelia in Finland), to be able to assess change in the prevalence of disease; in some countries such as Switzerland, the communities have been smaller, so that only changes in risk factors are assessed as main objectives. Some countries, such as Norway and Yugoslavia, have had problems finding a reference area. The emphasis in scope and content has also varied a great deal. Some programmes, such as in the German Democratic Republic, have placed more emphasis on the role of health services, and others on the role of community organizations, such as in the Federal Republic of Germany. Table 1 summarizes the nine main programmes in the CCCCP.

In quasi-experimental designs, the assignment of the experimental and control units is not random, and both a biased sample (selection of study units) and biased selection of experimental and reference units are possible. Random selection is not always possible. For instance, in the North Karelia project, the intervention area was identified by petition of the entire population (North Karelia County). The only choice was then the selection of a reference area and another county was chosen (12).

The design used to evaluate the effect of the programme on risk-factor levels has usually been the separate-sample pretest-posttest control group design presented by Campbell & Stanley (13). Separate cross-sectional samples are drawn from the same populations, one in the intervention area and another in the reference area, before and after the programme.

The results in the nine countries included in CCCCP are encouraging, and they are presented briefly here in text and tables summarized from the CCCCP report (11).

Finland: North Karelia

The major objective of the programme in North Karelia was to reduce mortality and morbidity rates for coronary heart disease and related major cardiovascular diseases in the whole population, but with special emphasis on middle-aged men. Primary prevention was emphasized through attempts to reduce the levels of the critical risk factors, especially by effecting general changes in lifestyle. The comprehensive educational and service-oriented programme to modify the risk-factor profile of the population was based on local community action and the local service structure and attempted to encourage lifestyles that reduce risk-factor levels and promote health. Practical skills were taught, social support for the changes was

Table 1. Summary of the comprehensive cardiovascular community control programmes

Intervention area(s)	Type of community (N = size of population)	Reference community(ies)	Evaluation criteria	Starting year	Evaluation year(s)	Type of intervention
Finland						
North Karelia	Whole county (N = 180 000)	County of Kuopio (N = 250 000)	Morbidity: AMI, stroke, cancer Mortality: all and cause-specific Disability: all and cause-specific Risk factors Lifestyles	1972	1977, 1982	Comprehensive community-based, emphasizing community organization, health centres, mass media
German Democratic Republic						
Schleiz	Whole district (N = 33 000)	District of Dippoldiswalde (N = 46 000)	Morbidity Mortality Risk factors	1976	1976, 1981	Comprehensive community-based emphasizing health services
Federal Republic of Germany						
Eberbach and Wiesloch	Towns of Eberbach (N = 16 000) and Wiesloch (N = 21 000)	Town of Neckargemünd (N = 15 000)	Mortality Morbidity (only infarction)	1976	1976, 1980, 1984	Screening, health education, community participation

397

Table 1 (contd)

Intervention area(s)	Type of community (N = size of population)	Reference community(ies)	Evaluation criteria	Starting year	Evaluation year(s)	Type of intervention
Hungary 17th district of Budapest, Pécs and Siklós	District of Budapest (N = 56 279) town of Pécs (N = 168 715) and rural area of Siklós (N = 49 258)	Other districts of Budapest (N = 194 751) town and rural area (N = 469 003)	Mortality Morbidity: AMI, stroke Risk factors Lifestyles	1976	1978, 1981, 1983	Screening, health education, etc.
Italy Martignacco	Town (N = 5 259)	San Giorgio di Nogaro (N = 7 S651)	Mortality Morbidity Risk factors Lifestyles	1977	1977, 1981, 1983	Health education, other community activities, etc.
Norway Finnmark and Tromsø	County of Finnmark (N = 80 000) and Tromsø municipality (N = 45 000)	None	Risk factors Lifestyles	1974	1974/1975 1977/1978 (Finnmark) 1977, 1979/1980 (Tromsø)	Screening, health education and counselling

Table 1 (contd)

Intervention area(s)	Type of community (N = size of population)	Reference community(ies)	Evaluation criteria	Starting year	Evaluation year(s)	Type of intervention
Switzerland Aarau and Nyon	Towns of Aarau (N = 16 000) and Nyon (N = 12 000)	Vevey (N = 12 000) and Solothurn (N = 16 000)	Risk factors Lifestyles	1977	1977, 1980	Health education, other community activities
Union of Soviet Socialist Republics Moscow, Kaunas, Minsk, Kharkov, Tashkent, Frunze	Cities: all men aged 40–59 years from randomly selected areas (N = 71 000)	Two comparable reference groups in each city (N > 3 000 in each group)	Mortality Morbidity Risk factors Invalidity	1977	1977, 1982	Primary and secondary prevention
Yugoslavia Novi Sad	City (N = 230 000)	None	Mortality Morbidity Risk factors Invalidity Lifestyles	1975	1976, 1984	Comprehensive community-based

Note. AMI = acute myocardial infarction.
Source: Puska, P. et al. *(11).*

provided and environmental modifications were implemented as part of the comprehensive mobilization of the community for change.

Changes in risk factors and health behaviour in the population were assessed by examining cross-sectional random samples of the middle-aged population. Changes in North Karelia were adjusted for equivalent changes in the matched reference area to assess the programme effect (showing the net change in North Karelia).

Major population surveys in North Karelia and the reference area were carried out in 1972, 1977 and 1982. Each survey included almost 10 000 subjects, and participation rates ranged from 80% to 94%. Disease rates in North Karelia were monitored according to WHO criteria, using special myocardial infarction and stroke registers that operate in the whole country. Developments in mortality and disability pensions in the two areas and in the whole country were assessed using data from the national register.

The results of the first five years of the project (12) were so encouraging that it was decided to continue the programme and to follow up the changes in risk factors and disease rates in the area. This was considered vital to learn about the long-term consequences of this type of activity. At the same time, however, the project has increasingly been associated with national applications of the results. Although in accordance with the original aims, this reduces the availability of reference areas for evaluation.

The changes in health behaviour and risk-factor levels from 1972 to 1982 are presented in Table 2. Significant net reductions for all the risk factors took place for men. For women, significant net reductions were found for blood pressure and dietary fat consumption.

From 1969 to 1982 mortality from coronary heart disease among the middle-aged male population in North Karelia decreased annually by 2.9% (reference 2.3%, nationally 2.0%). Most of this decrease occurred after 1973 (Table 3). From 1974 to 1979, when the initial net change in risk factors could begin to have an impact, mortality from coronary heart disease fell by 22% in North Karelia, 12% in the reference area and 11% in the rest of Finland. Mortality from coronary heart disease among women declined more in North Karelia than in the rest of Finland, but as there were fewer women in the sample, the statistical significance of the results for women is more uncertain.

The North Karelia project is continuing to promote these favourable developments. This is also considered important for purposes of national and international demonstration and training. It is also

400

important to continue to monitor the trends in risk factors and diseases to assess fully the long-term impact of the project. This is done using a method of monitoring trends and determinants in cardiovascular disease known as MONICA (14). Further, the scope of the project has been enlarged to include major related non-communicable diseases in an integrated way (by Finnish participation in the WHO countrywide integrated noncommunicable diseases intervention (CINDI) programme) and to emphasize the promotion of positive health. Since 1978, the project has also launched systematic and carefully evaluated programmes to influence the health behaviour and risk factors of children and adolescents (the North Karelia youth project).

Before 1977, the North Karelia project team did not try to promote changes in risk factors in the reference area or the rest of Finland. Nevertheless, the project already had substantial positive national publicity. After 1977, the project team began to apply the results nationally. Government committees on health education and hypertension recommended many experiences for national use and recommended the establishment of a new office for health education in the National Board of Health. The project's health education materials have been distributed nationwide in great numbers. A major national activity has been a series of national health education programmes on Finnish television carried out by the project since 1978. Antismoking legislation was introduced in 1977.

Lifestyle factors related to cardiovascular disease started to change in Finland as a whole, concomitant with these developments, and a favourable change in mortality rates from cardiovascular disease has been observed in Finland (Table 3). The mortality from coronary heart disease of men in Finland has decreased nationwide, and Finland is losing its status as the country with the highest mortality rate from coronary heart disease in the world. The experience and results support the idea that a well conceived comprehensive community-based programme can have a positive impact on life-styles and cardiovascular risk factors in a whole population, and that such a development is associated with reduced mortality rates from cardiovascular disease.

German Democratic Republic: Schleiz

Community-based intervention related to cardiovascular and non-communicable diseases for the population of the Schleiz district was

Table 2. Changes in the main target health behaviour and risk factors among men and women in North Karelia (NK) and the reference area Kuopio (KUO), according to cross-sectional population surveys in 1972, 1977 and 1982

A. Men, 30–59 years of age

Health behaviour and risk factors		1972	1977	1982	Difference 1972–1982	Net percentage change 1972–1982
Percentage	NK	52	44	38	− 14 (P<0.0001)	− 17 (P<0.0001)
of smokers	KUO	50	45	45	− 5 (P<0.001)	
Amount	NK	10.0	8.6	6.6	− 3.4 (P<0.0001)	− 28 (P<0.0001)
of smoking[a]	KUO	8.6	8.5	7.9	− 0.7 (NS)	
Fat consumed in milk and on bread	NK	83	59	54	− 29 (P<0.0001)	− 22 (P<0.0001)
(g per day)	KUO	72	62	61	− 11 (P<0.0001)	
Serum cholesterol	NK	7.1	6.7	6.3	− 0.8 (P<0.0001)	− 3 (P<0.0001)
(mmol/l)	KUO	6.8	6.7	6.3	− 0.5 (P<0.0001)	
Systolic blood pressure	NK	149	143	145	− 4 (P<0.0001)	− 4 (P<0.0001)
(mmHg)	KUO	146	146	147	+ 1 (NS)	

[a] Number of cigarettes, cigars and pipes smoked per day per subject (smokers and non-smokers taken together).

Note. NS = not significant.

planned and prepared from 1973 to 1975. To evaluate the results, the Dippoldswalde district was chosen as the reference area. The intervention was applied as part of the existing health care system.

To evaluate the effects of the programme, 673 people in each district were randomly recruited and examined in 1976 and 1981; the response rates ranged from 63% to about 90%. The surveys showed that cardiovascular risk factors were reduced in the intervention district compared with the reference district (Table 4).

The incidence rates of acute myocardial infarction and stroke in the two districts showed net changes of − 3.8% and − 5.9%,

B. Women, 30–59 years of age

Health behaviour and risk factors		1972	1977	1982	Difference 1972–1982	Net percentage change 1972–1982
Percentage	NK	10	10	17	+ 7 (P<0.0001)	+ 1 (NS)
of smokers	KUO	11	12	18	+ 7 (P<0.0001)	
Amount	NK	1.1	1.2	1.7	+ 0.6 (P<0.0001)	− 14 (NS)
of smoking[a]	KUO	1.2	1.4	1.9	+ 0.7 (P<0.0001)	
Fat consumed in milk and on bread	NK	45	31	28	− 17 (P<0.0001)	− 16 (P<0.0001)
(g per day)	KUO	39	33	29	− 10 (P<0.0001)	
Serum cholesterol	NK	7.0	6.6	6.2	− 0.8 (P<0.0001)	− 1 (NS)
(mmol/l)	KUO	6.8	6.5	6.0	− 0.8 (P<0.0001)	
Systolic blood pressure	NK	153	142	141	− 12 (P<0.0001)	− 5 (P<0.0001)
(mmHg)	KUO	147	144	143	− 4 (P<0.0001)	

[a] Number of cigarettes, cigars and pipes smoked per day per subject (smokers and non-smokers taken together).

Note. NS = not significant.

respectively. The incidence of fatal acute myocardial infarctions showed a net reduction, but there was a net increase in nonfatal events (Table 5). The incidence of cancer was reduced while there was a net increase in both fatal and nonfatal rates of diabetes. The evaluation of the Schleiz project also included gathering information on other experiences related to the project. A preliminary cost–benefit assessment revealed a favourable estimate similar to the findings of the North Karelia project.

After the implementation of the Schleiz project, a number of other national activities were launched in parallel. A major effort, and a

Table 3. Average annual regression-based decline in age-adjusted mortality from coronary heart disease in North Karelia, in the reference area and in Finland (excluding North Karelia)

| Area | Annual decline (%) | | | |
| | Men | | Women | |
	1969–1982	1974–1979	1969–1982	1974–1979
North Karelia	2.9	3.7	4.9	2.2
Reference area	2.3	1.9	4.1	1.8
Finland, excluding North Karelia	2.0[a]	1.7[b]	3.0[b]	1.2

[a] Difference from North Karelia in relation to random variation, $P < 0.0001$.
[b] Difference from North Karelia in relation to random variation, $P < 0.05$.

Table 4. Risk factor changes in the Schleiz project between 1976 and 1981

| Risk factor | Mean value in Schleiz in 1981 | | Net difference 1976–1981 | Net percentage change 1976–1981 |
	Men	Women		
Systolic blood pressure (mmHg)	136.5	137.2	− 5	− 3.6 ($P < 0.05$)
Diastolic blood pressure (mmHg)	84.5	84.9	− 5.5	− 6.2 ($P < 0.05$)
Serum cholesterol (mmol/litre)	5.9	5.7	−10.1	− 4.5 ($P < 0.05$)
Body mass index (kg/m^2)	25.4	25.0	− 1.2	− 4.9 ($P < 0.05$)
Number of cigarettes smoked per day	8.9	7.7	+ 0.8	+10.7 (NS)

Note. NS = not significant.

natural extension of the Schleiz project, is the integrated control programme of cardiovascular and other noncommunicable diseases. The main long-term objective — as in the Schleiz project — is the reduction of morbidity and/or mortality from cardiovascular and

Table 5. Incidence of cardiovascular disease in 1982 and net changes from 1976/1977 to 1981/1982 in Schleiz, according to the acute myocardial infarction (AMI) and stroke registers

Type of attack	AMI and stroke			AMI			Stroke		
	Incidence per 10 000 in 1982	Net change 1976/77–1981/82	Net percentage change 1976/77–1981/82	Incidence per 10 000 in 1982	Net change 1976/77–1981/82	Net percentage change 1976/77–1981/82	Incidence per 10 000 in 1982	Net change 1976/77–1981/82	Net percentage change 1976/77–1981/82
All	63.9	– 2.7	– 6.7	33.2	– 0.9	– 3.8	30.7	– 1.1	– 5.9
Fatal	38.3	– 9.7	– 33.1	15.3	– 6.1	– 41.2	23.0	– 3.3	– 23.9
Nonfatal	25.5	+ 7.1	+ 52.6	17.8	+ 4.8	+ 52.7	7.7	+ 2.2	+ 48.9

405

noncommunicable chronic diseases at younger and middle age. Thus, there has been a gradual development ultimately to implement coordinated, sustained and effective national control of cardio-vascular and related noncommunicable diseases.

Federal Republic of Germany: Eberbach-Wiesloch

The main aim of the project was to test whether communities, under the guidance of the medical profession, are able to take care of their own health problems without additional state support.

The promotion and maintenance of the interest of the population in the problems of cardiovascular diseases were successfully achieved. Self-sustainment was also achieved. The models developed seem to be satisfactorily transferable. This is proven by the absence of major obstacles to integrating the models in Wiesloch and by the quick spread of the Eberbach-Wiesloch programme to other towns in the Federal Republic of Germany — at present more than 20 towns.

Hungary: Budapest, Pécs and Siklós

The cardiovascular programme in Hungary started in Budapest in 1976. In 1982, the programme was extended to new areas and new subprogrammes were introduced. In addition to the Budapest programme, Pécs, a town in southern Hungary, and Siklós, a rural area in the same county, started a pilot project. The intervention has included special education courses for health workers, mass health education for the general population and for the population at special risk, and active and passive screening for cardiovascular disease and other chronic conditions.

No major evaluation results are yet available. Two-year changes of some risk factors, estimated by examining samples of the general population, showed satisfactory control of hypertensive people, but an increase in mean serum cholesterol and in the prevalence of obesity and smoking was recorded. The preliminary conclusion was that traditional health education through general practitioners and health workers has little effect on the levels of risk factors. The programme in Hungary continues and is being expanded. In 1982, the MONICA system was introduced and serves as a further tool for monitoring change. The programme among children has been continued. Based on the experience with the cardiovascular programme, Hungary has joined CINDI in an attempt to develop effective integrated measures to control cardiovascular diseases and related noncommunicable diseases.

Italy: Martignacco

The Martignacco community cardiovascular control project was established in 1977 as a pilot study in northern Italy to ascertain the feasibility, safety and efficacy of a comprehensive programme targeting the entire population and based on the current health and social service organization in the community.

The comprehensive intervention was based on three main strategies: a population strategy, mainly using educational activities to teach people about risk factors for cardiovascular disease and how these risks can be reduced; a strategy targeting individuals or specific groups at high risk; and a strategy for secondary prevention, to inhibit the progress and recurrence of disease when already established.

The evaluation goals were to assess feasibility, and the changes in the prevalence of risk factors, in cardiovascular disease incidence and in the probability of suffering a cardiovascular event or death. Table 6 summarizes the effects of the programme on risk-factor levels in Martignacco and in San Giorgio, a similar community selected as a reference area.

An estimate of the risk of coronary heart disease was also calculated, using a multiple logistic risk function with five factors. The analysis showed a significant net reduction in risk in Martignacco by an average of 61.9% in five years. The crude mean annual incidence of coronary heart disease and stroke from 1978–1983 is presented in Table 7, showing a favourable trend for the population of Martignacco, with the only exception being coronary heart disease among women.

Towards the end of the initial intervention period, the people of Martignacco particularly expressed their general acceptance of the project. Many expressed fear that the project might end and the whole community felt that continuation was important. A formal petition was then presented to the district administration and local health authorities late in 1983. The Council of Martignacco formally decided to continue and an agreement for a further five years was signed in 1984.

The continuation programme included implementation of the already established activities and several intensified intervention measures. The possibility of developing an integrated prevention programme for noncommunicable diseases in the area is also being examined. The evaluation of further developments is taking place in the framework of the MONICA project.

407

Table 6. Risk factor levels among men and women aged 40–59 years in Martignacco (M) and San Giorgio (SG) and the net change in Martignacco from 1977 to 1983

Risk factors	Men					Women				
	Mean value				Net percentage change	Mean value				Net percentage change
	1977		1983		1977–1983	1977		1983		1977–1983
	M	SG	M	SG	M	M	SG	M	SG	M
Systolic blood pressure (mmHg)	147	145	147	159	–9 (P < 0.0001)	144	136	146	152	–11 (P < 0.0001)
Diastolic blood pressure (mmHg)	93	92	90	96	–7 (P < 0.0001)	90	88	89	90	–4 (P < 0.05)
Serum cholesterol (mmol/litre)	5.8	5.5	5.9	6.0	–8 (P < 0.05)	5.8	5.5	6.1	5.9	–3 (NS)
Body mass index (kg/m²)	26.0	26.7	26.2	26.8	0 (NS)	26.4	26.5	26.6	26.6	0 (NS)
Number of cigarettes smoked per day per head of population	10.0	10.0	6.4	6.0	+ 4 (NS)	2.5	4.3	1.7	3.2	–7 (NS)
CHD risk estimate (age-standardized)	22.2	19.7	22.0	29.3	–50 (P < 0.0001)	5.7	4.1	7.0	6.5	–33 (P < 0.0001)

Note. NS = not significant. CHD = coronary heart disease.

Table 7. Crude mean annual incidence of coronary heart disease (CHD) and stroke per thousand population in 1978–1983 in the Martignacco project among men and women aged 40–59 years

Type of attack	Martignacco			San Giorgio		
	Men	Women	Total	Men	Women	Total
CHD						
Fatal	0.5	0.7	0.6	1.4	0.5	1.0
Nonfatal	1.3	0.7	1.0	3.1	0.3	1.7
Total	1.8	1.5	1.6	4.7	0.9	2.8
Stroke						
Fatal	0.7	0.0	0.3	1.0	0.9	0.9
Nonfatal	1.6	0.2	0.9	1.0	1.0	1.1
Total	2.3	0.2	1.2	2.1	1.9	2.0

Norway: Finnmark and Tromsø

The state Mass Radiography Service in Norway carried out screening studies in Finnmark, Sogn og Fjordane, and Oppland counties from 1974 to 1985. Special community-based activities were launched in Finnmark, and the study became linked to the CCCCP. The Tromsø heart study was initiated by the University of Tromsø and started in 1974 as a well planned epidemiological study. This study was associated with intervention measures in the city of Tromsø, and also linked up with the CCCCP. Both projects involved community-based interventions on risk factors for cardiovascular diseases and an assessment of changes, but they lacked formal reference areas.

The results in Finnmark based on data from two surveys *(15)* showed that over three years the average serum cholesterol level (cross-sectionally) decreased by about 0.3 mmol/litre. Cigarette consumption decreased by 12% for males and 4% for females. The joint decrease (improvement) in risk factors indicates a possible health benefit of about 20%, calculated in terms of myocardial infarction over ten years.

Although it is difficult to assess the extent to which the changes were caused by information because there was no formal reference area, the study team was satisfied with the experience. The intervention was feasible and it was likely that changes among people at high risk were at least partially a consequence of the intervention. Because

409

mortality and morbidity from cardiovascular diseases in Finnmark are being monitored, the study team hopes to demonstrate future changes in disease rates as a reflection of the observed changes in risk factors.

The primary objective of the Tromsø heart study was to try to explain the relatively high mortality figures for coronary heart disease, a major health problem in this sparsely populated area. Steps were taken at different levels to try to reduce the risk of coronary heart disease in the population studied. The programme was run in four nearby areas in and around Tromsø. No reference area was established. Two large surveys were performed between 1974 and 1979/1980, and at the beginning people identified by measuring the risk factors as being at high risk were sent to outpatient clinics for treatment.

There was a substantial reduction in the prevalence of smoking (from 57% to about 48%) in adult men (this was also observed in the country as a whole), a slight and unexplainable increase in systolic blood pressure (from 127 mmHg to 130 mmHg) and a marked reduction in serum cholesterol (from 6.6 mmol/litre to 5.9 mmol/litre). The changes were strongly related to people's educational level at the beginning of the study in 1974. One third of those surveyed reported changing their diet, and the proportion of those who reported exercising regularly increased from 24% to 35% in five years. Some preliminary observations have been made on mortality data. From 1976 to 1980 a clear decrease in the death rate from stroke was observed and a flattening out of the increasing death rate from coronary heart disease.

The study team felt that the programme was feasible, but the effects were difficult to assess, partly because of national developments in Norway that undoubtedly were substantially influenced by the fact that several studies were being carried out in the country.

Switzerland: national research programme 1A on the primary prevention of cardiovascular diseases

The main objectives of this national research programme were to evaluate ways of reducing known cardiovascular risk factors among the local populations of the two intervention communities compared with two "normal care" communities, and to provide tested cost-effective methods for nationwide use in the future control of cardiovascular disease (16). To achieve this, comparable communities of between 10 000 and 20 000 inhabitants were selected.

410

Three main principles of community-oriented health education guided all the local intervention methods: active participation of the population, mobilization of personal and community resources, and integration of the new programme into existing local health and social services. The evaluation was based on baseline and follow-up surveys of random samples of the population.

Risk factor levels were reduced in all four communities from 1977 to 1980 (Table 8). The reduction in smoking was significantly greater in the intervention communities than in the reference communities. Cost–benefit analysis showed that the health benefits through the reduction of risk factors well outweighed the programme costs.

The experience and results obtained in this programme suggested that such community cardiovascular control programmes are both feasible and effective in Switzerland. The programme team emphasized that the final report gives decision-makers in Switzerland the opportunity to determine whether future countrywide preventive efforts are warranted. The team is now involved in a number of national activities in the field of control of cardiovascular disease that take advantage of this experience.

USSR: population study on multifactorial prevention of cardiovascular disease

A study on the multifactorial prevention of cardiovascular disease was started in 1977 in six centres: Moscow, Kaunas (Lithuanian SSR), Minsk (Byelorussian SSR), Tashkent (Uzbek SSR), Frunze (Kirghiz SSR) and Kharkov (Ukrainian SSR). The study was conducted in three population groups: a group in which intensive prevention was carried out by specially trained personnel and two reference groups. In the reference groups, the preventive measures were carried out by physicians from the existing network of health services. The first reference group was surveyed completely. In the second reference group, only 10% random samples were surveyed at the beginning and end of the study.

During the first four years of follow-up in Moscow, the prevalence of arterial hypertension and mean levels of systolic and diastolic blood pressure decreased significantly. This was a result of the improved treatment of patients and a reduction in incidence. The number of patients with arterial hypertension receiving treatment doubled, and the number of patients treated effectively increased from 16% to 35%. The incidence of arterial hypertension in the

411

intervention group was significantly lower than that in the first reference group.

Both groups smoked fewer cigarettes per day during the four-year follow-up, but this reduction was only statistically significant in the intervention group. The mean number of cigarettes smoked per day decreased 1.6 cigarettes per day in the intervention group and 0.9 cigarettes per day in the reference group.

Yugoslavia: Novi Sad

A comprehensive intervention project was started in 1975 in Novi Sad, with no reference area. No final evaluation of the experience in Novi Sad is yet available, but the feasibility of the programme has been good. Several positive changes have been reported. In 1982, the projects reported greatly improved control of hypertension and a 3% drop in tobacco consumption. At that time the registers showed no

Table 8. Risk factor changes in the random population sample
aged 16–69 years (standardized by age and sex)
in the national research programme 1A

Risk factor	Intervention towns (N = 848)		Reference towns (N = 1358)		Net percentage change 1977/78– 1980/81
	1977/ 1978	1980/ 1981	1977/ 1978	1980/ 1981	
Regular smokers (%)	33	27	37	35	− 11 ($P < 0.05$)
Amount of tobacco consumed (g/day)	5.0	4.2	6.7	6.3	− 8 (NS)
Serum cholesterol (mmol/litre)	5.6	5.4	5.6	5.4	0 (NS)
Systolic blood pressure (mmHg)	123	126	125	122	+ 4 ($P < 0.001$)
Body mass index (kg/m²)	23.4	23.8	24.1	24.0	+ 2 ($P < 0.001$)

Note. NS = not significant.

412

changes in the incidence of acute myocardial infarction, but there has been a decline in mortality from myocardial infarction and stroke.

Other countries

Austria, Bulgaria, Czechoslovakia, Greece, Malta, Portugal, Romania and Sweden were also involved in CCCCP. These countries, however, had programmes that were smaller, started later or complied less with the CCCCP protocol than those reported above.

The Stanford three community study (17) was planned and launched in the United States at the same time as the North Karelia project, but had a more limited scope. It focused on a much smaller population, and used mainly mass media intervention over three years to effect risk factor and behaviour changes, followed by assessment of the possible changes in rates of disease.

The results from this study encouraged the Stanford centre to initiate a larger study in 1978, the five city project (18). Two larger cities were selected for educational intervention, and three were assigned as reference areas. As the total population of the five cities was about 350 000, significant reductions in morbidity and mortality could be anticipated if the study lasted nine years. Because a self-sustaining programme in the community was required and because of the success of the North Karelia project in using community organization, the aim was to enhance and systematize the programme of community organization in the five city project. Preliminary mid-course results on the reduction of risk factors were encouraging (19).

At the same time as the North Karelia project and the Stanford three community study, a third, even more restricted community-based intervention study of risk factors for coronary heart disease started in Jerusalem (20). This study, called the CHAD programme, was instituted in a family practice in a western area of Jerusalem in the early 1970s. Its effectiveness was evaluated by comparing the changes among about 500 subjects surveyed in 1970 and 1975 with those observed among 1500 subjects in an adjacent reference neighbourhood. The prevalence of hypertension decreased by 33%, hypercholesterolaemia by 31%, cigarette smoking by 23% (among men), and obesity by 13%. The results suggested that intervention centred on primary health care had an appreciable effect on cardiovascular risk factors.

Several additional community programmes or studies are being planned or are already under way on other continents. Many of them are in principle comparable to the CCCCP and to the North Karelia project. As in Europe, some communities are too small for measuring changes in disease rates and studies only focus on changes in behaviour and risk factors. Some do not have reference communities and some only assess the changes among the subjects initially examined (cohort analysis), as in the Stanford three community study or the CHAD programme in Jerusalem. The actual community settings and intervention approaches vary considerably in the different studies. Such programmes have been launched in Ireland (Kilkenny health project), the United Kingdom (Heartbeat Wales and Scottish heart health study), Cuba, the People's Republic of China, New South Wales in Australia, near Capetown in South Africa, and Minnesota, Rhode Island and Pennsylvania in the United States. The studies in Minnesota (21) and Rhode Island (22) are large, comprehensive and long term. The three studies in Stanford, Minnesota and Rhode Island are linked through their common United States Government funding and through a common methodology for evaluating the outcome.

The development of community cardiovascular control programmes in developing countries has been more limited, for several reasons. These programmes have emphasized primary health care and general government decisions for early prevention to avoid the epidemic of cardiovascular diseases experienced in the developed countries.

The experience gained in Europe and the rapid growth of new programmes in Europe and elsewhere have clearly demonstrated the feasibility of comprehensive community-based cardiovascular programmes. No implementation of a programme has failed. Obviously the degree of success in implementation depends on a number of factors: the awareness and motivation of the population, the enthusiasm, skills and resources of the project team, and general support from local, regional and national activities for health. It is also interesting that programmes have been successfully carried out in countries with quite different political systems and health care systems.

Effectiveness of the programmes
Table 9 summarizes the changes in risk factors in the main European programmes, provided by the principal investigators (11).

About half of the nine programmes report reductions in the main risk factors. None of the risk factors is easier to change than the others. On several occasions, the changes observed in risk factors

414

were substantial. For instance, the reductions observed in males in North Karelia in ten years were 36% for smoking, 11% for mean serum cholesterol level and 5% for mean diastolic blood pressure. Not surprisingly, the changes in biological risk factors (serum cholesterol and blood pressure) were much smaller than the changes in smoking. Changes in risk factors of this magnitude may be considered small for an individual, but they represent mean changes for the whole population and are thus important for disease rates in a population.

The "natural" change, as reflected in changes in the reference areas, varied in the different countries. In North Karelia, the levels of risk factors also declined somewhat in the reference area.

In addition to some of the other European programmes, similar changes in risk factors to those reported in North Karelia occurred in the Stanford three community study and the CHAD programme in Jerusalem. Given the similarities in underlying theory and in its application to entire communities, these experiences can be viewed as replicative, demonstrating the feasibility and, at least partially, indicating the effects and the ability to generalize this kind of approach.

The effects observed in the North Karelia project and some of the other successful programmes compare well with those observed in some recent multifactorial clinical trials such as the Multiple Risk Factor Intervention Trial (23) in the United States and the European

Table 9. Risk factor changes in the major European comprehensive cardiovascular community control programmes

Change	Number of programmes reporting changes in:		
	smoking	serum cholesterol levels	blood pressure
No net effect or a negative effect (if no reference: no change or a negative change)	1	2	2
A reduction, but no reference available	3	2	2
A nonsignificant net reduction	2	1	—
A significant net reduction	3	4	5

Collaborative Trial (24,25). Greater effects have been achieved only in smaller-scale intensive clinical trials with subjects at very high risk such as a study in Oslo (26). The community-based approach generally provides a much greater cost–benefit ratio, especially considering the cost per subject involved. Raising the general health level of lifestyles in a community may also prevent some of the possible psychological and emotional problems involved in intensive labelling of and intervention among subjects at high risk — in addition to the other advantages of the community-based approach.

Despite the clear success of the community programmes some of them failed to have positive effects on the targeted risk factors — at least during the evaluation period used. At this stage, it is very difficult to determine clearly which of the many potential determinants arising from either baseline factors or intervention methods are responsible for the favourable or unfavourable changes in risk factors obtained in different programmes, and what recommendations should be made for further replications elsewhere. A community programme ultimately tests whether a specific programme (which should be designed so that it can be applied on a larger scale) is feasible and effective under given conditions. The impact of various conditions in the community and of different components of the project on the successes and failures of a given programme can be evaluated only to a limited extent, and the present international experience can provide only very limited conclusions (11).

In the assessment of effect, the main emphasis has clearly been on changes in risk factors. Many of the communities used have been too small or the follow-up period too short to observe any disease-related effects. Nevertheless, the programmes that have reported clear changes in risk factors over a longer period have generally also reported changes in rates of cardiovascular disease (North Karelia, Schleiz, Martignacco). The ten-year disease changes in North Karelia especially strongly suggest that the cardiovascular trends in a community respond to the changes in risk factors initiated by the intervention.

Community Control of Cardiovascular Disease: Future Direction and Prospects

The results of community cardiovascular programmes confirm that the strategy of targeting the entire population has been correct. It is important to realize, however, that the activities implemented in a community do not maintain themselves. In North Karelia, for instance, the greatest change in risk-factor-related behaviour occurred during the first five years. No further decreases in blood pressure occurred afterwards (Table 3). An analysis of the effects of hypertension care even shows a deterioration, especially among middle-aged women between 1977 and 1982; this was followed by an increase in stroke mortality in middle-aged women between 1977/ 1978 and 1980/1981 (27). The lesson from this may be that, in addition to activities targeted at the whole population, special and continual attention should be paid to people with one or two recognized risk factors.

Studies have shown that mortality from disease is higher in lower social classes (see Chapter 5). Community control programmes have focused on changing health behaviour in entire populations and on organizing care for sick individuals. It is difficult to test the influence of changes in the socioeconomic pattern of a society on the reduction in the disability caused by cardiovascular disease. Little attention has been directed towards how community control programmes have succeeded in their goal of improving health equity in whole populations. In the North Karelia hypertension programme, care improved throughout the community (28). Dietary behaviour changed favourably: improvements were similar in different age, educational and occupational groups and in urban and rural populations (29).

Many community cardiovascular programmes have shifted from vertical programmes towards a more horizontal, integrated approach, thus enlarging their scope to cover other noncommunicable diseases (30). This is a natural and logical development, since such diseases share the same risk factors as cardiovascular diseases. The theory behind integrated programmes to control noncommunicable diseases has thus followed what is happening in practice. Activities already established at the level of the population have had a simultaneous effect on the onset of most other chronic diseases. The leading role of cardiovascular disease control programmes has been and will continue to be essential in developing integrated noncommunicable disease control programmes.

Risk factors for cardiovascular diseases already exist in developing countries; it is only a question of time before the consequences of unhealthy behaviour become a reality. Preventing this from happening in developing countries is a major challenge in the control of cardiovascular disease at the global level.

References

1. **Fejfar, Z. et al**. Cardiovascular diseases: care and prevention. Part I. *WHO chronicle*, **28**: 55–64 (1974).

2. **Keys, A**. *Coronary heart disease in seven countries*. New York, American Heart Association, 1970 (Monograph No. 29).

3. *Myocardial infarction community registers*. Copenhagen, WHO Regional Office for Europe, 1976 (Public Health in Europe No. 5).

4. **Ovcarov, V.K. & Bystrova, V.A**. Present trends in mortality in the age group 35–64 in selected developed countries between 1950–1973. *World health statistics quarterly*, **31**: 208–346 (1978).

5. **Pisa, Z. & Uemura, K**. Trends of mortality from ischaemic heart disease and other cardiovascular diseases in 27 countries, 1968–1977. *World health statistics quarterly*, **35**: 11–17 (1982).

6. **Dawber, T.R. et al**. Epidemiological approaches to heart disease. The Framingham Study. *American journal of public health*, **41**: 279–286 (1951).

7. **Pooling Project Research Group**. *Relationship of blood pressure, serum cholesterol, smoking habits, relative weight and ECG abnormalities to incidence of major coronary events: final report of the Pooling Project*. Dallas, American Heart Association, 1978 (Monograph No. 60).

8. **Inter-Society Commission for Heart Disease Resources**. Primary prevention of arteriosclerotic diseases. *Circulation*, **42**: 55–95 (1970).

9. **Kottke, T.E. et al**. Projected effects of high risk versus population based prevention strategies in coronary heart disease. *American journal of epidemiology*, **121**: 697–704 (1985).

10. **Rose, G**. Incubation period of coronary heart disease. *British medical journal*, **284**: 1600–1601 (1982).

11. **Puska, P. et al**. *Comprehensive cardiovascular community control programmes in Europe*. Copenhagen, WHO Regional Office for Europe, 1988 (EURO Reports and Studies No. 106).

12. **Puska, P. et al**. *Community control of cardiovascular diseases: evaluation of a comprehensive community programme for control of cardiovascular diseases in North Karelia, Finland,*

1972–1977. Copenhagen, WHO Regional Office for Europe, 1981.

13. **Campbell, D.T. & Stanley, J.C.** *Experimental and quasi-experimental designs for research.* Chicago, Rand McNally, 1963.

14. **WHO MONICA project principal investigators**. The World Health Organization MONICA project (monitoring trends and determinants in cardiovascular disease): a major international collaboration. *Journal of clinical epidemiology*, **41**(2): 105–114 (1988).

15. **Tretli, S. et al**. Intervention on cardiovascular disease risk factors in Finnmark County: changes after a period of three years. The Cardiovascular Diseases Study in Finnmark County, Norway. *Scandinavian journal of social medicine*, **13**: 1–13 (1985).

16. **Gutzwiller, F. et al**. Community-based primary prevention of cardiovascular disease in Switzerland: methods and results of the National Research Programme (NRP1A). *Preventive medicine*, **14**: 482–491 (1985).

17. **Farquhar, J.W. et al**. Community education for cardio-vascular health. *Lancet*, **1**: 1192–1195 (1977).

18. **Farquhar, J.W**. The community-based model of lifestyle intervention trials. *American journal of epidemiology*, **108**: 103–111 (1978).

19. **Farquhar, J.W. et al**. Risk factor reduction from community education: preliminary results of the Stanford Five City Project. *CVD epidemiological newsletter*, **35**: 48 (1984).

20. **Abrahamson, J.H. et al**. Evaluation of a community programme for the control of cardiovascular risk factors: the CHAD programme in Jerusalem. *Israeli journal of medical sciences*, **17**: 201–212 (1981).

21. **Jacobs, D.R., Jr. et al**. Community-wide prevention strategies: evaluation design of the Minnesota Heart Health Program. *Journal of chronic diseases*, **39**(10): 775–788 (1986).

22. **Lefebvre, R.C. et al**. Theory and delivery of health programming in the community: the Pawtucket Heart Health Programme. *Preventive medicine*, **16**(1): 80–95 (1987).

23. **Multiple Risk Factor Intervention Trial Research Group**. Multiple risk factor intervention trial. Risk factor changes and

mortality results. *Journal of the American Medical Association*, **248**: 1465–1477 (1982).

24. **Kornitzer, M. et al.** Belgian heart disease prevention project: incidence and mortality results. *Lancet*, **1**: 1066–1070 (1983).

25. **Rose, G. et al.** UK heart disease prevention project: incidence and mortality results. *Lancet*, **1**: 1062–1066 (1983).

26. **Hjerman, I. et al.** Effect of diet and smoking intervention on the incidence of coronary heart disease. Report from the Oslo study group of a randomized trial in healthy men. *Lancet*, **2**: 1303–1310 (1981).

27. **Tuomilehto, J. et al.** Effectiveness of treatment with anti-hypertensive drugs and trends in mortality from stroke in the community. *British medical journal*, **291**: 857–861 (1985).

28. **Nissinen, A. et al.** The influence of socioeconomic factors on blood pressure control during a community-based hypertension control programme. *Acta cardiologica*, **41**(2): 99–109 (1985).

29. **Pietinen, P. et al.** Dietary changes in the North Karelia Project (1972–1982). *Preventive medicine*, **17**: 183–193 (1988).

30. **Leparski, E. & Nüssel, E., ed.** *CINDI (countrywide integrated noncommunicable diseases intervention programme). Protocol and guidelines for monitoring and evaluation procedures.* Berlin (West), Springer Verlag, 1987.

18

Community psychiatry and health promotion research

Odd Steffen Dalgard,
Tom Sørensen & Sven Bjørk

This chapter deals with various aspects of health promotion and related research relevant to contemporary social psychiatry and community mental health. The findings and conclusions referred to, although emerging primarily from psychiatric epidemiology and preventive psychiatric research, supply potent guidelines for a more complete framework of mental health promotion that has already begun to influence health professionals, planners in different fields, public authorities and policy-makers, and community representatives.

Sharp demarcations between normal and abnormal are less appropriate in mental health than in somatic health. Mental health also has a broader scope for differences in interpretation and definition. For example, positive mental health status may be defined as the absence of impairing syptoms of stress or dysfunction, or as a state of being that expresses a richer vitality, creativity and active participation in life. The levels of functioning, in terms of coping with the stresses and strains of daily living, can be viewed as a continuum from the best to the worst. It therefore makes sense to examine the individual prerequisites and the environmental conditions that are most likely to influence the mental health of individuals, groups and communities.

The areas of mental health research most relevant to health promotion are: epidemiological surveys based on population studies; the assessment of environmental risk factors, including the social integration of local communities; living conditions and the quality of life; social networks and social support; stress; personal skills; and coping strategies. This chapter will attempt to highlight relevant research findings, especially those from Norway, though largely presenting international thinking in these areas. Mental health is approached from a systems perspective, viewing the different areas of study, from the environment at large to the individual, and moving from recent research findings to logical strategies for intervention and health promotion.

Epidemiology of Mental Health

From the point of view of research, epidemiology is the logical approach to community health and this also applies to mental health. Using descriptive, analytical and experimental epidemiology, the dimensions of the problem can be assessed, risk factors can be identified and programmes of health promotion can be tested.

This section explains how the epidemiological approach has been used in the mental health field. Most of the examples are drawn from the authors' own experience and research in Norway, which has roots in sociology as well as psychiatry.

Community mental health is at the crossroads between social, cultural and political processes at the community level, and family and small group processes at the individual level.

Incidence and prevalence of mental disorder as the basis
for mental health promotion

In a historical perspective, psychiatric treatment, service development and psychiatric epidemiology show mutual influences. The inclusion of neuroses and psychosomatic disorders and, later on, the development of extramural services have made it more urgent to survey the general population to ascertain the true prevalence of mental disorder.

The results of epidemiological studies of psychiatric cases have been an important part of the scientific basis for community mental health programmes. These studies showed that the proportion of the population with psychiatric problems was far greater than first supposed (1,2). Caplan (3) emphasized that it is the responsibility of community psychiatry to treat mental disorders within the confines of a community, including both current and potential cases.

In a review and reanalysis of the results of epidemiological studies of the true prevalence of psychiatric disorders among adults,

Dohrenwend *(4)* estimated this prevalence in the United States population to be 15–20% (periods from weeks to one year). These figures are similar to those in studies in Norway based on direct interviews with representative samples of the adult population. Dalgard *(5)*, using the same questionnaire as Leighton in Sterling County *(1)*, found a mean prevalence of 26% for different neighbourhoods in Oslo. With the same instrument, Sørensen *(6)* found a prevalence of 21.4% in a mixed rural and semirural district in the southern part of Norway. The magnitude of the problem was confirmed by Sørensen *(7)* in a survey of a population in northern Norway, where 25% had anxiety and depressive symptoms comparable to those seen in psychiatric cases.

Andersen *(8)*, using clinical evaluation, estimated the life prevalence of total psychiatric morbidity to be 17.7% in two contrasting communities in northern Norway. Fugelli *(9)*, a general practitioner for two small municipalities in northern Norway, estimated that the psychiatric morbidity was 31.3%. This was assessed by a general practice registration over a two-year period and examination of the total population. Although the studies referred to vary in cultural context, type of population and method of evaluation, this indicates the proportions of the problem.

The follow-up to the Sterling County study *(10)* shows that more than half of the people found to have anxiety and depression in the first study either never recovered during the eighteen-year follow-up period or had serious recurrences. This makes it clear that the high prevalence figures in this type of study do not represent mostly transient and mild cases. Psychiatric disorders are long-standing and a serious concern for public health; they are the most common cause of disability in Norway.

The mean prevalence of psychiatric disorder in Norway is about 20%. This raises the question of whether primary prevention is the ideal way to reduce prevalence. Using the follow-up to the Sterling County study, Leighton points out that primary prevention can easily be overrated. The results suggest that the high prevalence of depression and anxiety is much more a result of chronicity and relapse than of new cases. The incidence seems to be only 0.9% per year for these disorders. Even with 100% successful primary prevention programmes, it would be many years before an effect on prevalence was apparent. Leighton draws attention to a more complex multifaceted approach. Called target spectrum for the control and prevention of psychiatric disorders, its main elements are: treatment that reduces discomfort and disability, care that maximizes self-healing processes and spontaneous recovery, conditions that minimize the disabling effects of chronic psychiatric illness, actions to reduce the duration of illness, and actions focused on preventing relapse and initial occurrence.

Demographic variation

The above-mentioned studies indicate that the psychiatric morbidity of large heterogeneous populations will be about the same. But even studies using the same case-finding instruments find differences between smaller, more homogeneous communities.

In Dalgard's study (5) the prevalence of psychiatric morbidity in the different neighbourhoods varied from 13.5% to 34.5%. In Sørensen's study (6) of communities with differing proportions of long-distance commuters, prevalence ranged from 13.0% to 29.0%. Andersen (8) found 14.8% and 20.7% in two contrasting communities. Sørensen (7), however, registered only insignificant differences between four municipalities in northern Norway. In accordance with surveys in other countries, all the studies in Norway have found higher rates for women, with neuroses comprising the difference. This sex difference is highest among the population of Oslo (31.0% versus 18.8%) (5) and lowest in one of the rural communities in southern Norway (14.0% versus 12.0%) (6).

Age does not seem to show the same striking contrast as sex. Both Dalgard (5) and Sørensen (6) found the highest rates among middle-aged people, especially women. Sørensen (7) found no significant correlation with age. The correlation with socioeconomic status varies in these studies. In accordance with earlier studies in Scandinavia, Sorensen (6) found no consistent correlation with indicators of socioeconomic status such as occupation and education in a rural area in southern Norway. Dalgard (5) in Oslo and Sørensen (7) in a coastal district in northern Norway, however, have demonstrated a clear correspondence between psychiatric morbidity and lower social class, most clearly for men.

Environmental risk factors: social disintegration
and lack of social support

The step from descriptive epidemiology, which gives the rate and distribution of mental disorders in a community, to analytic epidemiology, which identifies factors of high risk, brings people closer to understanding the causal mechanisms. Nevertheless, simple linear

424

chains of causation are not likely to be found in the field of psychiatric epidemiology. Circular models, with positive and negative feedback loops, seem to fit the data better as is generally the case in the social sciences. It is therefore often difficult to distinguish between cause and effect. Full understanding of the etiological processes cannot be reached before prevention is undertaken. Hence, experimental epidemiology, which attempts to manipulate the possible high-risk factors and assess the effects, is a logical way to obtain more concrete knowledge about causal processes. Based on this perspective, the research referred to below can only lead to tentative conclusions about high-risk factors.

One of the most publicized attempts to examine community mental health using psychiatric epidemiology was the studies by Alexander Leighton and collaborators (1,11). Interestingly, the authors conceive of the community as being more than an aggregate of smaller social units (which have been the main targets of earlier psychiatric research), and they diagnose the community as a whole. The central concept in this model is social disintegration, a situation that is considered to increase the risk of mental disorders.

A socially disintegrated community is falling apart. It is characterized by absence of local leadership, reduced social interaction, distrust between people, fragmentation of social networks and anti-social behaviour (1). The factors behind this process may be excessive migration, cultural confusion, secularization and poverty, usually in a destructively interactive process. In the study of Sterling County in Nova Scotia (1), a mainly rural or semirural area, the prevalence of mental disorders was found to be considerably higher in the disintegrated areas than in the well integrated areas. The authors explained these differences with a need–frustration model, assuming that the basic needs for love, recognition, self-realization and belonging to a moral order could not be fulfilled in a disintegrated community.

Dalgard (5,12) examined the relationship between the qualities of different neighbourhoods and mental health in Oslo. To the extent that comparisons can be made between rural Canada and Oslo, the hypothesis linking mental disorders to social disintegration was supported.

Dalgard interviewed about 1000 adults, randomly selected from five types of neighbourhood, and used a shortened version of Leighton's questionnaire to measure their mental health. The highest prevalence of psychiatric morbidity was found in a new satellite town on the outskirts of Oslo, and the lowest prevalence was found in the well established, stable neighbourhoods that had mainly one-family homes, also located on the periphery of the city. The prevalence in the central areas of the city was intermediate to the other two. This pattern did not change when variables such as age, sex, education, marital status, income and migratory status were controlled for, using multivariate statistical methods.

The new satellite town differed in various ways from the other neighbourhoods, especially from the area with the lowest prevalence of mental disorders. This applied to characteristics at both macro and micro levels. Typical of the new satellite town were a high resident turnover, lack of collective resources such as private and public services and recreational opportunities, and extensive economic problems. Also, social networks were poor and people had relatively low self-esteem.

Even if the combination of poor social network and poor mental health could be explained partly by selective migration, there was a causal connection between the characteristics of the neighbourhood as a whole and fragmented social networks, which led to an increased risk of mental disorders. Instead of increasing the risk of mental disorders by itself, poor social networks seemed to influence mental health chiefly by interacting with other environmental factors. In the neighbourhood with the highest prevalence, people also had the least supportive relationships with other people, and poor social networks seemed to increase the risk of mental disorder more than in the well integrated neighbourhoods. Hence, the socially underprivileged and disintegrated neighbourhood of the new satellite town seemed to have a doubly negative effect on mental health. The social characteristics of the area made it difficult to maintain and establish supportive social networks, and the neighbourhood provided more than its share of social stressors and frustrations, making social support from other people especially important in preventing mental health problems.

The environment and individual coping
Pursuing health promotion at the level of the individual requires a thorough understanding of the dynamics that operate and influence patterns of health and disorder in individuals. Environmental stress is a key concept. The stressors may be part of the external environment and may express themselves as new physical, social, economic or

426

cultural conditions that represent demands for change and adaptation. Disturbances in a society may fragment the social network structure of the local communities, and thereby increase the vulnerability of the individual to stressful life changes. These are demands for adaptation that threaten the coping capacity of individuals and are not the usual stresses and strains of daily life.

Psychosocial stresses relevant to mental health can be divided into three types: the frustration of needs caused by understimulation and lack of opportunities for self-realization, self-determination and belonging; excess external demands on the internal capacity for change, through stressful life events; and stress as an internal event, such as a psychodynamic conflict representing irreconcilable demands on the person's psyche. This last type is usually related to some kind of idiosyncratic vulnerablility of the personality. The first type has been dealt with previously in this chapter. The second type is reflected in life events research, an area of substantial recent interest. Life events are stressful life changes such as separation and divorce, the death of a spouse and conflict at work. An area associated with these recent life events is problems of a more chronic nature, such as economic problems, housing difficulties, long-term illness in the immediate family and long-term interpersonal conflicts. Life events are short-term distinct stress factors; chronic problems are longer term and are rarely distinct, as they usually overlap and are connected with several areas in a person's life.

Early research by Holmes & Rahe *(13)* considered life events in terms of an objective stress load that did not take into account the subjective experience and the contribution of the individual to the pattern of life events reported. More recent research *(14–16)*, however, emphasizes the role of perception and individual vulnerability. The same stressors will obvioulsy mean different things to different people, and to the same person at different times. It is also debatable whether stressful life events are important sources of learning and personal growth *(17)* which, even through periods of personal crisis can provide a powerful impetus for change, and strengthen coping reservoirs.

Coping is a key concept in health promotion. Coping is how people handle the stressful events they experience or situations they are brought into or have created. Coping depends on adaptability, the inherent ability to adapt to change, and on mastery, the individual ability to create and recreate personal reality.

There are three kinds of coping: attempting to change the situation that caused the stress, controlling the emotional response to the event, and attempting to control the meaning of the event (reframing).

The first is active, problem-solving coping and may be expressed in a variety of ways, ranging from seeking more information about the problem and solving it (such as by support from one's social network), to actively eliminating or neutralizing the stressor. Controlling the emotional response reflects a symptom-oriented approach, which may be adequate, depending on the person and the situation. Psychological defence mechanisms are important here. Controlling the meaning of an event implies altering one's subjective experience of the event and reflects the role of perception and the extent to which this is open to manipulation (18).

Preliminary results from a ten-year follow-up of the study in Oslo (5) seem to indicate that coping resources are strongly related to a person's level of self-esteem and to previous experience with the problem or similar problems. Accepting the need to view change and challenges in a positive way mentally seems equally important (19). This ability, or mind-set, again seems to be related to self-esteem and one's internal belief system. Do I believe in my ability to deal with this crisis? Do I view problems as defeats, or as challenges to be overcome?

Mental Health Promotion: Methods and Evaluation

Psychosocial processes that represent a threat to mental health may take place on different social levels. Accordingly, intervention to reverse the processes may be directed towards social units of different size and order. The community at large, the local community, the neighbourbood, the group or the individual may be the target for intervention. Whereas health promotion is related mainly to programmes involving populations as a whole in the context of their everyday lives (20), prevention involves programmes for people at risk of specific diseases. Nevertheless, they are not always easy to distinguish. To the extent that activities are directed at the causes of health, rather than the causes of disease (another characteristic of health promotion) among high-risk groups in the population, this work also includes elements of health promotion. Some projects attempting to promote mental health that emphasize the importance of social integration and social support for mental health will be

428

briefly described in the following section. In most of the projects, serious efforts have been made to evaluate systematically the impact of intervention on mental health outcome. Unfortunately, such evaluation is rare in this field.

The community level
In Nova Scotia, Leighton and collaborators have not only provided deeper insight into the relationship between social processes and mental health; they have also contributed to a community development project with the objectives of improving the general quality of life of the population and enhancing mental health status over a period of time.

The project took place in one of the most disintegrated settlements, which had been the focus of an intensive case study (11,21). This settlement had a high prevalance of mental disorders and people suffered from numerous social deprivations and limitations, including underemployment, shortage of capital and credit, illiteracy, hostile interpersonal relations, broken homes, weak social organizations and a reputation for being undependable.

The settlement had attracted the attention of county authorities and the psychiatric research team, and the team was aksed to recommend remedial steps. Three recommendations were made; it was emphasized that all three steps were necessary:

— increase social integration through improved patterns of social support and mutual aid;
— increase cognitive assests through greater educational opportunities; and
— increase economic resources.

Through the concerted effort of different authorities, the three steps were implemented and things began to change in the settlement. A few years later the standard of living had improved, unemployment had dropped, the level of education among children had increased and people's relationships were better. When a new epidemiological survey was carried out ten years later, the previously high prevalence of mental disorder in this settlement had been reduced to the same level as that for the county as a whole. Even if this outstanding example of experimental epidemiology supports the hypothesis about social integration and mental health, it does not prove it. The authors (11) emphasized that this was only one case study, and the apparent

429

support this gave the hypothesis could have been a result of chance. Nevertheless, the study has contributed to new thinking in mental health promotion, particularly by illustrating how psychiatric epidemiology, combined with more intensive population studies can be useful in evaluating intervention.

The neighbourhood level

In mental health research, and in health promotion, it is necessary to define communities by their physical boundaries and architectural infrastructures. Two obvious urban definitions, therefore, are the city and the neighbourhood. Interest has grown in the expanded concept of health within the urban context — a trend expressed in the WHO Healthy Cities project, a multidisciplinary and intersectoral approach to health planning in cities (22–24).

At the neighbourhood level, as at the community level, a central principle in mental health promotion is to involve people in a common effort to improve their environment. If the mental health worker participates, it is as a catalyst, withdrawing from the process when people can run the projects themselves. One of the new satellite towns in Oslo, very similar to the one described earlier, had a very high rate of mental disorders, and a project was undertaken to improve the physical surroundings. The main idea was to transform the uncultivated fields of grass around the high-rise buildings into a park, with trees, flowers and places for adults to garden or just sit and relax, and areas where younger people could play or arrange sports activities. To get people involved, a pamphlet was produced with information about the project and an invitation to submit concrete ideas, using pictures and maps, about what people thought could be done. Pamphlets were sent to all the households in the neighbourhood, and many people returned them with concrete proposals. Not as many were willing to take part in the practical work, but there were enough to carry out the project. The result was improved surroundings, which provided better opportunites for relaxation and recreation and thus for more social interaction. It is not known whether the mental health status of the people has improved, but the wellbeing of the neighbourhood has probably been somewhat improved.

The group level

Based on the assumption that social disintegration and lack of supportive social networks have a negative impact on mental health, several projects have been carried out in Oslo to improve mental

430

health by stimulating social networks. In one of these projects, the target group was a psychiatric high-risk group. The project was closely related to the psychiatric survey in Oslo referred to previously *(5,12)*, as this survey identified a high-risk group suitable for intervention.

The survey had already shown that people in this new satellite town, and especially those with a poor social network, were at increased risk of mental disorder. A subsequent study of a subsample of this survey indicated that middle-aged women, both in well established and in new satellite towns, were overrepresented among the people with poor mental health who did not get professional help *(25)*.

The combined results of these two studies made the authors choose middle-aged women (45–55 years old) with a poor social network, low quality of life, high score on stress symptoms and living in a satellite town, as the target for their intervention programme *(26)*. This high-risk group was not likely to attract attention from the psychiatric services, which became an extra reason for offering them the programme.

A new epidemiological survey determined which women took part in the programme, including a representative sample of all women aged 45–55 living in a new satellite town. From a sample of 318, a subgroup of 100 was selected, comprising women with a poor social network, low quality of life and high level of stress symptoms. This group was then randomly divided into an experimental group (N = 26) and a control group (N = 29). The size of the groups was somewhat reduced by refusal to participate or by migration. Evaluation took place after six months, one year and three years.

The goal of the programme was to strengthen the social network of these women and thereby improve their quality of life and mental health. The women were invited to take part in weekly group activities for one year guided by two research psychologists. There were three types of group, all including 5–7 women from the sample: a social activity group, a physical training group and a porcelain painting group. Professional instructors were also assigned to the latter two groups.

The group activity was intended to expose the women to other women in similar life situations in a friendly and warm atmosphere, providing them with opportunities for making new friends. It was hoped that sharing the same kind of life situation would enable the

431

women to develop a group identity and mutual social support. It soon became obvious, however, that substantial effort by the researchers was necessary to help these women to make friends and to overcome their passivity. This was not surprising, as relatively isolated women in a city such as Oslo would be expected to have problems making new friends and acquaintances, and it was not just that they lacked opportunities to meet people.

The programme succeeded in significantly improving the social network and quality of life of the women in the experimental group during the study, compared with the control group. There was little difference between the psychiatric symptoms of the two groups at the end of the study, but after three years the experimental group had a lower mean symptom score than the control group. The women who were most active in the group meetings benefited most from the programme.

The individual level
It seems natural to consider health promotion in terms of intervention that can help people to cope better. For people subjected to increasing environmental stress, this may mean improving their consciousness of the importance of developing coping strategies. These may include helping people to view change and challenges in a more positive light, helping them to develop stronger and more flexible social networks designed to act as buffers against stress in a preventive way, and expanding their coping resources, both instrumentally and emotionally.

Finally, research indicates that much can be done within the family to improve the conditions that affect young children. Many of these conditions operate structurally and are not always readily subject to intervention. Nevertheless, mental health promotion must try to meet the basic requirements for normal psychosocial development, including a warm and accepting environment with stable parents (or parent substitutes), who are sensitive to children's emotional needs, and who provide appropriate conversation and opportunities for play, consistent discipline, supervision, and support (27). In addition, it must be possible to increase autonomy and independence, to express emotion and learn adaptively from adults who are good role models (19). Adequate interaction with other children and adults outside the home (including relatives, friends and neighbours) and suitable learning opportunities are also important.

The continuity of relationships with parents is especially important in the first few years of life. Brown & Harris (14) have demonstrated how early losses through separation or death create vulnerability to later depression. In a world with increasingly rapid social change, there are an increasing number of family breakups. Adult reactions to family breakups are well documented in mortality and morbidity statistics. The reactions of children have been insufficiently explored (27).

The effects of environmental conditions on the psychological development of children deserve the utmost interest from both researchers and policy-makers. The promotion of mental health should then be viewed in the context of a social system and in a generational context. Coping patterns are established in early childhood.

The Environment, the Individual and Mental Health Promotion

Interaction between individuals and the environment

The authors have given examples of mental health promotion at the community, neighbourbood, group and individual levels. The common denominator is that efforts are made to stimulate interaction between individuals and a social environment that develops supportive structures and enhances the fulfilment of basic psychosocial needs. In community development, people have been encouraged to take part in various organizations and activities to improve their social environment according to their own perception of their needs. In the neighbourhood examples, people were invited to pool their efforts to improve specific aspects of their environment, by joining ad hoc action committees. The groups for middle-aged women in the satellite town were specifically designed to stimulate social networks by gathering relatively lonely women into activities of common interest. Even when working with individuals, mental health promotion should strengthen coping abilities and improve social integration, in contrast to psychiatric treatment, which is mainly concerned with symptoms and pathology.

The dialectic interaction between individuals and the environment, which is the basis for the examples of mental health promotion presented, is best described by circular feedback processes rather than

433

by linear models of causation. The individual in this context is typically conceived of both as the subject and as the object, implying that intervention presupposes active participation and is not limited to mere manipulation of the environment. Social participation itself is considered to have health-promoting effects.

Fulfilment of needs

The basic psychosocial needs to be met in a healthy society were the centre of interest for Leighton's ideas about community development and mental health promotion. The main needs, which also correspond with Maslow's thinking, seem to be: the need for love and friendship, the need for recognition and respect, and the need for challenge and stimulation.

The frustration of these needs that occurs in the socially disinte-grated community increases the risk of mental disorder, whereas fulfilment of the needs not only prevents mental disorder, but also positively enhances mental health. These basic psychosocial needs are given priority in all the examples of mental health promotion presented. Working together for a common purpose in various types of organization or activity group enhances friendship and a sense of belonging. When participating individuals are given the opportunity to contribute their interests and skills, the needs for recognition, respect and challenge are met.

Strengthening of coping

Strengthening individual coping may be approached in different ways in mental health promotion. In the examples given, the goal has been to strengthen coping abilities by increasing social support and by influencing the individual directly. In community development, it was essential to improve cognitive assets by providing educational opportunities in addition to improving the pattern of social support. In neighbourhood and group intervention programmes, improving social skills on the individual level was as important as group formation to the success of the programme.

People have greatly varying coping abilities and potential, which means that not everyone can benefit from the same type of programme. It is then necessary to adjust mental health promotion programmes to the special needs and coping abilities of certain weak groups, to ensure that they are not left out. Long-term psychiatric patients are an example of this, as they are quite often too weak in social skills to function in an ordinary group. Group leaders with professional training will then be necessary. If the positive aspects of mental health are kept in focus, and not the psychiatric symptoms, this will still be health promotion and not treatment.

The need for research

The basis for successful mental health promotion programmes is, of course, understanding the interaction between individuals and the environment in terms of mental health. This insight has mostly been provided by epidemiological studies and surveys of mental health in various populations. More research of this type is necessary: for instance, in terms of community diagnosis research, where risk factors and health-promoting factors are analysed in relation to mental disorder and mental wellbeing.

Even if more research of this type is necessary for mental health promotion, it is also important to stress that more is known than is put into practice. Researchers should analyse why the available knowledge does not lead to action, rather than increasing knowledge further. Another important subject is the systematic evaluation of programme development and its impact on mental health in various population groups.

Because of the close interaction between mental health and somatic health, both must be included in epidemiological research and programme evaluation. Consequently, the authors are now conducting a community diagnosis study in a section of Oslo and contrasting rural areas in northern Norway, to identify environmental and lifestyle risk factors for mental and somatic health. The next step will be to advise politicians about what can be done in terms of health promotion and, one hopes, to evaluate the impact of the actions taken.

Strategies for mental health promotion

Political and legal measures and direct community work by mental health workers in cooperation with other agencies may be used to promote mental health. One of the major tasks of the agents of mental health promotion is to make politicians aware of the relationship between environment and mental health, and of possible preventive measures. One example of such work is the recommendations of the survey described previously that analysed the relationship between mental health and the types of neighbourhbood in Oslo (5).

The poorly integrated new satellite town, which had an excess of mental health problems, stimulated the following guidelines for planning new neighbourhoods:

— develop the housing areas in stages;

435

- arrange for the necessary public and private services before people move in;
- vary the age composition;
- avoid concentrating people with special problems in certain blocks;
- build neighbourhoods of limited ("human") size;
- vary the types of housing, allowing for a multigenerational community;
- provide special houses and/or flats for collective activities and social interaction;
- establish recreation areas for different age groups;
- promote neighbourhood organizations responsible for various social activities in the area; and
- encourage future inhabitants to participate in planning new neighbourhoods.

These recommendations and similar recommendations from other professional groups seem to have had some impact on the planning of new neighbourhoods in Oslo.

The acceptable standards of the physical environment are often regulated by law to prevent somatic ill health. The increasing interest in mental health and the social environment has stimulated the development of regulations in this field also. An example of this is the Worker Protection and Working Environment Act in Norway, which sets standards not only for the physical environment but also for the psychosocial environment. In the future it is likely that such legal regulation of the environment, for example in planning new housing areas, will be increasingly important for mental health promotion.

The decentralization of political and economic power seems important to be able to plan and regulate the environment according to people's needs. If the distance is great between the people who suffer from poor environmental conditions and the people who have the power to make changes, it is less likely that change will occur, and alienation rather than social integration is the consequence. It is thus a positive sign that a relatively big city such as Oslo is now going to be divided into a number of smaller units with a certain amount of political and financial autonomy. This means that neighbourhoods such as the new satellite town will be given more authority to solve their own problems. The local mental health centre will also have a better opportunity to engage in health promotion. In this context the mental health centre should strive towards a strategic network position *(28)*, working through agencies and individuals that are the most important in influencing people's living conditions and lifestyles. Besides other professionals in health-related fields, this includes representatives from politics, economics, culture and religion.

References

1. **Leighton, D.C. et al.** *The character of danger. Psychiatric symptoms in selected communities.* New York, Basic Books, 1963.
2. **Srole, L. et al.** *Mental health in the metropolis. The midtown Manhattan study I.* New York, McGraw-Hill, 1962.
3. **Caplan, G.** Community psychiatry: the changing role of the psychiatrist. *In*: Goldston, S.E., ed. *Concepts of community psychiatry.* Washington, DC, US Government Printing Office, 1965 (Public Health Service Publication No. 1319).
4. **Dohrenwend, B.P. et al.** *Mental illness in the United States. Epidemiological estimates.* New York, Praeger, 1980.
5. **Dalgard, O.S.** *Bomiljø og psykisk helse* [Home environment and psychological health]. Oslo, Universitetsforlaget, 1980.
6. **Sørensen, T.** *Pendling, lokalmiljø og mental helse* [Commuting, the local environment and mental health]. Thesis, Institute of Psychiatry, Oslo University, 1979.
7. **Sørensen, T.** *Mental helse i Nordkyst* [Mental health on the north coast]. Bodø, Nordland Fylkeskommune, Fylkeshelsesjefen,1987.
8. **Andersen, T.** *Ill health in two contrasting societies.* Tromsø, Institute of Community Medicine, University of Tromsø, 1978.
9. **Fugelli, P.** *Helsetilstand og helsetjeneste på Værøy og Røst.* [Health status and health services on Værøy and Røst]. Oslo, Universitetsforlaget, 1978.
10. **Murphy, J.M. et al.** Diagnosis and outcome: depression and anxiety in a general population. *Psychological medicine,* **16**: 117–126 (1986).
11. **Leighton, A.H. & Murphy, J.M.** Primary prevention of psychiatric disorders. *Acta psychiatrica scandinavica,* **76**: (Suppl. 337): 7–13 (1987).

12. **Dalgard, O.S.** Living conditions, social network and mental health. *In*: Isacsson, S.O. & Janzon, L., ed. *Social support: health and disease.* Stockholm, Almqvist & Wiksell, 1986.

13. **Holmes, T.H. & Rahe, R.H.** The social readjustment scale. *Journal of psychosomatic research.* **11**: 213–218 (1967).

14. **Brown, G.W. & Harris, T.** *Social origins of depression: a study of psychiatric disorder in women.* London, Tavistock Publications, 1978.

15. **Paykel, E.S. et al.** Scaling of life events. *Archives of general psychiatry,* **25**: 340–347 (1971).

16. **Paykel, E.S.** Methodological aspects of life events research. *Journal of psychosomatic research,* **27**: 341–352 (1983).

17. **Lazarus, R.S. & Launier, R.** Stress-related transactions between person and environment. *In:* Pervin, L.A. & Lewis, M., ed. *Perspectives in interactional psychology.* New York, Plenum Press, 1978.

18. **Pearlin, L.I. & Schooler, C.** The structure of coping. *Journal of health and social behaviour,* **19**: 2–21 (1982).

19. **Bjørk, S.** Sosialt nettverk, stress og mestring [Social network, stress and mastery]. *In:* Dalgard, O.S. & Sørensen, T., ed. *Sosialt nettverk og psykisk helse* [Social network and psychological health]. Oslo, Tano Forlag, 1988.

20. **Kickbusch, I.** Health promotion: a global perspective. *Canadian journal of public health,* **77**: 321–326 (1986).

21. **Leighton, A.H.** Poverty and social change. *Scientific american,* **212**: 21–24 (1965).

22. **Hancock, T. & Duhl, L.** *Promoting health in the urban context.* Copenhagen, FADL, 1988 (WHO Healthy Cities Papers No. 1).

23. **WHO Healthy Cities Project Office.** *Five-year planning framework.* Copenhagen, FADL, 1988 (WHO Healthy Cities Papers No. 2).

24. **WHO Healthy Cities Project Office.** *A guide to assessing healthy cities.* Copenhagen, FADL, 1988 (WHO Healthy Cities Papers No. 3).

25. **Anstorp, T. et al.** *Hvorfor søker de ikke hjelp* [Why don't they seek help]? Thesis, Oslo Institute of Psychology, Oslo University, 1979.

26. **Dalgard, O.S.** Epidemiology as basis for preventive intervention. *Acta psychiatrica Belgica,* **86**: 470–475 (1986).

27. **Brogren, P.-O**. *Promotion of mental health*. Gothenburg, Nordic School of Public Health, 1985 (Rapport NHV 1985:3).
28. **Sørensen, T. et al**. Desentralisert psykiatri i nettverksperspektiv [Decentralized psychiatry in a network perspective]. *In:* Dalgard, O.S. & Sørensen, T., ed. *Sosialt nettverk og psykisk helse*. [Social network and psychological health]. Oslo, Tano Forlag, 1988.

19

The role of community groups and voluntary organizations in health promotion

*Alf Trojan, Helmut Hildebrandt,
Christiane Deneke & Michael Faltis*[a]

Some places and institutions in the community are particularly interesting as settings for health promotion. Some have untapped resources, such as medical and allied health professionals who should become more involved in health promotion in the future: examples are health services and hospitals. Some settings have health-damaging effects that can best be fought on the spot: this applies partly to schools and particularly to workplaces. These institutions are well established and many different interventions have been developed to improve people's health in these settings.

Community groups and voluntary organizations are far less known as a setting for health promotion because:

— they belong to the lay system and are not regarded as a resource for activities and intervention relevant to health;

— they seem to have no clear health-damaging effects (although working for or participating in community groups may be very demanding or even stressful); and

[a] The project *Gemeindebezogene Netzwerkförderung* is funded by the Federal Ministry for Research and Technology, Germany. The authors would like to thank Ina Schweigert, Volker Enkerts, Ruth Halves, Martina Mahnke and other colleagues for their valuable help.

— many of these groups, organizations and associations are neither known to the public nor to researchers and politicians because the groups are overshadowed by the large institutions of society.

A profoundly important explanation of why the significance of community groups and voluntary organizations for health remained undiscovered for a long time is the dominance of the medical disease model, with its overemphasis on natural sciences, on technological methods in diagnosis and therapy, and on the professional work of medical doctors and allied health professionals.

We can only adequately appreciate the relevance to health of community groups if a social model of health becomes more widely known and accepted. Research findings in medical sociology and social epidemiology, as well as some important innovative strategies of WHO, have led to a new positive and socioecological concept of health. Health promotion takes up these new empirical and theoretical developments in social epidemiology and other health sciences, and provides an umbrella concept for activities, action programmes and policies in support of the goal of health for all *(1–3)*.

It is not difficult to relate the principles of health promotion to community groups and similar small networks:

— most community groups actually support or wish to support emotional and social wellbeing, personal growth, and their members' or clients' feeling of self-esteem;
— community groups try to shape or change the physical, social and political living conditions that commonly cause social problems and diseases;
— community groups, which often belong to grassroots movements, are indicators of the many forms of mutual help, of social and political participation, and of involvement of the local population in its own affairs; and
— community groups are a means of enabling and empowering people to increase control over, and to improve, their health.

Assuming that community groups can significantly promote health may sound completely plausible to the sympathetic observer or supporter of new and old local groups, organizations, associations and initiatives. For sceptical or even critical health professionals or politicians, however, plausibility alone is not enough. They would

442

presumably like to know what is meant by community or voluntary organizations and similar groups, what evidence there is on the quantitative and qualitative aspects of the significance of these groups for health, and what action is required in this recently discovered and previously relatively neglected field of health promotion.

Research on the Voluntary Non-profit Sector

A statement made in 1911 stressed the importance of conducting research on associations in what is now termed the voluntary non-profit sector *(4)*:

> It is a fundamental task of sociology to study those structures that are conventionally dubbed 'social', i.e. all that lies in the gap between the politically organized or recognized powers — state, municipality and established church on the one side — and the natural community of the family on the other. Thus, essentially: a sociology of associations in the widest sense of the word ... *(4)*.

The statement did not, however, lead to substantial interest in empirical studies. Moreover, all attempts to classify organizations, groups, initiatives and associations remained unsatisfactory *(5–7)*. It is thus nearly impossible to give a systematic and comprehensive overview of the available knowledge in this area. Nevertheless, we will try to present the most relevant studies to review the topics of research and the foci that have been chosen.

Voluntary work and voluntary action

Voluntary work is defined mostly as "unpaid work for any organization or for people other than relatives and friends" *(8)*. Many voluntary (or nongovernmental) organizations (or societies, groups, associations), however, have paid staff, mostly for administrative and secretarial work. Newton *(9)* reported that about one quarter of the organizations surveyed had paid staff.

The boundaries between the statutory services and the voluntary agencies that get about 90% of their income from tax money are even more difficult to draw *(10)*. Consequently, most of the research focuses on the relationship of voluntary organizations to official (formal) institutions and government bodies. This also applies to recently emerging new social initiatives *(11)*, which are mostly a mixture of voluntary unpaid and professional paid work — the new welfare mix.

Voluntary action groups do not concentrate on providing services, but on pressure group and lobbying activities *(12)*.

Quantitative aspects

Hatch *(8)* reported that 10% of the population of the United States and 15% of the population of the United Kingdom had taken part in nonreligious voluntary activity in the previous year, suggesting considerable undeveloped potential. The prevalence of voluntary organizations in different cities has been reported as:

— 20 per 1000 inhabitants in a small town in the United States *(13)*;

— 10 per 1000 in Geneva, Switzerland *(14)*;

— 5 per 1000 in Paris, France *(14)*;

— 1–2 per 1000 in three small towns in the United Kingdom *(15)*;

— 2 politically active voluntary organizations per 1000 voters in Birmingham, United Kingdom *(9)*; and

— 25 per 1000 in Leon, Mexico and Neuquen, Argentina *(16,17)*.

The relatively small difference in different places and at different times is striking, because the studies varied considerably in the definitions and methods used to identify voluntary associations *(18,19)*. All authors were convinced that their rates were too low, mainly because they could not (and therefore did not try to) find the more informally organized groups.

Meister *(14)* concludes from his comparison of Geneva and Paris that: "Swiss decentralization and great liberalism may help explain why citizens of Geneva constitute more social, educative and community groups.". For further studies from France see Ferrand-Bechmann,[a] Roudet *(20)* and Trojan *(21)*; for an international comparison, Bauer & Thränhardt *(22)*.

Functions

Newton *(9)* wrote:

> From Marx and de Tocqueville to Truman and Dahl, political scientists have argued that [organized groups and associations of the nineteenth and twentieth centuries] play a crucial role in the politics of

---

[a] **Ferrand-Bechmann, D**. *Moderniser le bénevolat*, 1986.

industrial societies, and from Weber and Dürkheim to Wright Mills and Kornhauser, sociologists have pointed to their crucial role in social and political systems. Writers as diverse as Simmel, Lipset, Tönnies, Laski, Parsons, Mills, Arendt, Cole, Dahrendorf and Riesman agree that groups are in fact, or could be in theory, absolutely vital in maintaining social and political stability, bringing about peaceful political change, protecting democracy, reducing the intensity and violence of political conflict, acting as channels of communication, giving citizens a sense of belonging and control, helping to integrate society, and bringing about a whole host of other social and political processes which are essential to the political and social health of any large scale society.

Koldewyn *(17)* gave an account similarly evocative of the concept of healthy public policy by mentioning the following five functions of voluntary associations in two South American cities:

(1) organization of community services ...; (2) solving of middle class housing and consumer problems ...; (3) improvement of agricultural production and industrial planning; (4) development of expressive and recreational opportunities; (5) creation of neighbourhood, parent and cultural activity groups that strive for community improvement.

Voluntary organizations thus have secondary or latent functions for health *(14)*. It is interesting, however, that only 1% of the 4264 voluntary organizations in Birmingham were classified as being relevant to health *(9)*.

A more comprehensive review of the functions of voluntary associations was published by Amis & Stern *(5)*, and in the report of the Wolfenden Committee *(15)*. This report has been criticized because it almost exclusively concentrated on the more traditional voluntary organizations and the committee said very little about self-help and community initiatives *(23,24)*. We will therefore address studies of more recent types of voluntary action.

Community work and community involvement

In Great Britain the notion of community groups (or associations) is closely connected with the expansion of new housing areas and municipal housing after the First World War. The word neighbourhood is sometimes used instead of community, particularly in the United States. Community work is the most commonly used umbrella term for a wide range of activities such as community (or urban) development, community organization, community service or action.

All these usually refer to the common aim of meeting community needs *(25)*.

Leat *(26)* compiled research on community involvement and found it impossible to distinguish studies of community development from those of community action. Her research directory included:

— services providing or involving volunteers, and voluntary groups and organizations within the spheres of social service, health, probation and aftercare, education, law, local government and the environment;
— the involvement of family, friends and neighbours in providing services;
— self-help and neighbourhood groups; and
— community action and pressure group activity of all kinds.

Most studies in this area are case studies or other small-scale research. One interesting qualitative study *(25)* summarizes the objectives of a community association as aiming:

— to promote the spirit of community
— to provide opportunities for leisure-time occupation
— to see that gaps in community services are filled
— to manage the community centre
— to provide a basis and training for democracy
— to bring together other organizations in the neighbourhood
— to bring individuals together
— to provide a corporate voice for the neighbourhood.

In the United States, White *(27)* studied advisory neighbourhood commissions, and identified their five major functions as: advising on policy, dealing with service complaints, co-production, providing services and regulating the quality of life. She regards such neighbourhood participation as a new form of "urban politics in a time of social change".

A similar framework taken from political science, and a corresponding focus, are particularly prominent in Newton's study on voluntary organizations in Birmingham *(9)*, in Baer's research on political interest groups *(28)* and a report on citizen initiatives in the Federal Republic of Germany by Helm *(29)*. Freudenberg *(30)* and Bachrach & Zautra *(31)* surveyed organized citizen action for environmental health in the United States.

446

Based on two studies conducted in Northern Ireland, Griffiths *(24)* highlights the contrasting features of community action organizations (which are based locally, supposedly operate democratically and rely on self-help or minimal aid strategy) and voluntary organizations (which are often entrepreneurial enterprises with a managerial structure and provide services on an altruistic or welfare basis to others). Griffiths believes, however, that this distinction is not so clear-cut as it may appear, and gives examples where one type of organization has the major characteristics of the other type.

Self-help and mutual aid

Mutual aid groups exist for many diseases and conditions. In a narrow sense the concept refers to small groups, and many studies have especially emphasized groups with diseases and physical problems *(32–35)*. Self-help groups are undoubtedly part of the voluntary sector, but not all voluntary and community organizations are necessarily self-help or mutual aid groups. Nevertheless, mutual aid and self-help have become so popular that the terms are sometimes used to cover almost the whole range of nongovernmental and non-profit organizations; Vilmar & Runge *(36)* have tried to portray the great variety and complexity of social self-help groups.

A very broad approach was also used in Romeder's study *(37)* on self-help groups in Canada. This study mainly included people with individual problems or diseases, while a study in Great Britain *(23)* on self-help in the inner city described 30 community initiatives, such as playgroups, tenants' associations and clubs for older people, which can promote prevention and health. The characteristic features of self-help were compared with the data on community groups, and Knight & Hayes *(23)* concluded that "community initiatives have some but not all of the characteristics of self-help".

There is also some quantitative evidence on the degree to which voluntary community organizations overlap with self-help and mutual aid. Meister *(19)* found that 15% of these organizations in Paris and 23% in Geneva were oriented towards mutual help. Koldewyn *(16,17)* classified about 20% of the voluntary organizations in his two studies as being community service and mutual aid organizations (disregarding his category "neighbourhood commissions and school support groups"). About the same percentage of groups considered themselves self-help organizations in our study (see below).

Health action and community health initiatives

The self-help literature usually refers to self-help groups as being a resource for coping better with disease, but there is almost no literature that discusses the potential of the voluntary sector for prevention and health promotion, except for some new approaches in the Federal Republic of Germany and Great Britain.

One empirical study was carried out in the Mettmann district *(38)*. The study — which was more qualitative than quantitative — focused on organizations in the areas of health, sports and youth, on programmes of the health insurance schemes and on adult education. The organizations studied, though not part of the statutory services, are mostly highly organized and form the core membership of regional health education associations. The goal was to improve cooperation and coordination between the different organizations involved in health education and disease prevention, but this proved to be nearly impossible.

The London Community Health Resource Unit and the Community Health Initiatives Resource Unit have stimulated research with the following results:

— report of a conference *(39)*;
— various editions of (London) *Health action network*, directories of new community health initiatives, pressure groups, or campaigns; and
— a collection of interesting case studies *(40)*.

The most striking theme to emerge in the last of these *(40)* was how the boundaries of health and sickness are constantly being assessed and redrawn. This may equally apply to health promotion as a practical and political concept.

Survey of Community Organizations in Hamburg

Our current project *Gemeindebezogene Netzwerkförderung* (community-based promotion of health-related social networks) is based on a survey of community organizations in Hamburg. It has taken questions and suggestions from the above-mentioned research and pursued them further. It is the only known study that has systematically and comprehensively examined the significance of community organizations for health.

448

We prefer to use the term community organization instead of voluntary or self-help organization (or group or association) because it has neither the philanthropic connotation provided by the word voluntary nor the (false) suggestion of complete autonomy associated with self-help. Further, the word community emphasizes that the local level is the most important arena for any type of health promotion activity that is done neither to nor for people but with them.

Community organizations as social networks

Social networks are seen as an important resource for prevention (41). In social epidemiological research they are taken as the informal structure for coping with health hazards and stress. Badura (42) distinguishes between personal, social and institutional resources. The focus of interest is social resources. Other names for this are secondary networks, community networks, and small non-professional or informal networks. All these concepts remain poorly defined and overlap considerably. Hamburg & Killilea (43) use the concept of informal social support systems. This includes families and relatives, neighbours, self-help groups and community organizations. We focus on community organizations, or networks within the community.

Most studies of informal social support systems focus on ego-centred social networks: the individual is the centre of the network. In our research, however, we have concentrated on organized networks in the community. These community organizations are not centred around a particular person but instead around a task or common interest; we therefore call them task-oriented or interest-oriented social networks. Individuals and their networks were not the subject of the survey; they are, however, important targets of the activities of community organizations. Another difference in focus is that we have looked at the outward-oriented goals and effects of social networks, while most research, and especially that conducted by community psychologists, looks at the effects on the central person, who is usually a person in need.

Social networks have functions that are relevant to health (44–48). These health-relevant functions can be summarized in the concepts social support, social action, network promotion and empowerment. The section in this chapter on results provides information on the operationalization of these concepts and the degree to which these functions are fulfilled by community organizations. Table 1 gives an overview of health promotion structures in the informal and formal sectors.

Scope and procedure of the Hamburg survey

The survey was to include all organizations in the informal sector. A great variety of directories, pamphlets and newspapers provided the addresses of about 1700 organizations, associations and citizens' initiatives. The large number of addresses was a remarkable result in itself, and it shows the quantitative importance of this research field.

Between May 1986 and August 1986 we sent questionnaires to these 1700 community organizations. The first part of the questionnaire determined whether respondents fulfilled the selection criteria: nongovernmental, non-profit, no restrictions on access, not primarily cure-oriented or therapy-oriented, and not temporary but permanent activities.

A number of areas, such as sports clubs, and parish and senior citizens' clubs, were excluded although they fulfilled the criteria, as

Table 1. Examples of health-related structures in the
formal and informal sectors

Informal sector	Formal sector
Personal networks: family, household, neighbours, colleagues, friends	**Other political sectors and areas of intervention:** education; social, youth, cultural, sports departments; traffic policy; town planning; workplace
Community networks (grassroots, non-profit): local consumer organizations, citizen's advice centres, local resource centres, infant schools, youth groups or clubs, women's centres, self-help groups, community action groups, citizens' initiatives, multicultural groups, charitable organizations, health service initiatives, self-help organizations, community care centres	**Public health service:** decentralized, municipal departments of health and the environment **Associations for health education (Germany) including as members:** health insurance schemes, professional bodies and chambers, local authorities, pharmaceutical industry, subgroups of political parties, trade unions

they would have required special research instruments; 1163 community organizations were included in the survey.

Response rate and representativeness

A total of 473 (41%) of the questionnaires were returned. Respondents and nonrespondents were compared by: postal code (the part of Hamburg in which they were located) and main activity area (this information was recognizable from organization names in most cases). There were no significant differences between respondents and nonrespondents in these two parameters, except that a higher proportion of organizations in the illness and psychosocial problems area responded than did those in other activity areas.

Relevance to health

Most of the organizations surveyed were involved in activities that are directly or indirectly related to health. We used two criteria to differentiate groups that were more involved in health from those that were less involved: whether health was a goal of their activities; and whether the group was motivated to perform health-related activities in the future.

A total of 309 organizations (65% of the respondents) declared that health was either a primary or secondary goal of their activities (and were referred to as health-related organizations). About two thirds of these health-related organizations would be interested in expanding their health promotion activities, if time and money were available (we refer to them as highly motivated health-related organizations). Some 23% of the 309 health-related community organizations did not indicate that they were prepared to expand their health-related activities. These organizations, however, may also be relevant for health promotion. First, the attitudes and goals of organizations change over time and, second, the goal of health would probably be more intensely pursued if sufficient incentives and assistance were offered.

Of the 473 respondents, 35% declared that health was not a goal of their work. These organizations were eliminated from the following analysis. The result of a corresponding question showed, however, that a large majority of these organizations consider their work relevant for the health of their users and/or of society. Half of the respondents that had neither health goals nor self-reported health effects provide some sort of social support. According to social

451

epidemiological findings, this is important for neutralizing and buffering stress, and therefore for preserving health.

Results

Characteristics of the health-related community organizations (N = 309)

Activity areas. The areas of activity were numerous (Table 2). Virtually no organizations engaged in only one activity. Social activities were recorded most frequently.

Self-concepts. It is not appropriate to subsume all the organizations under self-help, as only about one fifth considered themselves self-help groups or associations for mutual aid. Help for others explicitly prevailed over self-help; only 26% felt that they belonged to the self-help movement. A total of 72% sympathized with one or more social movements. Between 11% and 17% of the respondents felt close to one of the following movements: citizens' initiatives, health, environment, peace, alternative, women, youth and human rights.

Only 14% of the organizations considered themselves to be part of the official care system, 26% complementary and 21% alternative, while 39% said that they had nothing to do with the care system.

Target groups. Each organization reported an average of four to five target groups (Table 3). Not all of these target groups can be reached equally well; there has been less success in reaching immigrants, addicts, unemployed people, disabled people, chronically ill people and others in need of care. Less than one third of the organizations that had tried to reach out to these groups considered that they had been successful or very successful. More than half the organizations had been successful or very successful in reaching out to women, parents, couples, families, children, youth and employed people.

The large proportion of organizations targeting the general public can be explained in two ways. First, it is necessary to target the public on a large scale to reach eventual users or supporters of the organizations; second, it indicates that organizations do not select specific target groups or problems but are oriented towards the general public in a community.

Work methods. The methods of work reflected the diversity of activity areas and orientations. An average of five to six different

452

Table 2. Activity areas covered by 309 health-related community organizations (more than one choice possible)

Activity area	Proportion of organization covering this area (%)
Social work	46
Psychosocial	42
Hobby or leisure	30
Nutrition or good health	26
Education	25
Environment	25
Training or adult education	23
Community work	22
Disease	20
Addiction	18
Sociocultural	18
Workplace	17
Peace	16
Human rights	15
Religion	12
Third world	11
Arts	11
Consumer rights, sciences, housing and others	23

Table 3. Target groups of 309 health-related community organizations

Target groups	Percentage of organizations aiming at these groups as:	
	main target group	one of many target groups
General public	38	60
Parents, couples or families	9	49
Youth	10	46
Elderly	6	39
Children	8	39
Immigrants	4	38
Disabled	6	38
Women	6	36
Unemployed	2	28
Ill or in need of care	4	28
Addicts	5	27
Employed	1	25
Poor	1	22

methods of work were reported; four of these were related to users or user groups. Personal services were the most common: individual consultation (83%), leisure activities (64%), practical help (60%), nursing or education (51%) and care (17%). About half of the organizations offered courses, social group work and study groups. Public relations was the most important non-user-oriented method (72%), while 36% reported protest action and 34% lobbying or committee work.

Health-related functions of community organizations

Health goals. Health was a central goal of one third of the health-related organizations. Almost all organizations reported that their activities affected the health of their users, and almost three quarters believed that they had an impact on the health of society in general. Other health-related goals were: educating for more health-conscious behaviour (40%), developing a holistic health concept (37%), and conveying a healthier perception of the body and sensuality (35%).

Main hypotheses of the survey. Our basic thesis is that task oriented social networks or community organizations have important functions for people's wellbeing, and are a hidden health promotion system (adopted from Levin & Idler's notion *(49)* of the hidden health care system). This general idea was divided into the following four research hypotheses.

1. Community organizations are a source of social support for the community and for the target groups of their activities.

2. Community organizations carry out social action to fight health problems and threats to health.

3. Community organizations promote the development of other (smaller) social networks.

4. Community organizations are a means of empowerment.

The following paragraphs will examine the degree to which the hypotheses were confirmed by the results.

Social support. The following actions were counted as forms of social support (including emotional, informational, practical and material support) *(50)*:

— relief by conversation;

— contributing to the self-recognition of people who have been "thrown off the track";

454

— offering sympathy, understanding and emotional support for people in need;

— helping with information or advice in cases of personal crisis, disease or other problems;

— informing people about social causes of diseases or health threats and how to cope with them;

— strengthening practical skills;

— assisting other people in difficult tasks (such as completing forms);

— helping people to obtain financial or material benefits (such a clothing, housing and furnishing); and

— helping people in trouble in other ways.

Almost all of the health-related organizations reported having at least one out of these nine possible social support goals. A total of 75% indicated that they were successful or very successful in reaching at least one goal (3–5 goals: 30%; 6–9 goals: 17%); partly attained and unattained social support goals were not considered.

Social action for better health. Health is a social category that depends on social support for the individual and on good living conditions: an environment without pollution, a workplace without toxic substances, a society that enables the development of self-esteem, and many other factors. Organizations reported social actions directed towards improving: working conditions (19%), the environment (32%) and the conditions of life in general (41%). Only those who mentioned these social actions to be half or most of their work were considered. This hypothesis was less strongly confirmed than the first hypothesis.

Network promotion. Community organizations want to support personal networks. Items of support for personal networks were: providing relief for or strengthening families and partnerships, enabling friendships, organizing mutual aid, and increasing social contacts and communication in the community. Some 34% reported three or more of these activities; 80% mentioned at least one activity.

But task-oriented networks were supported as well, and 63% of the organizations granted immediate and obvious support, even to groups not belonging to the same organization. Support was most frequently offered in the form of advice, followed by providing space free of charge. Some 78% of the organizations tried to start new networks or groups. New groups actually emerged less frequently (65%). Thus, the organizations substantially contribute to preserving and further developing this important sector of society.

Empowerment. People who see themselves and their lives dominated by the decisions of others and who have learnt that they can do virtually nothing to change their situation are not very likely to try to control and to improve their health. Referring to the research on the locus of control, Rappaport *(51)* proposed a strategy of empowerment for those in need (see also Berger & Neuhaus *(52))*. The intensification of empowerment, social activation and not being completely dependent on others higher in the hierarchy is decisive for good health. The neglect of this factor has been a major reason for the failure of many health education programmes; they have not strengthened people, but have kept them dependent and thus made them even more helpless. The indicators for empowerment that we used were: strengthening self-esteem, developing skills for self-help and standing up for one's rights, encouraging the afflicted to collaborate for their common interests, and mobilizing citizen participation in politics and in decision-making bodies.

These items were to show the level to which organizations strove to emancipate their target groups of users or clients. Some 44% of the organizations mentioned three or more of these activities, while 85% mentioned at least one activity.

Summary

Between 75% and 85% of all health-related community organizations provide social support, carry out health-related social actions, promote other small networks and try to empower people. These activities are central to health promotion as defined in a WHO discussion paper on the concepts and principles of health promotion *(3)*. Community organizations (task-oriented networks) are a hidden health promotion system. To a great extent, therefore, promoting health means strengthening community organizations.

The structural and organizational characteristics, cooperation, participation and demands for support of the community organizations are not described here.[a] A summary of the results (Fig. 1)

---

[a] **Deneke, C. et al**. *Community organizations in Hamburg and their significance for health,* 1987 (unpublished paper).

shows that community organizations are understaffed, underpaid and underfinanced; work under insecure conditions; use a large proportion of their time for cooperating and gathering information; and have a wide range of needs, such as support from local authorities, help with public relations, a voice in public bodies, and organizational and personal counselling and supervision.

These social networks have important empowering, supporting and health-promoting functions, but need empowerment and support from public bodies. Health promotion activity has to take into account the possibilities and limits of the supportive and innovative potential of community organizations to improve the health of the community and its population.

Recommendations for Policy

Our survey was influenced partly by the changing focus of social epidemiological research from stress to social support and social networks. Our framework also stems from the international discussions about health promotion and a new public health, largely generated and organized by WHO.

In November 1986, a local conference in Hamburg convened about 3000 people from community organizations and some formal institutions to discuss the results of our study with the responding community organizations and other interested people. The conference, entitled "Health is more" (53), confirmed the main results of the survey. Community organizations — regardless of their main activity area — are generally interested in action for health; many of them would like to intensify their health-related activities and their cooperation with formal institutions; most of them need support for their present tasks and to extend health promotion activities.

One result of the conference was that the local health authorities became more interested in this research and in the potential for strengthening health promotion activities in the community. They requested a report on the significance of community organizations for health, and some policy proposals. The following summarizes our recommendations to the health authorities in Hamburg (54). These recommendations are based on the five action areas of the Ottawa Charter for Health Promotion (2): build healthy public policy, create supportive environments, strengthen community action, develop personal skills, and reorient health services. They are not only useful but also required for putting health promotion into practice.

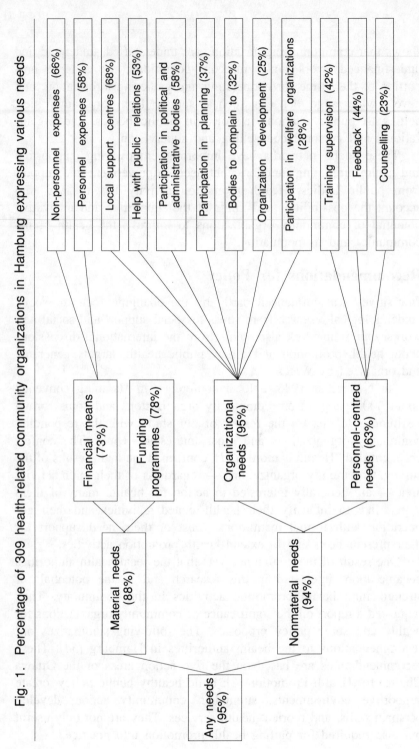

Fig. 1. Percentage of 309 health-related community organizations in Hamburg expressing various needs

Non-personnel expenses (66%)

Personnel expenses (58%)

Local support centres (68%)

Help with public relations (53%)

Participation in political and administrative bodies (58%)

Participation in planning (37%)

Bodies to complain to (32%)

Organization development (25%)

Participation in welfare organizations (28%)

Training supervision (42%)

Feedback (44%)

Counselling (23%)

Financial means (73%)

Funding programmes (78%)

Organizational needs (95%)

Personnel-centred needs (63%)

Material needs (88%)

Nonmaterial needs (94%)

Any needs (95%)

Community organizations and their actions are an expression of a community's needs and problems, but also of its strengths and potential. By providing support or by applying political pressure, community organizations contribute to all the areas of the Ottawa Charter.

Recommendations

Local action and resource centres for health promotion
Independent local action and resource centres for health promotion should be created as intermediary structures between the big social institutions and municipal governments on the one hand, and social networks and grassroots organizations on the other. They should:

— enable and initiate health-related activities of community organizations and other local initiatives;

— mediate between informal social networks at the grassroots level and the health authorities or other formal institutions; and

— advocate and support healthy public policy, for example, by organizing campaigns against toxic hazards or improving the quality of food.

This mediating body between the informal and the formal sector would have bridging and buffering functions. It also represents the infrastructure necessary to promote networks at the community level.

Some health promotion activities that might result from the work of such an action and resource centre for health promotion are:

— neighbourhood forums and discussions on health-threatening living conditions (such as toxic emissions or traffic hazards) and how to counteract these and protect oneself;

— initiatives to improve the quality of meals being served to children in kindergartens and schools or to adults in workplaces;

— health fairs that bring groups together and promote the exchange of opinions and ideas; and

— working groups on specific topics and health problems, such as toxic hazards, AIDS, radioactive contamination, urban planning, conditions in schools and the specific problems of ethnic minorities.

459

A local action and resource centre for health promotion could meet the majority of needs and requests expressed in our survey. Out of 247 community organizations that said that they directly or indirectly were involved in health:

— 78% felt that new health knowledge should be transferred from research and demonstration projects to independent institutions and initiatives;

— 74% would like a forum to foster the exchange of experience and information on questions of health and social support;

— 70% asked for suggestions for health-related activities and health-promoting activities;

— 69% would like more surveys on the health problems that upset people or put them under pressure;

— 65% would like official institutions to cooperate more closely with community organizations and initiatives; and

— 60% stated that more organizational support was necessary for health-related activities or projects.

Putting health on the agenda of community organizations

A special programme could help to spread the idea of health promotion to a wider public and to reach grassroots groups interested in carrying out specific health promotion activities. Based on the experience with such programmes in Canada, a fund should be created. The money could come from sources such as public bodies, health insurance schemes, interested sectors of industry, social foundations, churches and unemployment agencies.

The programme should enable non-profit community groups to conduct projects they cannot finance themselves, increasing public participation in health promotion and enabling these groups to develop health promotion programmes in accordance with the needs of their target population. About half of all community organizations would like to develop more health-related activities if they had more money and other resources.

This programme could be an incentive for innovation and new ideas. Special topics or areas such as unemployment, toxic hazards, community development and nutrition could be emphasized for a certain period *(55)*.

460

Opening health institutions for community participation
Although this is beyond the scope of our research, the formal sector
needs:
— to decentralize health authorities down to the district level (in
  Hamburg these institutions have just been renamed *Gesund-
  heits- und Umweltämter* — departments for health and the
  environment);
— to establish health bureaux as places where people with health
  problems can go, and as a starting point for health-related
  community work and long-term planning for a healthy community;
— to create posts for health counsellors or prevention advocates
  in these bureaux, to gather information on local health
  problems and needs, and to give this information to the
  appropriate authorities and political institutions;
— to increase community participation by reserving more seats
  in local health councils or committees for ordinary citizens,
  self-help groups, independent associations or other health-
  related grassroots initiatives, thus improving direct democracy at the local level.

Conclusion

The responsibility for health promotion has to be shared among many
agencies: community groups as well as formal institutions. The
public health service and the proposed local action and resource
centres for health promotion could play a key role as coordinators,
facilitators, catalysts and agents of change.

If health promotion is to become a joint endeavour not only for
people but with them, and if the idea of community participation is to
be put into practice as a basic principle of health promotion, community groups and similar social networks are a central setting and an
important resource in the process of enabling people to increase
control over, and to improve their health.

References

1. **Anderson, R**. *Health promotion: an overview*. Edinburgh,
    Scottish Health Education Group, 1984 (European Monographs
    in Health Education Research, No. 6).

2. Ottawa Charter for Health Promotion. *Health promotion*, **1**(4): iii–v (1986).

3. Health promotion: a discussion document on the concept and principles. *Health promotion*, **1**(1): 73–76 (1986).

4. **Weber, M**. Geschäftsbericht, Verhandlungen des 1. deutschen Soziologentages 1910 in Frankfurt (English translation). *Journal of voluntary action research*, **1**: 20–23 (1972).

5. **Amis, W.D. & Stern, S.E**. A critical examination of theory and functions of voluntary associations. *Journal of voluntary action research*, **3–4**: 91–99 (1974).

6. **Hougland, J.G., Jr**. Toward a participation-based typology of voluntary organizations. *Journal of voluntary action research*, **8**: 84–92 (1979).

7. **Smith, D.H**. Dimensions and categories of voluntary organizations/NGOs. *Journal of voluntary action research*. **2**: 116–120 (1973).

8. **Hatch, S**. *Voluntary work: a report of a survey*. London, Voluntary Organizations Research Unit, 1978 (Occasional Papers Series).

9. **Newton, K**. Voluntary organizations in a British city: the political and organizational characteristics of 4264 voluntary organizations in Birmingham. *Journal of voluntary action research*, **4**: 43–62 (1975).

10. **Kramer, R**. *Voluntary agencies in the welfare state*. Berkeley, CA, University of California Press, 1981.

11. **Jarre, D. & Pavelka, F., ed**. *New social initiatives in European countries*. Report on an expert meeting on Established Social Services versus New Social Initiatives — Conflict, Change, and Cooperation. Frankfurt, German Association for Public and Private Welfare, 1984.

12. **Humble, S., ed**. *Research into voluntary action 1977–1980 — a directory*. Berkhamsted, Volunteer Centre, 1981.

13. **Warner, W.L. & Lunt, P.S**. *The social life of a modern community*. New Haven, CT, Yale University Press, 1941.

14. **Meister, A**. A comparative note on the prevalence of voluntary associations in Geneva and Paris. *Journal of voluntary action research*, **1**: 42–45 (1972).

15. **Wolfenden Committee**. *The future of voluntary organizations*. London, Croom Helm, 1978.

16. **Koldewyn, P**. Voluntary associations in Neuquen, Argentina. *Journal of voluntary action research*, **13**: 38–54 (1984).

17. **Koldewyn, P**. Mexican voluntary associations: a community study. *Journal of voluntary action research*, **15**: 46–64 (1986).

18. **Drake, G.F**. Social class and organizational dynamic. A study of voluntary organizations in a Colombian city. *Journal of voluntary action research*, **1**: 46–52 (1972).

19. **Meister, A**. *Participation, associations, development and change*. New Brunswick, NJ, Transaction Books, 1984.

20. **Roudet, B**. *La Commune et ses associations: Meylan (Isère)*. Corenc, Centre d'études des solidarités sociales, 1983.

21. **Trojan, A**. Groupes de Santé: the users' movement in France. *In*: Hatch, S. & Kickbusch, I., ed. *Self-help and health in Europe: new approaches to health care*. Copenhagen, WHO Regional Office for Europe, 1983, pp. 43–57.

22. **Bauer, R. & Thränhardt, A.M**. Verbandliche Wohlfahrts-pflege im internationalen Vergleich. Opladen, Westdeutscher Verlag, 1987.

23. **Knight, B. & Hayes, R**. *Self-help in the inner city*. London, London Voluntary Service Council, 1981.

24. **Griffiths, H**. Community action and voluntary organization. *Journal of voluntary action research*, **8**: 36–46 (1979).

25. **Twelvetrees, A.C**. *Community associations and centres: a comparative study*. Oxford, Pergamon Press, 1976.

26. **Leat, D**. *Research into community involvement 1974–1988*. Berkhamsted, Volunteer Centre, 1977.

27. **White, L.G**. Functions of neighbourhood advisory groups. *Journal of voluntary action research*, **10**: 27–39 (1981).

28. **Baer, A.M**. The development of political interest groups in a local environment: evidence from a British new town. *Journal of voluntary action research*, **8**: 57–66 (1979).

29. **Helm, J.A**. Citizen initiatives and the growth of voluntary action in West Germany. *Journal of voluntary action research*, **10**: 49–61 (1981).

30. **Freudenberg, N**. Citizen action for environmental health: report on a survey of community organizations. *American journal of public health*, **74**: 444–448 (1984).

31. **Bachrach, K.M. & Zautra, A.J.** Coping with a community stressor: the threat of a hazardous waste facility. *Journal of health and social behavior*, **26**: 127–141 (1985).

32. **Hatch. S. & Kickbusch, I., ed.** *Self-help and health in Europe: new approaches in health care.* Copenhagen, WHO Regional Office for Europe, 1983.

33. **Levy, L.** Mutual support groups in Great Britain — a survey. *Social science and medicine*, **16**: 1265–1275 (1982).

34. **Trojan, A., ed.** *Wissen ist Macht — Eigenständig durch Selbsthilfe in Gruppen.* Frankfurt, Fischer, 1986.

35. **Trojan, A.** Benefits of self-help groups. A survey of 232 members from 65 disease-related groups. *Social science and medicine*, **29**: 225–232 (1989).

36. **Vilmar, F. & Runge, B. ed.** *Auf dem Weg zur Selbsthilfe-gesellschaft?: 40 000 Selbsthilfegruppen: Gesamtüberblick, Politische Theorie und Handlungsvorschläge.* Essen, Klartext, 1986.

37. **Romeder, J.-M.** *Self-help groups in Canada.* Ottawa. Program Information Unit, Social Service Development and Grants Directorate, Department of National Health and Welfare, 1982.

38. **von Ferber, C., ed.** *Gesundheitsselbsthilfe und professionelle Dienstleistungen: Soziologische Grundlagen einer bürger-orientierten Gesundheitspolitik/hrg. v. Forschungsverbund Laienpotential, Patientenaktivierung und Gesundheitsselbst-hilfe.* Berlin (West), Springer Verlag, 1987.

39. **Somerville, G.** *Community development in health: addressing the confusions.* Report of a conference organized by the King's Fund in collaboration with the London Community Health Resource Unit. London, King's Fund Centre, 1984.

40. **Kenner, C.** *Whose needs count? Community action for health.* Written for Community Health Initiatives Resource Unit, National Council of Voluntary Organizations. London, Bedford Square Press, 1986.

41. **Caplan, G.** *Principles of preventive psychiatry.* New York, Basic Books, 1964.

42. **Badura, B.** *Soziale Unterstützung und chronische Krankheit.* Frankfurt, Suhrkamp, 1981.

43. **Hamburg, B.A. & Killilea, M.** Relation of social support, stress, illness and use of health services. *In*: Office of Assistant

Secretary for Health and Surgeon General. *Healthy people. The Surgeon General's report on health promotion and disease prevention*. Washington, DC, US Government Printing Office, 1979, pp. 253–276 (DHEW Publication No. (PHS) 79-55071A).

44. **Berkman, L.F. & Syme, S.L.** Social networks, host resistance, and mortality: a nine-year follow-up study of Alameda County residents. *American journal of epidemiology*, **109**: 186–204 (1979).

45. **Blazer, D.G.** Social support and mortality in an elderly community population. *American journal of epidemiology*, **115**: 684–694 (1982).

46. **House, J.S. et al.** The association of social relationships and activities with mortality: prospective evidence from the Tecumseh Community Health Study. *American journal of epidemiology*, **116**: 123–140 (1982).

47. **Trojan, A. et al.** Selbsthilfe, Netzwerkforschung und Gesundheitsförderung. Grundlagen gemeindebezogener Netzwerkförderung als Präventionsstrategie. **In**: Keupp, H. & Röhrle, B., ed. *Soziale Netzwerke*. Frankfurt, Campus, 1987, pp. 297–317.

48. **Welin, L. et al.** Prospective study of social influences on mortality. The study of men born in 1913 and 1923. *Lancet*, **1**: 915–918 (1985).

49. **Levin, L.S. & Idler**, E.L. *The hidden health care system: mediating structures and medicine*. Cambridge, MA, Ballinger, 1981.

50. **Veiel, V.O.E.** Dimensions of social support. *Social psychiatry*, **20**: 165–172 (1985).

51. **Rappaport, J**. In praise of paradox: a social policy of empowerment over prevention. *American journal of community psychology*, **9**: 1–25 (1981).

52. **Berger, P.L. & Neuhaus, R.I**. *To empower people. The role of mediating structures in public policy*. Washington, DC, American Enterprise Institute for Public Policy Research, 1977 (AEI-Studies 139).

53. **Enkerts, V. & Schweigert, I., ed**. *Gesundheit ist mehr! Soziale Netzwerke für eine lebenswerte Zukunft*. Hamburg, Ergebnisse, 1988.

54. **Trojan, A. et al**. *Gesundheitsförderung im informellen Bereich*. Hamburg, Gesundheitsbehörde der Freien und Hansestadt Hamburg, 1987.

465

55. **Hildebrandt, H**. *Lust am Leben. Gesundheitsförderung mit Jugendlichen. Ein Aktions- und Ideenbuch für die Jugendarbeit*. Frankfurt, Brandes & Apsel, 1987.

20

Health promotion through self-help: the contribution of self-help groups

Ann Richardson

Self-help groups (also known as patient support groups) are no longer uncharted territory. For many years, people were aware that groups were developing in Europe and North America, but there was little systematic knowledge about their operation or effectiveness; this is no longer so. Research from disparate countries and disciplines has created a wealth of knowledge about these groups and their contribution to coping with disease. This chapter attempts to distil some of this knowledge. It is not a review of the growing literature in this field, although a bibliography is appended for those who wish to read further in this area.

Self-help Groups

People in self-help groups have a common problem and come together to do something about it. The groups range from well known and long established organizations such as Alcoholics Anonymous to new and small groups formed around rare and little known diseases and disabilities. All these groups can significantly contribute to health promotion. They deal with every aspect of health — mental, social and physical wellbeing — and can help at every stage, from prevention to day-to-day health care and rehabilitation. They tend to incorporate a holistic approach to individual problems; a person is not viewed as someone with a particular disease that needs treatment, but as an individual with wide-ranging needs for care and attention.

There are few hard data on the number and distribution of groups in various countries at present or in the past, primarily because groups are difficult to define and categorize. There is no simple register of the organizations that could appropriately be labelled self-help. Further, while new groups form every week, existing groups also disband. Nevertheless, the number of groups clearly increased in the mid-1970s, and this continued well into the 1980s, and there is no evidence of any current decline.

It is not clear why self-help groups have proliferated. Some people attribute this growth to an upsurge of interest in lay health care and to antipathy to professional dominance in health care delivery. Although the former is undoubtedly a factor, many people choose to combine self-help and professional help and are not hostile to the contribution of professionals. More important, however, this does not explain the initial movement towards increased lay health care. Many subtle factors were at work, including changes in the number of people with certain chronic diseases, changes in attitudes towards the role of lay people in the control and care of disease, and changing economic and social patterns that made organizing easier. To some extent, self-help groups replaced other forms of social network, such as the extended family and closely knit communities. Successful groups also provided suitable models for new ones to develop.

Self-help groups are particularly appropriate for people suffering from chronic diseases. Chronic disease creates a new and permanent state of being. Sufferers must learn to cope not only with new symptoms but also with a new sense of identity. They may also need to make substantial changes in lifestyle and living conditions. Self-help groups provide patients with an opportunity to meet and learn from one another over time, both about how to detect and control symptoms and about how to cope with their new situation. People who have had a disease for some time provide a useful model for those who are new to it, offering reassurance that it is possible to live and cope with the disease.

The Impact of Self-help Groups

Self-help groups function at two different levels. They deal with the social and health needs of their members, but also with broader

468

policies on and the delivery of health care. These groups usually have substantial and beneficial effects on their members, providing an important source of social and emotional support to members with many different diseases and problems. Groups help to improve members' sense of identity and to overcome loneliness and isolation through shared social activities. Participation plays a crucial role in enabling some members to cope with and to accept the nature of their disease. Some members become empowered, improving their capacity to look after their own health and to promote the health of others.

Self-help groups are an important source of information and advice, both for coping directly with a particular disease and for other sources of help. They increase members' awareness of both the quantity and the quality of external help and therefore improve members' ability to exercise informed choice. Some groups also provide services to their members, from small casual exchanges (such as babysitting) to more substantial help (such as care centres for people with a disease, or specialized counselling arrangements). These services may differ from equivalent traditional services in content and style. It is notable that, in some cases, these new services are then taken over by statutory service providers.

Not all the effects of support groups, of course, are positive. Some groups create a bond between members, but isolate them from the wider community. Groups also tend to create great expectations among members, which are not always fulfilled. Sometimes group discussions can seem unrealistic, so that suggestions are not followed up at home. Some groups tend to develop a single-factor etiology for a disease, leading to an inappropriately narrow approach.

It is important not to generalize too freely about the effect of groups on members. This impact differs enormously according to the nature of the disease. Benefits also vary according to the stage in the disease at which a member takes part, and the degree of stigma attached to the disease.

Many groups seek to extend their focus beyond their members to engender greater public awareness of their members' disease in particular and of their health needs in general. In some cases, the problem must be demystified; in others, public or private resources must be focused on the disease. Some groups raise funds for further research on prevention or cure. Evidence about the wider impact of these groups is regrettably modest. A long time span is necessary and cultural changes are highly subtle. The impact varies notably between countries, and is affected both by particular health care arrangements and by local values and norms.

The wider activities of self-help groups affect health professionals. Through involvement in a group, some professionals become considerably more knowledgeable about the group and about the disease around which it was formed. They also learn a great deal about members' problems and views. While some professionals increasingly support these groups, others feel that self-help groups obtain public resources at the expense of other broader activities for health promotion.

Self-help groups mobilize new resources to provide health care. They foster a new kind of volunteer, providing help to others who have the particular disease or condition. In some countries, groups also find new ways of perceiving needs for care and organizing around them. Because groups focus clearly on single diseases, they tend to ignore strict professional and institutional boundaries. Groups press for services to be integrated around their disease, forming new coalitions of interested lay and professional people.

Participation and Involvement

Self-help groups do not all function the same way. The activities of groups and their longevity vary substantially. Their functions often change over time in response to perceived changes in needs or expectations. New groups often concentrate on the somatic aspects of a disease and then broaden to focus on wider improvements in health. Groups also change in response to the changing concerns of members; the interests of older members, for instance, are often quite different from those of younger ones.

People are involved at different levels within groups, depending on what individual people want and what they are able to do. Some want to be highly active, others simply want to attend meetings, and others do not want to participate actively but want to know the group is there. Group leadership can be crucial here, as a strong charismatic leader can generate an enthusiastic membership. Although the concept of reciprocity underlies the development of support groups, actual reciprocity is clearly uneven, both within individual groups and between groups. Serial reciprocity, whereby help received is paid back to others over time, may be one way that groups retain a reciprocal element.

470

Who joins self-help groups? Considerable evidence indicates that people who take part differ systematically from people who do not. Joiners tend to be middle class, educated, female, elderly and not from ethnic minorities or rural areas. They also tend to be socially competent, having both experience in expressing their needs and a sense of confidence in their ability to solve problems themselves. Not all joiners directly suffer from a disease; relatives and other well-wishers sometimes join, and people who no longer have the disease can also remain active.

There are many obstacles to participation; the key one is not knowing that a group exists. In addition, however, people can have practical problems in getting out, such as lack of transport, money or a babysitter. Many of the diseases themselves hinder attendance, such as diseases that reduce mobility. Sometimes a spouse discourages attendance. People living in closely knit communities may fear the loss of anonymity. Incentives to join are reduced when other primary social networks exist.

The issue of uneven participation is complex. To the extent that it reflects unequal access to information about the existence and benefits of groups, it is a matter for concern. To the extent that it reflects differing personalities and tastes, it should not cause concern. Ultimately, it must be accepted that self-help is not a universal solution and that many people, with full knowledge and competence, do not choose to join groups.

Support for Self-help Groups

The issue of the best way to provide support to self-help groups is very lively in many countries. The number of self-help clearing-houses in Europe has grown considerably, particularly in the Federal Republic of Germany and in Great Britain. They channel information about the location of self-help groups and focus support for groups in the local area. They provide practical advice about publicity and premises and, in some cases, general support to group leaders or founders. They can help to establish groups and can stimulate local professionals to help groups. These clearing-houses also symbolize public interest in self-help.

National organizations also support local groups, which are more familiar with the disease around which their groups are formed. Some governments have provided financial support to national specialist organizations. Specialist community workers employed by such organizations can increase participation in groups and promote new groups. Nevertheless, specialists at the centre can get out of touch with local groups and become unrepresentative. National organizations can also influence the climate of opinion in which local groups operate.

Professionals have a sensitive role in self-help groups. Some argue that professionals inevitably use groups to pursue their own professional aims. Group members are often deferential to professionals, despite the ethos of equality. Further, professionals may call attention to their presence, often unintentionally. Nevertheless, professionals can refer potential members to groups and provide other kinds of practical assistance. There is a strong case for giving health professionals some training in self-help support. Encouraging people to recognize their own competence and to reject the traditional role of patient requires very special skills.

The Future

Crystal-ball gazing is a notoriously hazardous activity, but the role of self-help groups will probably remain very much the same. Some groups will decline, new groups will emerge and some existing groups will be strengthened. With the growth of support from clearing-houses and professionals, the self-help phenomenon is likely to become more established.

New kinds of potential groups, however, are on the horizon: non-disease-specific groups for health promotion. The growing interest in expanding the role of lay people in health care and growing attention to health in its broadest sense will promote the growth of these groups. Many already focus on broad patient care or participation. They both reflect and foster a holistic approach to health. Self-help groups may stimulate this development as they begin to talk with and learn from one another. They will find a number of health issues of common concern: new coalitions may emerge.

The effect of new groups and those of longer duration will merit close attention. The new groups may positively affect people who take part, empowering people, extending their ability to promote their own health and that of others. Perhaps more significantly, they may affect broader service delivery, reorienting health services towards promoting health more generally. They may place health issues

472

firmly in the context of healthy public policy and remove them from the more restricted domain of the medical profession.

The role of national and international agencies presents difficult problems. The development of self-help groups presents a dilemma for public policy. On the one hand, groups can be viewed as solely private bodies: groups of people who find their mutual company congenial and derive benefits from taking part (as with a group of friends or a sporting club). On the other hand, they have an additional public function: contributing to the health of the population (as with programmes for health education). Self-help groups can then be interpreted either as a matter solely for the individual people involved or as a matter for social policy. The growth of attention given to self-help groups, from national governments as well as from WHO, suggests that the broader social interpretation is gaining influence.

The contribution of support groups to health promotion needs to be recognized and applauded. Given that professionals tend to receive great attention in the health care system, the balance must be corrected in favour of the consumer. Policies that facilitate support groups and enable them to flourish in their particular localities are needed, both nationally and internationally. By promoting and encouraging the development of groups and individual participation in them, WHO and others can and should play a key role in promoting equality of access to such groups. The International Information Centre on Self-help and Health in Leuven (Belgium) has already substantially contributed here. By producing a widely read newsletter, organizing workshops and providing networks for both researchers and policy-makers, it has kept the needs of self-help firmly on the international agenda.

In reviewing the contribution of self-help groups to coping with chronic disease, it is necessary to be positive but cautious. These groups offer their individual members a great deal and may have a wider beneficial impact. They contribute significantly to promoting individual health care and a refreshing lay view of health care. Their holistic approach to individuals merits particular attention. They represent and encourage a wider view of health as a social idea.

Support groups do not function without problems, however, and it would be inappropriate to expect too much of them. They are not universally available, either in terms of every disease or of every country or local area. Not everyone finds them an appropriate solution to his or her needs for care. Self-help groups should be viewed as an important complement to existing systems of health and social care and not a substitute for them. Their contribution needs to be recognized but not exaggerated. Self-help groups must now be examined with due care and conjoined in the wider movement for health promotion.

Bibliography

Barath, A. Hypertension clubs in Croatia. *In*: Hatch, S. & Kickbusch, I., ed. *Self-help and health in Europe; new approaches in health care*. Copenhagen, WHO Regional Office for Europe, 1983.

van den Borne, M. *Nazorggroepen Kankerpatiënten: Frequentieverdeling can de Onderzoeksvariabelen* [Cancer patient aftercare groups: frequency distribution of research variables]. Tilburg, Catholic High School, 1982.

van den Borne, M. *Lotgenotencontact bij kankerpatiënten* [Mutual aid among cancer patients]. Assen, Van Gorcum, 1985.

van den Borne, M. et al. Self-help in cancer patients: a review of studies on the effects of contacts between fellow patients. *Patient education and counselling*, **8**: 367–385 (1986).

Branckaerts, J. *A directory of generalised support systems for self-help in health and social welfare in Europe, the U.S.A., et al*. Leuven, Sociological Research Institute, Catholic University, 1985.

Branckaerts, J. et al. *Het zachte verzet* [The soft resistance]. Antwerp, Kluwer, 1982.

Bremer Shulte, M. *From polarization to collaboration in health care*. Maastricht, Interacademic Hospital Sciences Working Group, 1978.

Bremer Shulte, M. Patients in partnership with professionals: the duo approach. *Education for health*, **1**(2): 32–37 (1984).

Grünow, D. Formen sozialer Alltäglichkeit: Selbsthilfe in Gesundheitswesen. *In*: Badura, B. & v. Ferber, C. ed. *Selbsthilfe und Selbstorganization im gesundheitswesen*. Munich, Oldenburg, pp. 125–146.

Grünow, D. et al. *Gesundheitsselbsthilfe im Alltag: Ergebnisse einer repräsentativen Haushaltsbefragung über gesundheitsbezogene Selbsthilfeerfahrungen und Potentiale.* Stuttgart, Enke-Verlag, 1983.

Hatch, S. & Hinton, T. *Self-help in practice.* Sheffield, University of Sheffield, Joint Unit for Social Services Research, 1986 (Social Services Monographs: Research in Practice).

Hatch, S. & Kickbusch, I., ed. *Self-help and health in Europe: new approaches to health care.* Copenhagen, WHO Regional Office for Europe, 1983.

Humble, S. *Voluntary action in the 1980s.* Berkhamsted, Volunteer Centre, 1982.

Levin, L. et al. *Self-care: lay initiatives in health.* London, Croom Helm, 1977.

Levin, L.S. & Idler, E.L. *The hidden health care system: mediating structures and medicine.* Cambridge, MA, Bollinger, 1981.

Richardson, A. & Goodman, M. *Self-help and social care: mutual aid organizations in practice.* London, PSI, 1983.

Richardson, A. *Working with self-help groups.* London, Bedford Square Press, 1984.

Trojan, A., ed. *Wissen ist Macht – Eigenständig durch Selbsthilfe in Gruppen.* Frankfurt, Fischer, 1986.

Trojan, A. & Kickbusch, I., ed. *Gemeinsam sind wir stärker: Selbsthilfegruppen und Gesundheit: Selbstdarstellungen — Analysen — Forschungsergebnisse.* Frankfurt, Fischer Taschenbuch Verlag, 1981.

Vincent, J. *Constraints on the stability and longevity of self-help groups in the field of health care*: report to the Department of Health and Social Security. Loughborough, Centre for Research in Social Policy, Loughborough University, 1986.

Vincent, J. & Webb, A. The mirror of research. *In*: Landau-North, M. & Duddy, S., ed. *Self-help through the looking glass.* Leicester, Rural Press, 1985.

21

Citizen participation in community health: principles for effective partnerships

Neil Bracht

Citizen participation is a fundamental aspect of civic life and democratic tradition. Citizen involvement in various social, economic and cultural activities reflects the demands, expectations and aspirations that naturally arise in human societies. Many improvements in community life, including the enhancement of public health, result from the direct concern and action of citizens. Historical studies *(1)* of organized social life reveal that there are distinct urban and rural forms of social change and creativity. Complex urban environments often develop more formal avenues and infrastructures through which citizen involvement is mediated and realized. Rural villages or small towns more frequently have informal, ad hoc approaches. Regardless of geographic and structural determinants, citizen involvement or participation (these terms are used interchangeably here) is widely observed and documented and appears to be encouraged as a social norm of community life.

Perceptions of the social benefit of citizen participation are also widespread. Surveys in the United States document high rates of volunteer involvement and successful civic action projects *(2,3)*. Official government bulletins *(4)* often espouse the benefits of active citizen participation. Documents sponsored by WHO *(5–8)* recommend wider use of strategies to increase citizen participation. Chavis et al. *(9)* suggest that "creating partnership and linkages between social scientists and citizens can improve the quality of research, enhance the potential for its utilization and help people help themselves". Many volunteer health, social service and sports associations depend entirely on active citizen support. Greater employee participation is commonly reported in managerial decisions and quality control strategies at the workplace. Occasionally, in a twist of political irony, federal governments mandate requirements for citizen participation in local or regional programmes to obtain a consumer perspective *(10,11)*.

Citizen participation embraces many forms of citizen action and community problem-solving, including self-help groups. I define it as the process of taking part (voluntarily) in either formal or informal activities, programmes and/or discussions to bring about a planned change or improvement in community life, services and/or resources.

The results of citizen involvement are measurable, as are the variables associated with participation itself, including: opportunity for and level of decision-making or advising, amount and duration of time devoted to goal-directed activities, representativeness of the citizen and leader groups that are formed, degree of local ownership perceived and/or achieved, satisfaction with the processes of participation, and assessment of achievement and long-term maintenance of goals. Citizen participation can be theoretically seen as a dependent variable when the causes of participation are identified or as an independent variable when the consequences of participation are analysed *(12)*. Green *(13)* notes, however, that "the principle of participation has not been systematically codified in health education with a cohesive set of constructs, definitions and propositions, but even in its crude form it serves to explain a wide range of behavioural phenomena in health. . . ".

This chapter reviews what has been learned about citizen participation, particularly in health and social service programmes. Key principles and practices are presented as a guide to effecting citizen involvement, including the newer partnership and intersectoral strategies for health *(14–17)*. The references provided can assist readers in pursuing selected content areas. An extensive search of the literature reveals that organizing citizen groups for planned social change is a common approach in community-wide improvement activities and usually represents the efforts of local organizers, advocates or government sponsors to harness citizen interest and action. There is also much undocumented evidence about spontaneous citizen action such as grassroots social movements and/or mutual aid groups achieving important social goals (see Chapter 20).

This chapter focuses primarily on planned, systematic efforts that mobilize citizen energy towards health promotion, health policy and prevention programmes. There is substantial research describing the art and science required to make such efforts successful. Fortunately, as there is much interest in community-wide approaches to changes in health promotion and lifestyle policies, several texts and guides *(18–21)* have developed and improved the theory and principles of community organization. Progress has also been made in understanding the application of these principles to programme-specific health intervention and health promotion projects *(22–25)*.

Results from these reported studies, along with the plethora of current communitywide intervention projects in both North America and Europe, provide additional evidence of the feasibility of combining traditional strategies for community organization and citizen participation with the newer principles and techniques of social marketing, social learning and diffusion theories. The Institute for Health Promotion in Wales has an information base for 125 health promotion programmes in 30 countries. Wider environmental, intersectoral and policy applications (beyond intervention to change risk factors) are also developing through WHO initiatives such as the Healthy Cities project *(14,16,26–28)*. Community projects sponsored by the Kaiser Foundation in the United States reflect a wide range of targets for health and social intervention such as drug abuse, accident preventinon and pregnancy prevention. Programmes are also being developed in Latin America.

Programmes for social and community intervention in mental health and community psychology show promising short-term results but need more citizen and consumer involvement *(29)*:

> Needed for the next generation of social and community interventions are fewer individual and more collective efforts designed in concert with the groups and communities we seek to assist. Designing and conducting such programs with greater ecological sensitivity to issues of process and context will help insure that effective interventions endure after initial results have been published.

The content and perspective of this chapter are drawn principally from experiences and research findings in North America and northern Europe. Other applications of approaches towards citizen participation should be approached cautiously. Literature on community development and anthropology suggests that there are various cross-cultural styles (some passive, others more active) of coping with and responding to perceived community problems or opportunities. Almond & Verba *(30)* studied what citizens did to influence government and found differences in whether people preferred to act alone or work with others. Organizing informal groups or activating friends appeared to be more common in the United States and the United Kingdom, while direct work through political parties was preferred in other countries.

Citizen Participation

While citizen involvement may be desirable and frequently appropriate, studies of citizen participation in community development programmes show a mixed record of success *(31–33)*. Voth & Jackson *(12)* cite anecdotal evidence of citizens spontaneously mobilizing and achieving important objectives, but conclude that: "the citizen participation process cannot easily be stimulated or managed for policy purposes. Furthermore, the proportion of citizens involved may be limited and these may be primarily community elites.". In the United Kingdom, a number of groups attempt to participate in planning and setting objectives for health services, but "two groups with the least involvement are the work force and the community" *(34)*. Representatives from 26 European countries, Australia and Canada concluded that *(35)*:

> ... decisions are too readily and too frequently left in the hands of professionals only, with too little attention being given to educating, or allowing lay people to participate in the creation, implementation and evaluation of health promotion, disease prevention, treatment and support programmes.

There are exceptions to these negative assessments. The Vännäs project *(36)* tried to incorporate community and consumer expectations into changes implemented at a local primary care centre. Citizen involvement in neighbourhood health centres in the United States has generally been successful *(37,38)*. Simmons *(39)* and Cleary et al. *(40)* document several successful health education projects involving citizen action. Citizen health commissions in Cuba and consumer health cooperatives in Japan offer additional examples of successful citizen involvement.

Several researchers have studied the characteristics and motivations of people who actively participate in formal or voluntary associations. Wandersman & Giarmartino *(41)* found that people who were concerned about their neighbourhood, who had more experience in community leadership and who felt that competent colleagues could be enlisted in the project were more likely to participate. Smith *(42)* noted distinct differences in social class in that the participants he studied generally had higher socioeconomic status. More recent studies *(2)* show a wider spread of participation by age, sex and race. Young adults (14 to 17 years) contribute more volunteer work than any other age group, but one in four people over 75 years is still active in volunteer programmes. Some 38% of racial or national minorities and 40% of those characterized as poor volunteer and participate in community activities in the United States. More and more men report participating in volunteer activity but women still predominate (45% male versus 51% female) *(3)*.

Studies of community organization suggest additional variables to be considered in promoting or facilitating citizen participation. Zurcher *(43)* found that if health and welfare issues were to be successfully resolved, the early stages of community activation required orientation and information sessions about the scope of local issues and about the efficacy of cooperative action. Spergel *(44)* believes an important element in successful citizen participation is the ability of the organizing group(s) to offer specific rewards or benefits to the people involved. The benefits obtained in local health projects can either be instrumental, through actual improvement in personal or environmental health, or expressive, through feelings of pride in community health or recognition by others of successful efforts.

Voth & Jackson *(12)* have summarized the factors contributing to successful citizen participation:

— the sponsoring group or agency must operate in good faith;
— the authority of citizen groups must be clearly defined and resources must be available; and
— citizen groups must be able to create, sustain and control an effective organization.

Eight years of intensive experience with three distinct communities and their citizen boards in the Minnesota Heart Health Program *(15)* suggest six additional factors for successful citizen activation:

— early and extensive knowledge of community history, organizational resources, influence structures and interorganizational networks;

481

— commitment of project sponsors to partnership and/or local ownership from the beginning of a project;
— clearly stated roles and time commitments for community participants;
— the building of planned reinforcement (recognition) of citizen participants into programnme development and design;
— early identification and open discussion of forces resistant to change in the community;
— timely use of strategies for conflict resolution.

Citizen involvement in planning for community change is a way of:

— pretesting the feasibility and acceptability of new programmes or ideas;
— gaining broad citizen support and volunteer effort;
— incorporating local values, attitudes and symbols into implementation plans;
— gaining access to the resources of local leaders and technical skills not otherwise available;
— incorporating lay viewpoints into programme delivery;
— developing local skills and competence for future community development or opportunities;
— forcing coordination between loosely structured agencies and organizations, both public and private;
— mediating conflicts between political factions and special interest groups; and
— ensuring local ownership and long-term maintenance.

Citizen Involvement in Health Promotion

Is citizen involvement necessary to achieve health promotion goals? Can citizen input be bypassed or ignored without negative consequences? The research base for these questions is not readily available. More frequently, local or national values or political considerations determine whether citizens are actively engaged in social change.

Citizen involvement in change runs the gamut of manipulation and tokenism to actual control. Various levels of citizen participation are shown in Fig. 1. In most social action projects and movements

482

there is a middle range of involvement. Some partnership arrangement of citizens (usually initiated by a core group of community leaders) is combined with the knowledge and talents of vested agents for change and government experts. This has been particularly true of demonstration projects in chronic disease prevention during the last 10–15 years, beginning largely with the North Karelia project in Finland. Cardiovascular disease programmes in the United States (such as Stanford, Pawtucket and Minnesota) recognize that behaviour is strongly influenced by the larger social environment and the underlying values and norms of the community. Such basic change in the behaviour, value and norms of the community can occur only through the active participation of community residents and organizations. Citizen action is the key to realizing the social and health goals of many prevention-oriented projects.

But which models or approaches to citizen involvement are effective? Much of community organization theory (46) suggests that the impetus for community change comes from grassroots groups with change primarily directed by citizens. Realistically, social improvements are governed by many external factors, organizations and policies, and grassroots influence is only one albeit important factor in change. Few communities are independent of larger regional, national and international social and economic influences. Social planning models and advocacy models are also used. Petersson[a] has analysed the relationship between top-down and bottom-up strategies in Sweden and has found that there is close cooperation between people at the top of bureaucratic power and the local citizens and groups without a formal power base.

Another important avenue for citizen influence is modifying organizational goals and services. Aldrich (47) believes that "organizations that produce goods, deliver services, maintain order or challenge the established order are the fundamental building blocks of modern societies and must stand at the center of the analysis of social change". Community organizations and their leaders can be conceptualized as forming interorganizational networks or loosely coupled systems. Aldrich identifies the linking pin organization as a type especially geared to citizen involvement. Such an organization has extensive and overlapping ties to different parts of organizational

---

[a] **Petersson, B**. *Health policies development and local implementation — how to keep head and tail together*. Paper presented at the National Conference on Healthy States, Brisbane, Queensland, Australia, 13–14 April 1988.

Fig. 1. Eight rungs on a ladder of citizen participation

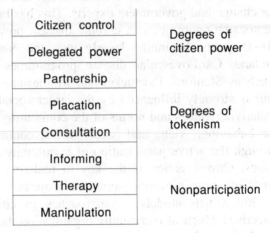

Citizen control	Degrees of citizen power
Delegated power	
Partnership	
Placation	Degrees of tokenism
Consultation	
Informing	
Therapy	Nonparticipation
Manipulation	

Source: Arnstein, S. *(45)*.

networks and can play a central role in integrating and coordinating them. Since health promotion and wellness systems are not well established, linking pin organizations have a good chance of survival because they are moving into an unoccupied niche. This type of organization may also develop a creative approach or form that has some advantage over existing groups or strategies.

In Minnesota, citizen advisory boards were developed in the three demonstration communities to build a partnership strategy between the university and the community *(15)*. These boards have now developed into non-profit independent organizations overseeing and expanding health promotion activities. The original functions of the university as an advisory board changed over time as local responsibility grew. The initial functions of the citizen advisory board in 1983 were envisaged as being:

— to facilitate links between the heart health programme and other community organizations and institutional sectors in order to involve them in education programmes;

— to establish and help coordinate the projects of community volunteer task forces staffed by heart health personnel;

484

— to provide advice to the university and the heart health director regarding major project initiatives; and

— to develop sustained community support for the project and for heart health, including the continuation of successful project initiatives after project funding ceases.

The final statement of the mission and goals of the citizen board in 1987 was:

> Bloomington Heart and Health Program, Inc. is a community health education program aimed at reducing levels of heart disease and promoting health.
>
> The program will:
>
> — provide opportunities for people to adopt healthy lifestyles in eating patterns, smoking cessation, physical activity and weight control;
>
> — advocate changes in the physical and social environment; and
>
> — coordinate with and support efforts of other community groups.

The more recent mission and goals include a name change in one community to reflect better the board's growing desire to expand health promotion beyond heart health activities. Recent evaluations within the programme reveal that the retention of founding members on these boards for a seven-year period was over 50%.

Such semi-independent boards might initially seem out of place in countries with social democratic traditions and highly structured systems of health care. Semi-autonomous community health boards, councils or coalitions can add another layer to an already complex system of health services. While this may be an organizational disadvantage in one sense, the advantage is that citizen boards represent a more neutral arena for community health promotion. In this partnership model, health professionals (the "experts") stretch to work with citizens. Control and programme direction is better balanced, and delegated power for long-term maintenance is possible.

In the North Karelia project, the public health services provide the professional and technical services required for intervention in cardiovascular disease risk, but a citizen advisory group and associated voluntary organizations have played a major linking pin role in programme dissemination, education and support (by petitioning government). The Pawtucket *(48)* and Pennsylvanian *(25)* heart health projects in the United States have also used citizen involvement in conjunction with local professional services to achieve the desired goals of risk reduction in these communities.

Experiences from the Mon Valley Health and Welfare Project, in Pennsylvania, United States, have shown that the presence of consumer representatives on the management board does not automatically guarantee meaningful consumer participation in decision-making and planning. Pecarchik et al. *(49)*, who studied the history and outcomes of this project, report that:

> . . . the most productive role for the consumer in bringing about changes in the health care system may be one of provoking issues between the primary and secondary health care layers and using various techniques to move the two layers toward the resolution of these issues. Through committees and task forces broader community involvement is achieved, new members added over time and direct participation in decision-making can occur. In effect, the strength of committees lies in their being forums in which representatives of all sectors of the community can respond to issues pertaining to the care delivery system . . . the most salient factor in meaningful participation by the consumer membership is preparedness.

Interestingly, the partnership approach in this project led to better informed citizens who could use their improved technical skills in future involvement. This experience is similar to Freire's *(50)* concept of critical consciousness, in which people examine their world and take action to transform it.

In community-wide programmes of social and policy intervention, cooperation between the private, public and voluntary sectors is not only desired but required if goals for social and programme change are to be realized. Few citizens have the skill to design the sophisticated social marketing and media campaigns often necessary to make people aware of a programme. Technical and professional experts are usually needed, but few professionals are exposed to heavy smoke and chemical hazards at their workplaces. The consumer perspective can be beneficial to professionals and government experts who design intervention strategies. Cooperation and partnership between experts, consumers and community leaders is essential. This cooperation extends to research as well, including effective feedback and dissemination between scientist and citizen *(9)*:

> Despite the difficulties involved, we conclude that returning research to the community and facilitating its utilization can have important ethical, social and scientific benefits. It can enhance the quality and

486

applicability of research, provide an opportunity for hypothesis generation and hypothesis testing and facilitate planning and problem-solving by citizens. The process of returning research to the citizen has the potential for building a positive relationship between scientist and citizen.

Kettner et al. *(18)* prefer collaborative and educational strategies in initiating change. While specific changes might be achieved more quickly through conflict tactics, collaboratively or educationally achieved changes tend to persist. Kettner et al. do not preclude using conflict when other strategies have failed or when strong evidence suggests that collaboration and education will not get the job done. Effective efforts for social change may require a mix of strategies and intervention tactics, including a major emphasis on policy changes such as smoke-free environments. Comprehensive intersectoral health projects are well suited to embrace multiple methods of intervention that can produce broader synergistic effects.

Nix *(19)* has summarized several general principles of change that provide a useful perspective for people about to initiate community organization and citizen mobilization:

— people in social groups or systems in all times and places have both resisted and accepted change;
— change in one part of a social system requires change and adjustment in other parts of the system;
— all change has its costs; it is difficult to imagine a significant social or technical change that does not have both negative and positive effects;
— the cost of social change is differentially borne by the members and groups of a system;
— the solution of one problem usually produces other problems.

Process and Structure for Citizen Organizing

Metsch & Veney *(11)* suggest that "guidelines for implementing consumer participation in health must be program-specific and reflect program goals, settings and complexity". Experiences from chronic disease prevention programmes in North America and Europe, including recent comprehensive and intersectoral community-based health promotion efforts, suggest at least six specific stages for citizen involvement with an inevitable overlap between stages (Fig. 2).

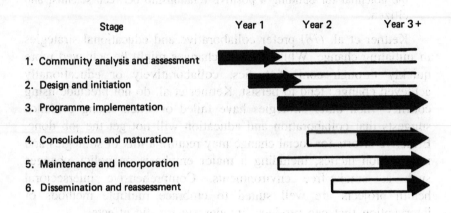

Fig. 2. Six-stage process of a typical community health promotion project

Stage	Year 1	Year 2	Year 3 +
1. Community analysis and assessment			
2. Design and initiation			
3. Programme implementation			
4. Consolidation and maturation			
5. Maintenance and incorporation			
6. Dissemination and reassessment			

Community analysis, for example, is a continuing process even after the initial assessment and profile of community needs are completed. Communities are dynamic entities, and continual updating of information, resources and interaction patterns is required. Occasionally, certain stages may be shortened if appropriate information already exists (community assessment can draw upon earlier studies and citizen work). Design and implementation are closely interrelated. Intervention projects must frequently be redesigned after initial pilot projects, citizen response or evaluation.

Structural considerations in facilitating citizen involvement surface quickly in any process of community action. The type of structure that best accommodates citizen involvement varies by community type and size, programme goals, past experiences and citizen preferences. The various organizing structures are shown in Fig. 3. A core group of concerned citizens usually initiates the action process. The group may select or identify a key person to coordinate the initial activities. This coordinator may be either a professional or a lay community leader. The group serves as a catalyst for assessing local needs and developing preliminary notions about what type of structure best accommodates citizen involvement. Task forces with delineated responsibilities usually carry out target activities with a goal of long-term incorporation or maintenance in the community.

Organizing structures

As shown in Fig. 3, there are at least six alternative structures for organizing community participation. The type used depends on community culture, history, capabilities and local preference for decision-making. Although the various structures are distinct, successful programmes are likely to use parts from several models. While it is necessary to assess each community and determine the best approaches, it is equally important to use whatever works. The alternative structures are briefly summarized below.

Coalition

Linked organizations and groups address community issues. The formation of a new community-wide coalition of groups and organizations is customary, although it is possible to interest an existing coalition in taking on a new community problem.

Leadership board or council

Existing leaders and/or community activists work together towards a common goal such as creating smoke-free environments or preventing accidents. The board usually includes leaders of diverse community groups who are identified as being necessary to achieve project goals. This model has been used successfully in the three-community Minnesota Heart Health Program.

Lead agency

A single community agency is identified as the primary liaison for health promotion activities in the community. This is useful when a community's political context, past history and/or available resources dictate the selection of a credible and well established agency, either public or private. In Pawtucket, the local hospital is used as principal community sponsor of heart health activities in collaboration with many other groups and organizations.

Grassroots

The informal structures of a community can be used to reach people who are not represented by formal structures, such as residents of

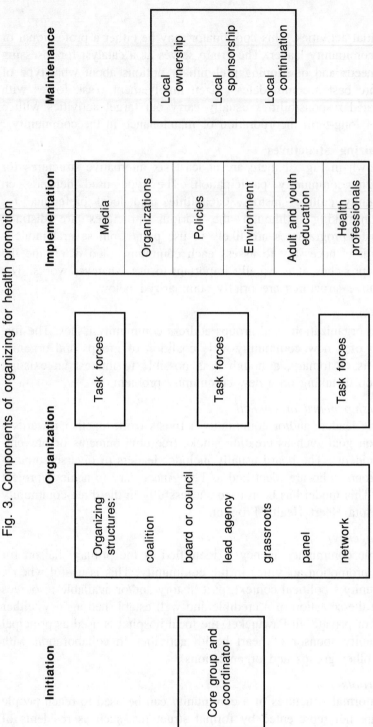

Fig. 3. Components of organizing for health promotion

blue-collar neighbourhoods, minority groups and residents of public housing. Mobilization occurs through direct involvement with residents, usually by educating individuals about a problem and producing enough concern to get people involved in addressing the problem. Some grassroots efforts evolve into consumer cooperatives in which local control is better achieved.

Citizen panels
New forms of citizen advocacy are emerging in partnership with bureaucratic organizations. These panels can be either appointed or elected and their task is limited in time. Usually the panel works closely with government bodies to shape programme policy and monitor programme performance.

Networks
Networks are less formal and hierarchical than coalitions, which tend to be directed by professionals. Networks bring together people who have a common commitment and who serve as catalysts to community action. Networks are best suited to short-term, well defined goals, in which collaborative action can be assured and long-term organizational resources and support are not of fundamental concern. Parents organizing against drunken driving or sports associations demanding improved safety in sports equipment are examples.

These models are not static and may evolve into new or modified citizen structures. Government bodies must be prepared to allow citizen groups to exercise control, and that includes the right to make changes and even mistakes in organizing and planning.

Citizen Participation and Government

This chapter began by reflecting on citizen participation as a fundamental component of democratic tradition and processes. Theorists of participatory democracy differ on the nature, scope and efficacy of citizens directly participating in political affairs. Some would limit participation to the minimum required to keep the electoral process operating. Others advocate creating a participatory society in which involvement in local public affairs is essential. As Pateman *(51)* observes:

. . . evidence supports the arguments of Rousseau, Mill and Cole that we do learn to participate by participating, and the feelings of political efficacy are more likely to be developed in a participatory environment. Furthermore, the evidence indicates that the experience of a participatory authority structure might also be effective in diminishing tendencies toward nondemocratic attitudes in the individual.

In this chapter, citizen participation has been examined in the context of the process of community development. In some societies, Nelson et al. *(52)* state that:

... community development is conceived as a function of government that necessitates the establishment of a department or bureau appropriately designated. It is, most certainly, a function of government but not one to be so easily delegated. In theory, when government is conceived as the servant of the governed, community development is the process whereby the governed make known their will to their chosen governors.

If citizen empowerment were widespread and social and community institutions were easily influenced through political processes, there would probably be less need for direct citizen mobilization and advocacy. Strategies for citizen participation are only one type of strategy for involvement and change, but they reflect a reawakening to the value of citizen talent, energy and competence. Government bodies alone have limited scope and ability to solve complex social, economic and environmental problems. New models for citizen participation are being developed and show promise of having an impact on policies and programmes *(53)*. Citizen participation and community organization as an active process "must permeate all relationships within the government and between specialized agencies and the people" *(52)*.

Active citizen involvement faces three distinct challenges. In some democratic societies, citizens feel that they are already participating in community life and social institutions through a political party or affiliated groups. Such citizens may already influence community goals and services as well as national programmes. Current involvement in the political process may make these citizens reluctant to participate in special projects they view as duplicative. Second, some see the process of citizen participation as cumbersome, slow and not cost-effective. In their view, response to social problems (and the resources required) is the legitimate domain of government (or cooperating volunteer organizations), and responsibility for programme improvements and special projects should be solely the business of elected officials and official agencies. Third, community priorities wax and wane. A coordinated national perspective (and resources) seems more efficient to some political theorists.

492

These reservations about citizen participation are valid. Despite these concerns and the difficulties involved, collaboration between government, private group and local citizen is desirable. As Cassell *(54)* concludes:

> Enhancing the social ties and connections among members of the community through participatory procedures can go far toward modifying those environmental factors which facilitate the occurrence of illness.

References

1. **Eisenstadt, S. & Schachar**, A. *Society, culture and urbanization.* Newbury Park, CA, Sage Publications, 1987.
2. *Report on model community programs: American Can.* Greenwich, CT, American Can Corporation, 1986.
3. *Americans volunteer 1985: an Independent Sector summary report.* Washington, DC, Independent Sector, 1986.
4. *What can be expected from health education programmes?* Strasbourg, Council of Europe, 1980.
5. Health promotion: a discussion document on the concept and principles. *Health promotion,* **1**(1): 73–76 (1986).
6. A framework for health promotion policy: a discussion document. *Health promotion,* **1**(3): 335–340 (1986).
7. Health promotion in action: practical ideas on programme implementation. *Health promotion,* **1**(2): 187–190 (1986).
8. **Leparski, E. & Nüssel, E. ed.** *CINDI (Countrywide integrated noncommunicable diseases intervention programme). Protocol and guidelines for monitoring and evaluation procedures.* Berlin (West), Springer Verlag 1987.
9. **Chavis, D. et al**. Returning basic research to the community: relationship between scientist and citizen. *American psychologist,* **12**: 424–434 (1983).
10. **Macrina, D. & O'Rourke, T**. Citizen participation in health planning in the U.S. and the U.K.: implication for health education strategies. *International quarterly of community health education,* **7**(3): 225–238 (1986/1987).
11. **Metsch, J. & Veney, J**. Consumer participation and social accountability. *Medical care,* **14**(4): 283–293 (1976).
12. **Voth, D. & Jackson, V**. *Evaluating citizen participation: rural and urban community development.* Washington, DC, Center for Responsive Governance, 1981 (Working Paper Series).

13. **Green, L.** The theory of participation: a qualitative analysis of its expression in national and international health policies. *Advances in health education and promotion*, **1**: 211–236 (1986).

14. **Ashton, J. et al.** Healthy Cities — WHO's new public health initiative. *Health promotion*, **1**(3): 319–323 (1986).

15. **Carlaw, R.W. et al.** Organization for a community cardiovascular health program: experiences from the Minnesota Heart Health Program. *Health education quarterly*, **11**: 243–252 (1984).

16. **Hancock, T. & Duhl, L.** *Promoting health in the urban context.* Copenhagen, FADL, 1988 (WHO Healthy Cities Papers No. 1).

17. **MacNair, R.** *Community partnership organizations: a better way to gain participation in health programs.* Atlanta, GA, Centers for Disease Control, US Department of Health and Human Services, 1980.

18. **Kettner, P. et al.** *Initiating change in organizations and communities.* Monterey, CA, Brooks/Cole Publishing, 1985.

19. **Nix, H.** *The community and its involvement in the study planning action process.* Atlanta, GA, Centers for Disease Control, 1977 (DHEW Publication No. 78–8355).

20. **Rothman, J. et al.** *Changing organizations and community programs.* Beverly Hills, CA, Sage Publications, 1981 (Sage Human Service Guides, Vol. 20).

21. **Seidman, E. ed.** *Handbook of social intervention.* Beverly Hills, CA, Sage Publications, 1983.

22. **Finnegan, J. et al.** *Information campaigns: managing the process of social change. Sage annual review of communication research.* Newbury Park, CA, Sage Publications, Vol. 18, 1989.

23. **Matazarro, J. et al.** *Behavioral health: a handbook of health enhancement and disease prevention.* New York, Wiley, 1984.

24. **Puska, P. et al.** The community-based strategy to prevent coronary heart disease: conclusions from the ten years of the North Karelia project. *Annual review of public health*, **6**: 147–193 (1985).

25. **Stunkard, A. et al.** Mobilizing a community to promote health: the Pennsylvania County health improvement program (CHIP). *In*: Rosen, J. & Solomon L., ed. *Prevention in health*

psychology. Hanover, NH, University Press of New England, 1985, pp. 144–190.

26. *Intersectoral action for health: methods and experience in planning for health.* Gothenburg, Nordic School of Public Health, 1984.

27. **WHO Healthy Cities Project Office.** *Five-year planning framework.* Copenhagen, FADL, 1988 (WHO Healthy Cities Papers No. 2).

28. **WHO Healthy Cities Project Office.** *A guide to assessing healthy cities.* Copenhagen, FADL, 1988 (WHO Healthy Cities Papers No. 3).

29. **Gesten, E. & Jason, L.** Social and community interventions. *Annual review of psychology,* **38**: 427–460 (1987).

30. **Almond, G. & Verba, S.** *The civic culture: political attitudes and democracy in five nations.* Princeton, NJ, Princeton University Press, 1963.

31. **Gittel, M. et al.** *Limits to citizen participation.* Beverly Hills, CA, Sage Publications, 1980.

32. **Kweit, R. & Kweit, M.** *Implementing citizen participation in a bureaucratic society.* New York, Praeger, 1981.

33. **Moynihan, D.** *Maximum feasible misunderstanding.* New York, Free Press, 1969.

34. **Green, A.** Is there primary health care in the UK? *Health policy and planning,* **2**(2): 129–137 (1987).

35. *Primary health care in industrialized countries*: report on a WHO meeting. Copenhagen, WHO Regional Office for Europe, 1985 (EURO Reports and Studies No. 95).

36. **Westman, G. et al.** Initiating change in primary care, the Vännäs project. Its realization and evaluation. *Scandinavian journal of primary health care,* **5**: 27-34 (1987).

37. **Partridge, K. & White, P.** Community and professional participation in decision making at a health center. *Health service reports,* **87**(4): 336–342 (1972).

38. **Sparer, G. et al.** Consumer participation in OEO-assisted neighborhood health centers. *American journal of public health,* **60**(6): 1091–1102 (1970).

39. **Simmons, J.** Making health education work. *American journal of public health,* **65**(Suppl.): 1–49 (1975).

40. **Cleary et al**. *Advancing health through education: a case study approach*. Palo Alto, CA, Mayfield Publishing, 1985.

41. **Wandersman, A. & Giarmartino, G**. Community and individual difference characteristics as influences on initial participation. *American journal of community psychology*, **8**: 217–229 (1980).

42. **Smith, D.H**. Voluntary action and voluntary groups. *Annual review of sociology*, **1**: 247–270 (1975).

43. **Zurcher, L.A., Jr**. Stages of development of neighborhood action groups: the Topeka example. *In*: Spergel, I., ed. *Community organization: studies in constraint*. Beverly Hills, CA, Sage Publications, 1972.

44. **Spergel, I**. *Community problem-solving*. Chicago, University of Chicago Press, 1969.

45. **Arnstein, S**. A ladder of citizen participation. *American Institute of Planners journal*, **5**: 216–224 (1969).

46. **Cox, F. et al., ed**. *Strategies of community organization*, 3rd ed. Itasca, IL, F.E. Peacock Publishers, 1979.

47. **Aldrich, H**. *Organizations and environments*. Englewood Cliffs, NJ, Prentice-Hall, 1979.

48. **Lasater, T.M. et al**. The Pawtucket heart health program: prospects and process. *In*: Gordon, W. et al., ed. *Perspectives on behavioral medicine*. New York, Academic Press, 1988, Vol. 3, pp. 43–60.

49. **Pecarchik, R. et al**. Potential contribution of consumers to an integrated health care system. *Public health reports*, **91**(1): 73 (1976).

50. **Freire, P**. *Education for critical consciousness*. New York, Seabury Press, 1973.

51. **Pateman, C**. *Participation and democratic theory*. Cambridge, Cambridge University Press, 1970.

52. **Nelson, L. et al**. *Community structure and change*. New York, MacMillan, 1985.

53. **Crosby, N. et al**. Citizen panels: a new approach to citizen participation. *Public administration review*, **46**: 170–178 (1986).

54. **Cassel, J**. The contribution of the social environment to host resistance. *American journal of epidemiology*, **104**(2): 107–123 (1976).

496